1. When does a personality
disorder become a neurosis?

Dementia

To Julie and Karen

Student Psychiatry Today

A comprehensive textbook

ROBERT I. COHEN, MRCPsych

Senior Registrar in Psychiatry, The London Hospital, London

JEROME J. HART, MRCPsych

Senior Registrar in Psychiatry, The London Hospital, London

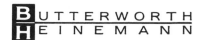

Butterworth-Heinemann Ltd
Linacre House, Jordan Hill, Oxford OX2 8DP

PART OF REED INTERNATIONAL BOOKS

OXFORD   LONDON   BOSTON
MUNICH   NEW DELHI   SINGAPORE   SYDNEY
TOKYO   TORONTO   WELLINGTON

First published 1988
Reprinted 1991, 1992

British Library Cataloguing in Publication Data
Student Psychiatry Today
1. Medicine. Psychiatry
I. Cohen, Robert I.   II. Hart, Jerome J.
616.89

ISBN 0 7506 0322 4

Printed and bound in Great Britain by
Billing & Sons Ltd, Worcester

CONTENTS

PREFACE

This book is primarily intended for medical students with little or no previous knowledge of the subject, although we hope that other undergraduates and trainees in related disciplines will find it useful. It covers all the major disorders encountered in adult psychiatry and also contains chapters on the subspecialities of child psychiatry, forensic psychiatry, psychiatry in the elderly and mental retardation.

The book has a number of aims, developed from an appreciation of the needs of students taught by the authors, and also based upon their comments and criticisms of existing texts. Although it is obviously impossible to write 'the ideal book' to meet everyone's requirements, this volume attempts to adhere to a number of common themes which students of psychiatry repeatedly ask for and subsequently value.

First, theories and concepts are expounded as clearly as possible, and then elaborated upon using a minimum of jargon. Second, where it is felt that they assist comprehension, flow charts and diagrams are used. Third, when technical terms are required, they are fully explained within the body of the text. To avoid repetition and to expand some definitions, a glossary of key terms is provided at the end of the book. Once a framework of understanding has been established, we have tried to present factual information in a concise, ordered yet readable fashion. This is assisted by the provision of a comprehensive summary at the end of most chapters. Finally, psychiatric phenomena and disorders are illustrated wherever possible with the use of vignettes and case histories.

At all times, we have attempted to give the reader a balanced view of causation and treatment, while demonstrating the relative values of a variety of therapeutic approaches used in the management of mental disorders. Throughout the text (with a few notable exceptions) we have used the male gender when referring to subjects and patients. This is done purely in the interests of uniformity and simplicity, and has no other significance.

Robert Cohen
Jerome Hart

ACKNOWLEDGEMENTS

We should like to thank the following people for their advice and comments in the preparation of this book:

Mr J. Carson, Dr C. I. Cohen, Dr R. Cook, Dr S.Y. Dunstan, Dr L. Fagin, Dr A. I. Garelick, Dr M. Goyal, Dr M. P. Joyston-Bechal, Dr G. M. Luyombya, Dr I. C. A. Moyes, Dr A. W. O'Halloran, Dr B. O'Neill, Dr C. M. Parkes, Dr J. M. Pfeffer, Dr I. Singh, Dr E. Stonehill, Dr J. Taylor and Dr G. Tufnell.

We also wish to express our gratitude to Julie Green for the line drawings and cover design, as well as to the many medical students at the London Hospital whose enthusiasm and interest inspired the creation of this work.

The tenth revision of *The International Classification of Diseases* (ICD 10) will be submitted to the World Health Assembly for endorsement in 1990. A draft of Chapter V (Mental, Behavioural and Developmental Disorders) has been prepared for field trials, from which extracts are reproduced throughout the text, by kind permission of the World Health Organization.

1

AN INTRODUCTION
TO PSYCHIATRY

There is an old story of two psychiatrists walking along a hospital corridor, who happen to meet a surgical colleague passing in the opposite direction. The surgeon smiles good naturedly, and after greeting them with a polite 'Good morning', continues on his way. Shortly afterwards, one psychiatrist turns to the other and is heard to ask 'I wonder what he meant by that?'

The caricature of the psychiatrist which this apocryphal tale depicts will perhaps strike a familiar chord with certain readers. In fact, it may not be too far removed from some of their own preconceived notions about the speciality and those who practise it. However, its portrayal as an esoteric discipline, peopled by eccentrics engaged in a perpetual struggle to probe the mysteries of the mind, is no more accurate or valid than other popular stereotypes. In essence, psychiatry is about people, not just about minds and mental illness, and it is the very nature and unique quality of the human condition which makes it such an exciting and stimulating branch of medicine. Certainly, psychiatry is not without its critics or opponents. It may infuriate the pedant who, like the words of the satirical song, cannot contend with people unless they are compartmentalised into 'little boxes'; it may terrify those who hide behind 'the white coat' and the veneer of professionalism in an attempt to deny their own fallibility; and finally, it may discomfort those who are forced to see their patients as human beings, rather than as mere repositories for the illnesses they suffer.

THE ROLE OF THE STUDENT IN PSYCHIATRY

On beginning their psychiatric attachment, students often find the experience both unfamiliar and daunting. They are frequently frustrated by their inability to understand certain concepts relating to the causation or treatment of mental disorder in ways with which they are already familiar. The human mind is too complex to be conceptualised in any one form, and many different perspectives of its functioning are possible, and indeed necessary, if those with psychological difficulties are to be offered effective help. Psychiatry therefore provides a constellation of viewpoints from which human behaviour can be more readily comprehended.

1

The student's understanding of psychiatry must extend beyond learning how to take a history and recognising abnormal features of the mental state *en route* to making a diagnosis. The need to consider the patient as a whole person, rather than simply as a disembodied 'disease' or 'illness', is of paramount importance, and any division between 'mind and body' is best regarded as purely artificial. Attention to psychological problems should therefore be viewed as an integral part of medical care, and not just in relation to psychiatry. Apparent abnormalities of behaviour or thinking need to be seen in the context of the patient's background, and should be considered according to the stresses imposed by his environment, his developmental history, and his physical and mental constitution. The student needs to develop a non-judgemental attitude towards patients, and attempt to understand their shortcomings and inadequacies with a sympathetic and open-minded approach.

At first, this may be hard to accomplish. The student encounters a clinical environment very different to that found on general medical or surgical wards. Not only do patients sometimes behave in an unpredictable, disturbed, non-communicative or overtly hostile manner, but also the relationships between staff are frequently perceived as being disconcertingly unstructured compared to the normal hierarchy found elsewhere in the hospital. Provided the student can overcome his initial fears and prejudices, the time spent in psychiatry provides an opportunity for the acquisition of good communication skills, as well as learning how to gather and interpret information involving a large number of variables. In addition, an appreciation of the importance of the doctor–patient relationship can be gained, particularly with regard to its bearing on therapeutic efficacy and outcome. Although only a minority of students will ultimately pursue a career in psychiatry, most will hopefully find the experience during their attachment both challenging and fulfilling, and of some benefit in their personal and professional lives.

THE CONCEPT OF MENTAL HEALTH AND ILLNESS

Most students entering psychiatry are already familiar with some of the concepts involved in the causation, diagnosis and management of physical illness. The latter is usually recognised as a pronounced deviation from the normal healthy state because it eventually produces symptoms, such as pain or difficulty with movement, which in some way inhibit function or cause subjective distress. Sometimes, a combination of symptoms result from a single cause (an underlying disease), the nature of which can be determined by physical examination or specific investigations. For example, a patient who complains of generalised itching, tiredness and abdominal pain may, on examination, have jaundiced skin and an enlarged liver. Biochemical tests of liver function and a biopsy of that organ might then confirm that the patient has cirrhosis.

Applying similar principles to psychiatry has a number of limitations. Differences between mental health and illness, and what is considered normal and abnormal in psychological terms, are not so easily determined as the clearer delineation between sickness and health which can more often be made in somatic medicine. Consequently, before considering some general aspects of causation and management in psychiatry, it is necessary to examine critically what is meant by mental illness.

When dealing with disorders in which disturbances of thought, perception, emotion, behaviour, intellect or personality are the presenting features, the psychiatrist is faced with a number of problems. First, there are considerable difficulties in defining both the qualitative and quantitative aspects of normal mental functioning. Few individuals are permanently content with life, emotionally stable all of the time or totally satisfied at work and with personal relationships. For most people, 'normality' needs to be considered along a continuum of 'self-fulfilment' in which such levels of perfection might only be achieved intermittently. Moreover, a broad range of emotional and behavioural responses can be observed among individuals in reaction to similar stimuli and circumstances. These will be further influenced by cultural factors and the social context in which they occur, so that the concept of 'normal mental functioning' is of necessity wide, and to some extent will also be dependent upon the perspective of the observer.

Attempting to define mental 'illness' is equally difficult, and efforts to do so in terms of demonstrating an underlying pathological process, or the existence of subjective distress, have a number of limitations. For example, senile dementia and schizophrenia are considered to be mental illnesses by most psychiatrists, because in both disorders there is evidence of a characteristic disturbance of some aspect of psychological function. However, although pathological changes within the brain are clearly evident in senile dementia, none can be consistently demonstrated in schizophrenia. Furthermore, suffering may be obvious in both conditions, although many patients with senile dementia appear content and blissfully unaware of their predicament, while some schizophrenics act with apparent indifference to their plight.

The problem of deciding whether or not someone is suffering from mental illness is of more than academic interest, since it can have important implications both therapeutically and legally. The latter may be an issue when considering the question of an individual's responsibility for his actions in a court of law, or when compulsory detention is contemplated for assessment or treatment in hospital (*see* Chapter 24).

MODELS IN PSYCHIATRY

Effective management in psychiatry, as in any branch of medicine, is contingent upon having a framework or model on which to base ideas and concepts concerning the evolution of disorders, their treatment and outcome. The **biological model** is founded upon reductionist principles, in which signs and symptoms of illness are attributable to a disease process within an organ or system of the body, and this in turn is explicable in terms of changes which occur at a cellular or molecular level. Genetic, biochemical and physiological factors are therefore identified as the causes of mental illness, and physical methods (such as drugs or electroconvulsive therapy (ECT)) are used as the mainstays of treatment. Consequently, mental disorders, irrespective of their mode of presentation, are seen as emanating directly or indirectly from cerebral dysfunction, and the distinction between mind and brain is considered of little practical importance. The limitations of this model are evident with regard to those psychiatric conditions (the functional disorders) which do not have a demonstrable underlying organic pathology. However, in view of past experience, some would argue that it is simply a matter of time before the appropriate agent, biochemical or physiological abnormality is detected to explain their causation.

The behavioural and social models adopt entirely different approaches to the causation and treatment of psychological symptoms. The **behavioural model** differs from the traditional biological model in that symptoms are regarded as 'learned habits' which can be eliminated with appropriate training (*see* Chapter 13). They are not attributed to any underlying pathology, so that removal of the symptoms removes the disorder. Again, notable discrepancies exist between theory and practice, in that although behavioural techniques may be highly effective in the treatment of certain conditions, such as phobias, they are of no use in eliminating the delusions and hallucinations of acute schizophrenia or severe depression.

The **social model** regards the individual as part of a social system in which mental disorder evolves in response to disruptive circumstances such as divorce, unemployment, bereavement or poor housing. Social or 'milieu' therapy focuses on altering the individual's relationship to the social system in which he lives. This is achieved through increasing self-awareness of the effect that environmental influences have on his well-being, and improving self-esteem by encouraging personal responsibility and enhancing his capacity to make satisfactory relationships. Similarly, within this model, it is sometimes helpful to view the family in terms of a social microcosm, in which the index patient is seen as part of a system which is ailing, so that recovery is contingent upon treating the family unit rather than the individual.

The **psychoanalytical model** is derived largely from analytical theory (*see* Chapter 13) in which all aspects of mental activity and subsequent behaviour are viewed as being influenced by an interplay between conflicting inborn drives and the demands of the outside world. Adult vulnerabilities to stress are seen as arising from developmental disturbances of the personality in the first few years of life, as well as from distorted child–parent relationships. The liaison between therapist and patient allows the feelings associated with these earlier relationships to be explored, so that the individual can gain an understanding of how past events influence his current behaviour and feelings, and thereby facilitate opportunities for change. Symptoms are therefore viewed as having meaning and need to be understood in order to be eliminated effectively.

It should be apparent that no single model provides a satisfactory explanation or solution to every psychological problem that is encountered. Which therapeutic approach (or approaches) to adopt is partly determined by the nature of the problem and the wishes of the patient, but is also a matter of clinical judgement. Consequently, it is important for the student to develop a firm grasp of the fundamental concepts of several models of causation and treatment, and to learn the feasibility, benefits and disadvantages of their clinical application. Adopting an **eclectic** approach to the evaluation and management of mental disorder requires due consideration to be given to the use of physical, behavioural, psychotherapeutic and social methods of treatment. However, effective therapy is not simply a matter of choosing the right technique for the presenting problem, but is also contingent upon adopting a humane approach, in which an appropriate sense of caring and compassion is displayed. Many people who seek help for emotional problems have already tried unsuccessfully to resolve their difficulties, and as a consequence feel demoralised, helpless or weakened by their abortive efforts.

AETIOLOGY

In all branches of medicine, aetiology (the study of causation) is the major determinant in the development of effective treatment. The various models that have been described reflect the complexities of establishing causation in psychiatry, since hereditary, physical, social and psychological factors would all appear to be involved in the evolution of mental disorder. In some conditions, cause and effect have a simple linear relationship; e.g. the mental retardation and physical abnormalities which occur in Down's syndrome can be attributed to a specific chromosomal defect. In other cases, a single cause may lead to several different effects, such as trauma to the head producing intellectual impairment, personality changes or symptoms of anxiety and depression. Furthermore, a combination of causes can sometimes produce a single effect, e.g. genetic factors and environmental stress are both thought to be involved in the development of schizophrenia.

Not all putative aetiological factors exert their effects within the same time interval. In the case of schizophrenia, genetic influences probably confer a vulnerability to develop the condition, and are known as **predisposing factors.** Stressors, such as adverse life events, occurring shortly before the onset of the illness are referred to as **precipitating factors**. Once the illness has developed, **perpetuating factors** may serve to prolong its course, as in the case of loss of self-confidence resulting from prolonged hospitalisation.

EPIDEMIOLOGY

Epidemiology is the study of how specific disorders are distributed throughout populations and the factors which influence that distribution. Information gained from epidemiological studies can be used to determine the incidence and prevalence of a disorder. The **incidence** is the number of new cases that occur within a given population over a specified period of time (e.g. the incidence of schizophrenia in Great Britain is 15–20 new cases per 100 000 population/year). The **prevalence** of a disorder is the total number of cases, both new and old, in a given population at any one time, often expressed as a percentage (the prevalence of schizophrenia in Great Britain is approximately 1% of the total population).

Epidemiological studies aid the identification of **risk factors** which increase the likelihood of the development of a disorder. These may include variables such as age, sex, socioeconomic class, marital status, ethnic origin and living environment (urban or rural). One result of epidemiological research has been to demonstrate that in some cases, the onset of illness appears to cluster around certain periods of an individual's life, often at a time when a major change or upset has been experienced. These changes, both adverse and favourable, are referred to as **life events** and include marriage, childbirth, bereavement, divorce, redundancy and moving house. Their impact on the development of illness will vary according to the individual's constitution and vulnerability to stress, his support system and the personal significance of the event. For example, depending upon the circumstances, pregnancy may either be viewed with great happiness or profound dismay, the latter being more likely to lead to the development of depressive symptoms.

The contribution of **genetic factors** to the development of mental disorder may also be determined by epidemiological means. The observation that certain disorders (such as schizophrenia) run in families suggests that genetic factors may play a part in their causation, although **family risk studies** alone cannot distinguish between the effects of heredity and the environment. The **clustering** of schizophrenia in families could occur for much the same reasons as the tendency for students of medicine to come from a medical background. To determine whether a true genetic influence exists, twin and adoption studies have been performed.

Twin Studies

When one member of a pair of identical (or monozygotic) twins suffers from a mental disorder, the other twin (who has an identical genetic make-up) would always be similarly affected if the condition is determined by genetic factors alone. Using schizophrenia as an example, this is not found to be the case, but the risk of the co-twin suffering from or developing the illness is still four times greater than when one of a pair of non-identical twins (who, like ordinary brothers and sisters, are heterozygotic) has schizophrenia. This finding lends considerable support to the concept of an inherited component in the illness. However, the most conclusive evidence for a genetic influence is provided by adoption studies, which exclude any possible environmental effect that may originate from living with a mentally disordered relative.

Adoption Studies

Children of schizophrenics, who were adopted away in the first few weeks of life to families with no schizophrenic member, were compared with a control group of adopted children whose biological parents did not have the illness. The findings were significant — about 10% of those children whose natural parent was schizophrenic developed the condition while living with their adoptive families, whereas there were no diagnosed cases in the control group.

To summarise, support for an inherited component exists if the risk of the identical co-twin suffering from or developing the condition (expressed as the concordance rate) is appreciably higher than with non-identical twin pairs. Similarly, close relatives of patients who suffer from disorders such as schizophrenia or depression, have an increased risk (compared with the general population) of developing the illness themselves. However, not only genetic factors are involved, since identical twins are not always similarly affected. This suggests that where genetic influences are thought to operate, a **vulnerability** to develop the disorder is inherited, rather than the condition itself, and that certain **environmental factors** (such as adverse life events) need to be present before the illness becomes manifest.

DIAGNOSIS AND CLASSIFICATION IN PSYCHIATRY

Although some mental disorders are attributable to demonstrable structural or physiological changes within the brain or other organs of the body (*see below*), several others (such as schizophrenia or mania) are not, and therefore cannot be verified or refuted by specific pathological, radiological or other investigations. In such disorders, direct observations of behaviour and information gained from other people are of some value, but **diagnosis** often rests upon evidence of current or past symptoms that the patient has reported. Consequently, diagnostic accuracy will depend upon a host of variables, including the consistency of what the patient says and how he behaves at different interviews, the manner in which questions are put to him (e.g. open-ended or direct), the interpretation made and the importance ascribed by the examiner to the answers given.

The significance of accurate and comprehensive history-taking and mental state examination is self-evident, but even so, diagnostic reliability based upon unstructured interview techniques remains low. Therefore, it is not uncommon to encounter patients who have had several admissions to hospital with a different diagnosis made each time, even though their symptomatology remained constant throughout. Standardised interview schedules (such as the **present state examination**) help to overcome some of these problems by ensuring that all possible phenomena are elicited, and by leaving the interpretation of the results to a computer program. The major drawbacks of such an instrument are that it is time-consuming and requires the interviewer to have special training, thereby limiting its use in everyday practice.

Classification Systems

By identifying and systematically grouping patients or conditions with similar clinical features, **classification** helps in the planning of appropriate treatment and predicting the outcome of psychiatric disorder. Mental disorder is commonly differentiated into mental illness, mental retardation and personality disorder (*see* Chapters 3 and 18). In **mental retardation**, features of the disorder have been constantly present from birth or a very early age. Evidence of **personality disorder** is usually apparent in one form or another from childhood or adolescence onwards, whereas in **mental illness** there is frequently an identifiable onset, preceded by a recognised period of normal functioning. Sometimes, difficulties in differentiation can arise, e.g. if illness has persisted for many years (as may occur in chronic schizophrenia), and no independent history of earlier behaviour is available. Furthermore, it is possible for mental illness to develop in someone with an underlying personality disorder or who is mentally retarded, and similarly mental retardation and personality disorder can coexist.

Mental illnesses may be classified in a number of ways. It is common practice initially to differentiate between those disorders which can be attributed to a demonstrable structural or physiological abnormality of the brain or other body organ, and those which cannot. The former are known as **organic disorders**, and where possible, treatment of mental symptoms is that of the underlying pathology or physiological disturbance (*see* Chapter 9). The latter group (which includes schizophrenia and the affective disorders) in some cases reflect a probable abnormality of brain function, but since no clear underlying pathology (such as a tumour or infection) is demonstrable, they are referred to as **functional disorders**.

The original distinction between functional and organic disorders was made at a time when organicity was determined either with the naked eye or by light microscopy. During the twentieth century, a few 'functional disorders' have been demonstrated to have an organic basis, and as knowledge in fields such as biochemistry and neurophysiology increases, similar theories of causation have been advanced for many others, where abnormalities are proposed to exist at a molecular level. For example, one theory suggests that schizophrenia is related to an excess of the neurotransmitter dopamine, acting at certain strategic locations within the brain (*see* Chapter 8). Nevertheless, because of the relative inaccessibility of the brain and the paucity of post-mortem material, many of these theories are based upon indirect measures of cerebral function, so that the treatment of functional disorders remains largely empirical.

Mental illnesses are also classified according to qualitative differences. When impairment of mental functioning occurs to the extent that the sufferer is unable to meet the demands of everyday life and no longer maintains adequate contact with reality (e.g. due to delusional beliefs or hallucinatory experiences), both functional and organic disorders are referred to as **psychoses** (*see* p. 126). Other disorders, in which contact with reality is maintained and psychological dysfunction is seen as an accentuation of the normal reaction to the stresses or strains of everyday living, are sometimes termed **neuroses** (*see* Chapter 4).

Although the terms psychosis and neurosis are widely employed, the student should be aware of several problems regarding their usage. In the first place, organic disorders, schizophrenia and certain mood disturbances can all fulfil the above criteria of a psychosis, but as they differ widely in other respects (i.e. with regard to aetiology, symptomatology and response to treatment), there is only a limited advantage in grouping them together in this way. Furthermore, the occurrence of neurotic symptoms in response to stress is sufficiently commonplace that it is sometimes difficult to regard the sufferer as being mentally ill. For example, bereavement is a state in which symptoms of anxiety and unhappiness usually occur, yet few would regard it as an illness, even though functional and emotional disability may be pronounced. Many view such 'symptoms' as nothing more than an understandable response to some difficulty or emotional conflict, which will resolve spontaneously when the problem has been removed. Finally, the terms psychosis and neurosis are sometimes used as synonyms for major and minor mental disorder respectively. However, any implication that neuroses are 'less severe' than psychoses does not take into account the degree of suffering experienced. In this respect, some neuroses are more severe than certain well-circumscribed psychoses.

Other **miscellaneous disorders** which are often treated by psychiatrists, such as substance abuse and eating and sexual disorders, do not fit clearly into any of the above categories and are therefore classified separately. A further grouping includes individuals who, in response to stress, may display symptoms indistinguishable from those found in neuroses or psychoses. However, unlike these conditions, the symptoms are marked by their brevity and usually dissipate rapidly once the source of stress is removed or resolved. They are therefore sometimes referred to as **adjustment disorders**.

Childhood psychiatric disorders are also classified separately, since most of them manifest as disturbances of behaviour which are unique to that age group (*see* Chapter 16).

ICD 9 and DSM III Systems of Classification

All systems of classification provide a framework for organising knowledge and offer a way of conveying 'shorthand' information between people, assuming that everyone attributes the same meaning to the terminology used. In order to do this, clear guidelines need to be established detailing which specific features should be present before a condition can be assigned to one particular category or another.

Two major classification systems attempt to improve diagnostic accuracy in psychiatric practice, but do so in contrasting ways. The **International Classification of Diseases**, currently in its ninth edition (ICD 9), seeks to standardise diagnosis using **descriptive definitions** of the major syndromes, as well as give some directives on differential diagnosis. Because the system is a compromise of classifications used in different countries, its definitions tend to be vague and somewhat imprecise. Nevertheless, it does provide a method of diagnostic coding which is understandable throughout the world. At the time of writing, ICD 10 is undergoing field trials. This will be a uniaxial classification system, making use of both operational criteria and descriptive definitions (*see below*).

The American Psychiatric Association has adopted a different system contained in the **Diagnostic and Statistical Manual of Mental Disorders**, currently in its third edition (DSM III), which has recently been revised and updated (DSM III-R). This relies upon **operational criteria** (rather than descriptive definitions) for diagnostic consistency. For each disorder, it clearly states which symptoms need to be present to fulfil the diagnosis, often quantifying the number necessary from a supplied list. Longitudinal criteria, that is the length of time for which symptoms need to be present, are also established, together with exclusion criteria. In order to convey a more complete picture of the individual, DSM III-R also records four additional types of information. These are details of associated personality and developmental disorders, related physical disorders, the severity of psychosocial stressors, and the highest level of social and occupational functioning in the previous 12 months. This is an example of **multiaxial classification** (a similar system being used in child psychiatry), and although extremely comprehensive, it is often considered too cumbersome for convenient everyday use. Despite the widespread use of DSM III-R in the UK for research purposes, ICD 9 remains at present the principal classification system used in clinical practice.

The Diagnostic Hierarchy

Conventionally, the diagnostic process progresses in a hierarchical fashion, and wherever possible, a single entity is used to explain all the symptoms elicited. For example, if a patient complains of feeling depressed and hearing voices, but is discovered to have a brain tumour, a diagnosis of an organic disorder would be made. Because organic conditions can account for any psychological symptom that might be encountered, the first step diagnostically is to exclude such a cause. If no organic aetiology can be elicited, then a diagnosis of schizophrenia is considered. Certain symptoms are held to be fundamental to this condition (see p. 131), since they rarely occur in any other disorder. If, for example, the patient were to complain of voices arguing about him in the third person, then, in the absence of an organic cause, a diagnosis of schizophrenia would be a strong probability.

Where no symptoms indicative of schizophrenia are elicited, the next diagnostic consideration is that of an affective illness. If the subject were to complain of low mood and voices referring to him in a derogatory fashion, addressing him by name or as 'you', then a diagnosis of a depressive psychosis would need to be contemplated. Finally, if the presenting symptoms do not fit within the framework of any of the above categories, they may be attributable to a neurotic disorder. Thus, a person who presented with feelings of anxiety and foreboding, and who was noted to be tremulous and sweating with a rapid pulse, would only be diagnosed as suffering from an anxiety state provided that organic causes (such as thyrotoxicosis) had been excluded, and other features indicative of schizophrenic or affective disorders had been ruled out. It follows that an organic state can include all the symptoms which are present in schizophrenia, affective or neurotic disorders, while diagnosing a neurotic disorder means that all higher categories have been excluded.

In practice, this process is not quite as straightforward as outlined here, since interforms (such as schizoaffective disorder) are now widely recognised as clinical entities (*see* p. 142). Furthermore, some symptoms may be attributed to other disorders (such as personality disorder, substance abuse or mental retardation), which do not fit into the traditional hierarchy outlined above.

Diagnostic Formulation

Many psychiatrists argue that clear diagnostic entities exist only in textbooks, and that in clinical practice, few patients fit neatly into one category or another. Consequently, this leads to unreliability in psychiatric diagnosis, and to unrealistic assumptions being made about disease categories. In addition, those who uphold the concept of **labelling theory** suggest that many of the psychiatric terms in current use, such as 'schizophrenia' or 'psychopathy', are merely pejorative and have little useful meaning, serving only to increase an individual's difficulties when he is labelled in this way. Although it is of vital importance to diagnose organic disorders and some major psychoses correctly, the value of labelling the neuroses is less evident (*see* Chapter 4). In fact, it is often more important to reassure people who are distressed as a result of life crises or relationship difficulties that they are not mentally ill, rather than to force them into Procrustean categories. (Procrustes was the mythical Greek robber who stretched his captives or cut their legs to make them fit his bed.) Furthermore, making a diagnosis of depressive illness or schizophrenia conveys nothing about the uniqueness of the individual, nor how interpersonal problems, personality factors, childhood experiences and life events may have contributed to his current state.

Because all of the above factors are important in deciding on appropriate management as well as predicting outcome, information is often conveyed by means of a **diagnostic formulation**. This represents a unique profile of the patient, summarising the salient features of the history and the current mental state, possible aetiological factors, the personality structure and the diagnosis or differential diagnosis. In addition, consideration is given to further investigations or information necessary to determine immediate and long-term management, as well as to the likely prognosis.

THE MULTIDISCIPLINARY APPROACH

Most psychiatric care is now based upon a multidisciplinary approach to treatment. Members of various disciplines meet regularly as a team, at which time patients' problems are discussed, information is exchanged and plans are formulated for both their immediate care and long-term management. The composition of the team varies, often depending upon availability of staff, but usually comprises a consultant psychiatrist (and occasionally a general practitioner), junior doctors, psychiatric nurses, a social worker, an occupational therapist, and a clinical psychologist. The advantages of such an approach are that it defines the role of each team member in the total care plan, and allows a sharing of the burden of responsibility. In addition, it creates a sense of cohesion among the disciplines and offers an opportunity for the acquisition of new skills, thereby increasing job satisfaction and self-worth among staff members. At a more practical level, it ensures that unnecessary duplication of work is avoided.

The training and responsibilities of all mental health workers are rapidly changing, with a resultant blurring of the boundaries relating to their roles and clinical obligations. Nevertheless, it is useful for the student in psychiatry to have some idea of the different skills that each member of the team can offer.

The Consultant Psychiatrist

In addition to those who seek help with subjective complaints of unhappiness or evidence of emotional distress, the psychiatrist is often asked to see people who show disturbance of function with regard to work, relationships or aspects of daily living, or who exhibit behaviour which is abnormal for them or outside socially acceptable limits. Of course, not every problem presented will be attributable to mental disorder. Some will result from social difficulties, while others may be due to previously undetected physical illness or perhaps considered as idiosyncratic behaviour.

The consultant psychiatrist's duties extend beyond providing a clinical service, and include administrative and managerial responsibilities. In addition to coordinating and integrating clinical aspects of both hospital and community-based services, consultants are concerned with securing resources and ensuring that they are implemented effectively. As a member of the multidisciplinary team, the consultant provides leadership by balancing directive and facilitatory roles, as well as by delegating responsibilities to others. At times, he will need to 'underwrite' other staff members' clinical decisions, and 'trouble-shoot' when things go wrong. Consultants also have a responsibility towards the Primary Care Team (*see* Chapter 14). In this respect, they not only provide a domiciliary assessment service for psychiatric problems in the community but, in many areas, regularly liaise face-to-face with general practitioners to discuss patients and their continuing management. Consultants undertake a commitment to teach junior medical staff, as well as members of other disciplines, and are also involved in the appointment of personnel.

The General Practitioner

The majority of people who have psychological problems are seen and treated by their general practitioner, and only a small proportion are referred to hospital psychiatrists. The role of the family doctor in psychiatric practice is dealt with in Chapters 5 and 13.

The Psychiatric Nurse

Psychiatric nursing is increasingly adopting a holistic view of patient care, and pursuing a 'problem-orientated' approach to management. Although continuing to perform the more traditional functions of general nursing, psychiatric nurses fulfil a number of additional roles. As members of the team who spend most time with the patient, they are in a position to develop a close therapeutic relationship with those under their care. In addition to providing support and comfort for the acutely disturbed or distressed, many nurses are actively involved in individual or group psychotherapy and behaviour modification programmes. Accurate observation of patients on the ward by the nursing staff not only provides important diagnostic information, but is also essential in monitoring the response to treatment.

The nurse's skills as a teacher may be conveyed through example (by setting a standard for personal appearance, general demeanour and manner of communication), by encouraging participation (such as involving patients in domestic chores on the ward), as well as by using more didactic methods of imparting information. To an extent, the nurse also plays a parental role by acting as supporter, adviser and confidant, while working towards helping the patient achieve independence and self-sufficiency.

With the move toward community care, the function of the psychiatric nurse outside the hospital has become increasingly important. Community psychiatric nursing is mainly concerned with the follow-up of patients after discharge from hospital. This includes the supervision and administration of maintenance treatment (such as depot injections), support for the individual and his family, liaison with the general practitioner and hospital staff, as well as the early detection of deterioration to prevent relapse.

The Social Worker

Psychiatric social workers provide a link between the hospital and community-based social services or agencies which lend support and assistance to those in need of their help. Many have an attachment to general practices within the locality, and provide an important input to the Primary Care Team. In addition to performing social assessments and offering help with financial problems, the social worker also advises patients about welfare rights and accommodation difficulties. Some undertake individual, marital or group therapy, in conjunction with the medical and nursing staff. Occasionally, an approved social worker may be involved in making an application for the compulsory admission of a mentally disordered person to hospital under the Mental Health Act (*see* Chapter 24).

After-care following discharge from hospital is an important aspect of treatment, and the social worker is frequently involved in arranging the provision of services in the community or helping patients to find suitable accommodation (*see* Chapter 14).

The Occupational Therapist

The occupational therapist is concerned with the promotion and maintenance of maximum personal and functional independence for the patient, by providing an opportunity for people to relearn or acquire new skills related to all aspects of work, leisure and daily living (*see* Chapter 14). In the psychiatric field, the occupational therapist works mostly in task-orientated groups, for which patients are individually assessed according to specific disabilities. Treatment may involve re-education in skills associated with living in the community, such as personal care and self-maintenance, shopping, budgeting and general home management. Patients might also require training in social skills in order to promote self-confidence, improve their ability to form relationships and enhance their integration back into the community.

Occupational therapists will often be involved in various aspects of work rehabilitation, which include assessing present capabilities, as well as helping the individual to return to a previous job or to undergo retraining. In many psychiatric units, they also help in the management and assessment of patients in the industrial therapy workshop, where contracted work is graded according to individual ability. Where full-time employment is unlikely to be achieved, the occupational therapist has an equally important role in educating patients in the use of their leisure time. Emphasis is often placed on promoting individual creativity through the media of art, music, movement and drama groups. In all settings, the occupational therapist observes the relationships that develop between individuals, and utilises these to highlight difficulties and promote communication skills.

The Clinical Psychologist

Psychology is the scientific study of mental processes and behaviour, and the work of the clinical psychologist involves assessment and treatment in a number of areas. These include estimating intellectual functioning, offering behavioural and cognitive therapies for the treatment of specific disorders, and assisting with the implementation and supervision of rehabilitation programmes. The latter aim to improve social functioning and self-care abilities for those with chronic mental disorders. The clinical psychologist is also concerned with assessing personality and clarifying the relationship between specific behavioural patterns and cerebral dysfunction. An increasingly important role is undertaken in the speciality of mental retardation where, in addition to utilising specific psychological techniques, the clinical psychologist acts as a coordinator and facilitator within the multidisciplinary team. In some areas, they also function as members of the Primary Care Team, through their attachment to local general practices.

REFERENCES AND FURTHER READING

American Psychiatric Association (1987). *Diagnostic and Statistical Manual of Mental Disorders*, 3rd rv, edn. Washington DC: APA.

Clare, A. W. (1980). *Psychiatry in Dissent*, 2nd edn. London: Tavistock.

Hill, P., Murray, R., Thorley, A., eds (1986). *Essentials of Postgraduate Psychiatry*, 2nd edn. London: Grune and Stratton.

Hollyman, J. A., Hemsi, L. (1983). What do psychiatrists understand by formulation? *Bulletin of the Royal College of Psychiatrists*; **7**: 140–3.

Wing, J. K., Cooper, J. E., Sartorius, N. (1974). *The Measurement and Classification of Psychiatric Symptoms*. Cambridge: Cambridge University Press.

World Health Organization (1977). *Manual of the International Statistical Classificaion of Diseases, Injuries and Causes of Death*, 9th edn. Geneva: WHO.

World Health Organization (1987). Tenth revision of *The International Classification of Diseases*, Chapter V (F): Mental, Behavioural and Developmental Disorders, Clinical Descriptions and Diagnostic Guidelines. 1987 Draft for field trials. Geneva: WHO.

2

THE PSYCHIATRIC HISTORY AND MENTAL STATE EXAMINATION

As with other skills in medicine, proficiency in psychiatric history-taking and examination of the mental state is only acquired through practice. The **history** will contain details of events and symptoms experienced by the subject prior to the interview. The **mental state** is concerned with the subject's appearance and behaviour during the consultation, as well as any symptoms and signs reported or elicited at that time.

THE PSYCHIATRIC HISTORY

On being introduced to psychiatry, students often feel daunted by the numerous questions that have to be asked and the amount of information that needs to be collected. However, as their knowledge of the subject increases and their clinical experience develops, they become better at recognising diagnostic clues and consequently are able to be more directive in their line of enquiry. Despite this, the likelihood of a psychiatric case in finals is for many an alarming prospect.

Although there is no short cut to proficiency, the clerking of patients in psychiatry would be a more profitable exercise for most students if, in addition to knowing the right questions to ask, they understood the reasons for asking them. Consequently, in addition to providing a framework for history-taking and mental state examination, each section also contains a brief note on the relevance of the information gained towards either reaching a diagnosis, formulating management plans or assessing prognosis. (Asterisked questions in this chapter are taken from the *Present State Examination*, and are reproduced by kind permission of the Cambridge University Press.)

1. General Information

This should include:

(a) name and address of informant
(b) age and sex

(c) marital status
(d) occupation
(e) country of origin
(f) religion
(g) patient status (in- or outpatient, informal or detained)

Whenever presenting a history verbally or in written form, it is always a good idea to make a concise opening statement which contains all the demographic information relating to the subject. For example, 'The patient I should like to present is Mr John Smith, a 44-year-old accountant married with two children, who is British born and Roman Catholic, and has been a voluntary inpatient on Lavender Ward at St Dibble's Hospital since the 3rd of this month.'

2. Presenting Complaint(s)/Reason for Referral

A brief note should be recorded as to the subject's **main complaint(s)**, where possible using the informant's own words. For example, it is incorrect to report that 'The patient complains of depressive symptoms' when he actually stated 'I feel sad and unable to enjoy myself'. In addition, it should be determined how the person's lifestyle is affected by the presenting problem(s), such as through poor work performance or domestic conflict. By allowing the individual to say at an early stage how he is specifically troubled by his symptoms, the rest of the interview will seem more relevant to him and increases the likelihood of his cooperation. A useful way of opening the interview might be to ask:

* *Q: To begin with, I should like to get an idea of the sort of problems that have been troubling you recently. What have been the main difficulties?*

Sometimes a person will have been referred by another professional agency (such as a general practitioner or social worker) and may not have any specific complaints himself. In such cases, the **reason for the referral** should be clearly stated at the beginning of the history.

3. History of Present Condition

The **duration of symptoms** should be determined by asking when the subject last felt completely well or his usual self. An enquiry is then made into the **nature of each symptom**, the **chronological order** in which they developed, possible **precipitants** and evidence of any **aggravating or relieving factors** (which may include self-prescribed treatment or that administered by another doctor). Related disturbances in sleep, appetite, weight, energy or libido should also be noted. Certain symptoms may still be present at the time of interview, so that inevitably there will be some overlap between information recorded about the history of the present condition and that in the current mental state. A few specimen questions are shown below, with further examples given later in the section on the mental state examination.

ENQUIRIES ABOUT MOOD

Depression or elation
* Q: *Do you keep reasonably cheerful or have you been very depressed or low-spirited recently?*
* Q: *Have you sometimes felt particularly cheerful and on top of the world, without any reason?*

Anxiety
* Q: *Have there been times lately when you have been very anxious or frightened?*

Diurnal mood variation
* Q: *Is the depression worse at any particular time of day? (such as the afternoon, the evening or the morning).*

ALTERATION IN PHYSIOLOGICAL FUNCTIONS

Sleep
* Q: *Have you had any trouble getting off to sleep during the past month?*
* Q: *Do you wake early in the morning?*

Energy
* Q: *Do you seem to be slowed down in your movements, or to have too little energy recently?*
* Q: *Have you felt particularly full of energy lately? Do you find yourself extremely active but not getting tired?*

Appetite/weight
* Q: *What has your appetite been like recently?*
  Q: *Has there been a recent change in your weight?*

4. Family History

The problems experienced by people may be a reflection of their family background, arising from disturbed relationships in the past or present, or through genetic factors influencing the development of mental illness. Consequently, a detailed **family history** should be taken either from the subject or from a relative.

(a) Record the **family members**
(b) **Parents'** ages or their age at death and cause if known
(c) Parents' occupations
(d) Name, age, sex, occupation and marital status of **siblings** (noting adoptive, step- or half-siblings, stillbirths and deaths)
(e) Personality of siblings and parents, and their past and present relationship to the patient
(f) Current mental and physical health of siblings and parents
(g) **Home atmosphere** and **degree of closeness** of the family
(h) Any **family history of mental or physical illness** (including grandparents, uncles, aunts, etc.). This should encompass psychiatric illness, substance abuse, personality disorder, suicide and self-harm, mental impairment and neurological disorders, such as epilepsy. Details of hospitalisation, treatment and outcome should be noted.

5. Past Psychiatric History

Information about **past psychiatric disorders** can be extremely important and helpful in reaching a diagnosis, formulating a management plan and predicting outcome, especially in recurrent or relapsing conditions such as depression or schizophrenia. However, each new admission should also be evaluated independently of previous ones, as it is unwise automatically to assume that the diagnosis and treatment will be the same as before. This is because past information may be incomplete or incorrect, or the current condition unrelated to earlier illnesses.

The following data should be recorded for each admission or course of outpatient treatment:

(a) name of **hospital**, **date** and **duration of care**, informal or detained under the Mental Health Act
(b) **diagnosis** and possible **precipitants**
(c) **treatment** received
(d) **outcome**.

6. Past Medical History

A record should be made of any **physical illnesses**, **accidents** or **operations**, especially those serious enough to require hospital admission or treatment, since these constitute 'life events' which may precipitate or perpetuate mental illness. Furthermore, physical disorders can give rise to psychological symptoms and vice versa (*see* Chapter 15). **Drugs** prescribed for medical complaints may produce psychological effects, so that **all** medication taken by the patient (both past and present) must be noted.

7. Personal History

(a) EARLY DEVELOPMENT AND CHILDHOOD

Details of early development should be recorded and, where appropriate, need to include significant prenatal events, such as intrauterine infection. A history of birth injury or developmental delay may alert the examiner to the possibility that the subject is intellectually impaired. For example, abnormal behaviour in adult life can sometimes be attributed to mental illness, when in fact it may be a consequence of mental retardation.

In addition, many psychological problems which occur in adulthood, may have their roots in early life, so that some information is required about this period of development.

The following details should be elicited:

   i. problems during **pregnancy** and **birth** — infections, trauma, drugs, etc.
   ii. any delay in **developmental milestones**
   iii. periods of **separation** from parents or care givers — including those caused by illness, death or marital breakdown
   iv. overall impression of **happiness** and **domestic stability** as a child, i.e. frequency of moving house and changes in sleeping arrangements
   v. **emotional** and **functional disorders** of childhood — bed-wetting and soiling, sleep disorders, tantrums, nail-biting, food fads, stammering, fears and shyness
   vi. **physical health** during childhood.

(b) SCHOOLING

School is usually the first regular social activity that children experience outside the home, and consequently, behavioural difficulties or evidence of impaired intelligence may emerge for the first time. Levels of achievement and potential at school also provide a useful baseline for comparison with attainments in later adult life. For example, the diagnosis of schizophrenia might be supported by demonstrating a decline in an individual's overall level of functioning from his time at school. In addition, behaviour associated with certain personality disorders (such as psychopathy), may first become apparent at school age, as evidenced by persistent fighting or truanting.

Information should include:

    i. **ages** of starting and finishing at each school
    ii. **qualifications** attained
    iii. periods of **prolonged absence** and reasons, i.e. illness, school refusal or truanting
    iv. **relationships with peers and teachers** and general level of enjoyment at school
    v. **antisocial behaviour**.

(c) EMPLOYMENT

Mental illness, mental retardation, substance abuse and some types of personality disorder often affect the ability to function, and therefore the capacity to find a job or remain at work. In addition, problems associated with employment may in themselves be responsible for the development or exacerbation of psychological symptoms. It is therefore important not only to consider details of present employment, but also past jobs and the reasons for leaving them. The work history should include details of:

    i. **present employment**, its duration and level of satisfaction at work; future prospects
    ii. chronological record of **previous jobs** and reasons for leaving, e.g. seeking promotion, dismissal or redundancy
    iii. periods of **unemployment**.

(d) PSYCHOSEXUAL AND MARITAL HISTORY

Sexual difficulties may be a problem in their own right, or secondary to some other physical or psychological disorder. Mood disturbances in women are sometimes related to menstruation or certain methods of contraception, so that details of the menstrual history should also be taken.

Many people find it extremely difficult to discuss sexual problems, so that great sensitivity and tact are needed when enquiring into this area. A first interview may or may not be the most appropriate time to take a sexual history. The interviewer should note the subject's reactions to his enquiries and desist if he feels that further questions are likely to jeopardise the establishment of a therapeutic rapport. When confidence has been gained, the person may be much more forthcoming in his replies. Students should also remember that some people resent being asked questions of a highly personal nature by someone of the opposite sex, or who is considerably younger than themselves.

Because marital difficulties are a common source of stress, it is important to record particulars of all marriages, as well as other significant relationships, past and present. Details of any offspring should be noted, including step-children and half-siblings.

The following information is recorded:

i. **menstrual history** — including age of menarche/menopause or onset of puberty in males
ii. **sexual history** — attitudes to sex, sexual practices including masturbation and fantasies, onset of dating, age at first intercourse, contraception, and any homosexual activity or other deviations
iii. **recent sexual activity**, degree of satisfaction, sexual dysfunctions
iv. **marital history** — how long partners knew each other before marriage, length of engagement, age at marriage of each partner, periods of separation, divorce, details of other marriages or significant relationships
v. age, occupation and health of **spouse** — nature of the marital relationship
vi. age, sex and health of **children** and how patient relates to them
vii. details of any miscarriages, terminated pregnancies, stillbirths or death of children.

8. Social Circumstances

A great deal can be learned about an individual by discovering how he spends the day. Some objective measure of the impact presenting difficulties have on a person's life may be gained through determining his level of functioning by taking a social history.

In addition, adverse social circumstances may be a source of great stress and lead to the development of psychological problems. Difficulties with housing, finances or relationships can all be precipitating or perpetuating factors associated with mental illness. Details of leisure activities are an important way of assessing an individual's social skills.

Information about a person's criminal record or any pending court cases must also be recorded, as they may be relevant to diagnosis and management. Details of the consumption or abuse of alcohol and non-prescribed drugs should always be documented, including illicit substances and those bought over the counter.

A note should be made of:

(a) **accommodation** — type and quality of housing, members of household, security of tenure
(b) **financial circumstances** – source of income, outgoings, current difficulties
(c) **leisure** interests and hobbies

(d) **social relationships**, support network and degree of isolation
(e) **tobacco** and **alcohol** consumption, evidence of abuse
(f) **illicit drugs** — abuse and dependency
(g) **forensic history** — record of convictions, imprisonment, probation, pending court appearances.

9. Premorbid Personality

The assessment of the subject's personality prior to the onset of any current difficulties (premorbid) is best verified independently by a relative or close friend. This should include an appraisal of **character**, **predominant mood**, **attitudes** and **self-image**. Any marked discrepancy in personality from that currently observed might be indicative of the effects of psychiatric disturbance. Asking the patient the following questions may be helpful in determining premorbid personality (*see* Chapter 3).

(a) Affective
   Q: Would you normally describe yourself as a cheerful person or do you generally tend to be pessimistic about things?

(b) Histrionic (hysterical)
   Q: Do you usually like to be the centre of attention?

(c) Explosive
   Q: Do you frequently lose your temper?

(d) Asthenic
   Q: Do you often find it difficult to cope with the demands of everyday life?

(e) Obsessional (anankastic)
   Q: Do you normally like things in your life to be orderly?

(f) Paranoid
   Q: As a rule, are you mostly treated fairly or do you tend to feel picked on?

(g) Schizoid
   Q: Do you normally mix easily or do you prefer to be alone?

(h) Antisocial
   Q: Do you usually dislike being told what to do?

   Self-image
   Q: What do you normally think of yourself as a person?

10. Additional History from any Other Informant

Where appropriate, additional information should be obtained from an **independent source**, such as a relative or friend, especially if details in the patient's history are conflicting, incomplete or require corroboration.

THE MENTAL STATE EXAMINATION

Some aspects of the mental state will have been elicited during the course of history-taking, although to complete the examination, an additional systematic enquiry is usually necessary. This cannot always be achieved at one interview, e.g. if the patient is very anxious, disturbed or unresponsive. Under these circumstances, it may be necessary to see the individual more than once, or use information provided by others (such as ward staff or relatives) who have observed the subject in different settings.

1. Appearance and Behaviour

Many important clues about the subject's mental state may be gained by observing his **appearance** and **behaviour**. For example, manic patients might wear inappropriate forms of **dress** for the time of day or year, or clothes which are garishly coloured. In addition, their general demeanour is often overfamiliar or disinhibited, and may be associated with overactivity and restlessness. By contrast, depressed individuals sometimes reflect their mood by dressing in sombre clothes, while their **facial expression** and **posture** are similarly indicative of sadness and despondency.

Signs of **self-neglect** can occur as a result of alcohol or drug abuse, as well as in other psychiatric conditions such as dementia, depression or schizophrenia. The presence of persecutory ideas may render the subject's **manner** suspicious and uncooperative, while those who experience hallucinations might appear vague and preoccupied, with poor eye contact. Organic states can produce fluctuations in the **level of consciousness**, resulting in inattentiveness or at times obvious drowsiness.

Abnormal **motor behaviour** may be symptomatic of either functional or organic disorders, or a consequence of the drugs used to treat these conditions (*see* Chapters 8, 9, and 12).

The following should be noted:

(a) bodily proportions and posture
(b) dress and self-care
(c) facial characteristics
(d) overall impression of state of health
(e) social behaviour — rapport, degree of cooperation, eye contact, appropriateness of manner

(f) overall impression of orientation, attention and level of consciousness
(g) general level of motor activity
(h) motor disorders associated with functional and organic disorders — including mannerisms, stereotypies, echopraxia, echolalia, automatic obedience, perseveration, negativism, waxy flexibility, mitmachen, mitgehen, forced grasping, catalepsy, pseudo-parkinsonism, orofacial and tardive dyskinesia, tremor, chorea, athetoid movements, tics, stupor (*see* Glossary for a description of terms).

2. Mood

The **mood** of an individual is his prevailing emotional tone or feeling over a period of time. However, emotions can change throughout the day, and their expression in terms of observed behaviour at any given moment is reflected by the person's **affect**. For example, the prevailing mood of manic patients may be one of elation, but this is commonly interspersed with short-lived episodes of tearfulness and dejection, at which time the affect is one of sadness. The DSM III glossary of technical terms succinctly distinguishes between affect and mood by stating 'that affect is to weather as mood is to climate'.

Abnormalities of mood may manifest in a number of ways, some of which can coexist (e.g. it is possible to be simultaneously anxious and suspicious). The prevailing mood or affect can be described as:

(a) depressed (sad)
(b) suspicious
(c) angry/irritable
(d) anxious
(e) elated
(f) perplexed
(g) fearful
(h) normal.

A useful means of assessing mood is by asking an open question such as:

Q: How do you feel in yourself, what are your spirits like?

Emotion may be abnormally expressed in various forms. **Shallow** affect or **indifference** can be observed in certain personality disorders or dissociative states. **Incongruity** of affect might occur in acute schizophrenia, in which the patient displays emotions inappropriate to the situation, i.e. laughing at distressing news. **Blunting** or **flattening** of affect refers to the reduction or absence of emotional expression most commonly seen in chronic schizophrenia. Rapid fluctuations of emotion (**labile** affect) are a feature of certain personality types and functional or organic disorders.

The assessment of mood and affect includes the following:

(a) the quality of prevailing mood as described by the subject
(b) objective observation of emotional expression, e.g. general demeanour, tone of voice
(c) appropriateness, constancy and reactivity of affect — incongruity, blunting, lability, shallowness or indifference.

3. Speech

The form of speech in terms of its **pattern**, **quantity** and **rate** should be noted here, the content being considered later. Abnormal patterns of talk may indicate an underlying thought disorder, which can occur in organic, schizophrenic and affective psychoses. Pressure of speech and flight of ideas are characteristic of mania, while the profoundly depressed patient might demonstrate poverty and slowness of speech. It is useful to make a verbatim record of any interesting or unusual aspect of the subject's conversation, in addition to noting the following:

(a) **pattern** — spontaneity, coherence and rationality, appropriateness and directness (i.e. answering questions to the point or being discursive), disordered connections (e.g. thought disorder, flight of ideas), abnormal words, puns, rhymes
(b) **quantity** — normal, increased, decreased
(c) **rate** — fast, normal, slow.

4. Thought Content

Abnormalities of thought content include obsessive-compulsive ideas, phobias, depersonalisation and derealisation, suicidal thoughts, ideas of hopelessness, abnormal beliefs and abnormal interpretation of events. One or more 'open' questions are given below as a suggested means of eliciting each of these phenomena.

(a) OBSESSIVE-COMPULSIVE PHENOMENA

Obsessions are recurrent ideas, thoughts, images or impulses which enter the mind and are persistent, intrusive and unwelcome. Although they are recognised as a product of his own mind, the individual regards them as absurd and alien to his personality. Attempts are sometimes made to ignore or resist them.

* Q: *Do you get awful thoughts coming into your mind even when you try to keep them out?*
  Q: *Do you recognise them as your own thoughts (i.e a product of the subject's own mind) or are they someone else's?*

Compulsions (or rituals) are obsessional motor acts which, although voluntary, are performed with reluctance since they are regarded as absurd and alien to the personality. The act is therefore carried out with a sense of compulsion coupled with a desire to resist. If resistance is attempted, anxiety mounts and can only be reduced by yielding.

* Q: *Do you find that you have to keep on checking things that you know you have already done?*
* Q: *Do you spend a lot of time on personal cleanliness, like washing over and over even though you know you are clean?*

(b) PHOBIAS

A phobia is a fear which is out of proportion to the demands of the situation, so that it cannot be reasoned or explained away. It is beyond voluntary control, and leads to avoidance of the provoking stimulus.

* Q: *Do you have any special fears, like some people are scared of feathers or cats or spiders or birds?*
  Q: *Do you fear certain situations, for example being in a crowd, travelling alone, or eating in a public place such as a restaurant?*
* Q: *Do you avoid any of these situations because you know you will get anxious?*

(c) DEPERSONALISATION/DEREALISATION

Depersonalisation is an experience in which the subject feels 'as if' he is no longer real, which has an associated unpleasant quality. **Derealisation** is an accompanying symptom in which there is a feeling of unreality that relates to the environment ('as if' the world is not real). Neither of these phenomena are delusional beliefs, because the person is aware of the nature of the change he experiences.

* Q: *Have you had the feeling recently that things around you were unreal? (As though everything was an imitation of reality, like a stage set, with people acting instead of being themselves?)*
* Q: *Have you yourself felt unreal, that you were not a person, not in the living world?*

(d) SUICIDAL THOUGHTS AND IDEAS OF HOPELESSNESS

Occasional **suicidal thoughts** are not uncommon, especially in times of great stress, but in most cases they are fleeting and no serious degree of intent exists. Of much greater significance is the person who describes recurrent or persistent suicidal thoughts, plans or ideas.

Most people who are suicidal welcome the opportunity to share their burden with someone, although the manner in which enquiries are made is extremely important. Direct questions such as 'Do you feel like killing yourself?' should in the first instance be avoided, as they do not instil an impression of caring and compassion in the patient's mind. It might be more appropriate to start by asking tactfully:

* *Q: Have you felt that life wasn't worth living?*

If affirmative, this can be followed by:
* *Q: Did you ever feel like ending it all?*
* *Q: What did you think you might do?*
* *Q: Did you actually try?*

As part of the assessment of the degree of suicidal intent, **ideas of hopelessness** should always be sought, since their presence increases the likelihood of self-harm.

* *Q: How do you see the future?*
* *Q: Have you given up or does there still seem some reason for trying?*

(e) DELUSIONS AND ABNORMAL IDEAS

A **delusion** is a false belief which is unshakeably held, even in the face of evidence to the contrary, and is out of keeping with the individual's social and cultural background.

This last part of the definition is important, particularly when assessing people of different nationalities or cultures. For example, a belief in the 'voodoo' is commonplace in parts of the West Indies, so that mishappenings attributed to its influence would not necessarily be considered delusional in someone born and raised in that area.

Delusions can be described according to their **origin** (primary or secondary), their degree of **fixity** (full or partial) and their **content** (i.e. persecutory, grandiose, etc.).

A **primary (autochthonous) delusion** is one which appears suddenly in the mind, fully formed like a 'brain wave', so that its development is not understandable in terms of previous thoughts or other experiences. It is an important diagnostic feature of schizophrenia and is sometimes associated with a **delusional perception**, or **delusional mood** (these are discussed further in Chapter 8).

Secondary delusions can be understood as developing from other psychological experiences. For example, the elated mood in mania may give rise to grandiose delusions of great wealth or fame. On the other hand, the depressed person might develop false beliefs of ruination and worthlessness in the context of his altered mood. Hallucinations (*see later*) may also give rise to abnormal beliefs, as in the case of someone hearing voices insulting him, who subsequently develops persecutory delusions. The evolution of a number of secondary delusions which are interrelated can lead to the formation of a complex **delusional system**.

In **partial delusions** the abnormal belief is expressed with great conviction but is not firmly held, and may therefore be amenable to reason. This can occur at a stage prior to the development of the **full delusion**, or in the recovery phase of an illness where insight is being regained. In order to establish the fixity of delusions it is helpful to ask:

 * *Q: Even when you seem to be most convinced, do you really feel in the back of your mind that it might well not be true, that it might be imagination?*

Overvalued ideas differ from delusions in that they are intense false preoccupations which are not held with unshakeable conviction, but have usually been present for a long time and are often associated with marked emotional investment. For example, a man objected to his sister receiving an intramuscular injection while she was a patient in hospital, as he held the strong conviction that their mother's death from a brain tumour had been caused by similar means. After a series of discussions with staff, he eventually capitulated, but even so continued to feel uneasy about this form of treatment.

The classification of delusions according to content includes the following categories:

   i. delusions of the possession of thought (thought alienation) and passivity experiences
  ii. persecutory delusions
 iii. delusions of reference
 iv. grandiose delusions
   v. delusions of jealousy
 vi. erotic delusions
 vii. nihilistic delusions
viii. delusions of guilt and worthlessness
 ix. hypochondriacal delusions.

i. Delusions of the possession of thought (thought alienation) and passivity experiences

These are phenomena in which the subject has a delusional belief that thoughts, actions, emotions or sensations which he experiences are not his own, and are being imposed on him by some outside force or influence against his will. Consequently, the subject is seemingly passive as he takes no active part in their generation. Under certain circumstances they are diagnostic of schizophrenia, and are discussed in further detail in Chapter 8.

In **thought insertion**, the individual experiences thoughts that he does not recognise as a product of his own mind, and which he believes have been put there by some outside force or agency.

In **thought withdrawal**, the individual experiences his thoughts as being taken out of his mind against his will by some external force or agency. Objectively, this might be apparent by the patient stopping short in mid-sentence. Afterwards he may describe a frightening experience of his mind having been completely emptied of all thoughts (**thought block**) so that it contained absolutely nothing. This is not to be confused with the common experience of momentary interruption in the stream of thought, when one cannot think of what to say next.

In **thought broadcast**, the subject experiences his unspoken thoughts as being known to, or shared by those around him, so that he believes that they are not contained within his own mind.

A general screening question would be:

* Q: *Can you think quite clearly or is there any interference with your thoughts?*

Thought insertion

* Q: *Are thoughts put into your head which you know are not your own? How do you know they are not your own? Where do they come from?*

Thought withdrawal

* Q: *Do your thoughts ever seem to be taken out of your head, as though some external person or force were removing them?*

Thought block

* Q: *Do you ever experience your thoughts stopping quite unexpectedly so that there are none left in your mind, even when your thoughts were flowing freely before?*

Thought broadcast

> *Q: Are your thoughts ever broadcast so that others can share them
> and know what you are thinking, even when they are not in the same
> room? How do you explain this?*

Made feelings are feelings or emotions that are experienced which the
individual does not recognise as his own, but are attributed to some
external force and are felt to be imposed upon him.

Made impulses: the individual has the experience of being overcome by
a sudden impulse that he believes is derived from some external influence,
and on which he subsequently acts.

Made acts: the subject experiences his actions as being under the
control of an external influence that initiates and directs the movements
throughout. He feels like a robot, the passive observer of his own actions.

Somatic passivity: the subject believes that he is a passive and reluctant
recipient of bodily sensations imposed upon him by some external
influence.

Passivity experiences of feelings impulses actions and sensations

> * *Q: Do you feel under the control of some force or power other than
> yourself? (As though you were a robot or a zombie without a will of
> your own?)*

Sometimes the experience of passivity may be described without
explanation, or attributed to X-rays, laser beams, hypnosis etc. On
occasion the subject may say that thoughts, emotions, impulses or actions
which he recognises as a product *of his own mind or volition* (i.e. not
experienced as alien in their origin) are being interfered with by an
external influence (a delusion of control).

ii. Persecutory delusions

Delusions of persecution involve the subject believing that he is being
followed, picked on, defamed, poisoned or conspired against by others,
who may or may not be known to him (*see* Chapter 8). They can render
the individual suspicious, uncooperative and at times dangerous, so that
great care must be taken when interviewing such people. Persecutory
delusions may occur in organic states, and functional disorders, such as
depression and schizophrenia.

> *Q: In general, do you feel people treat you fairly or unfairly?*
> * *Q: Is anyone deliberately trying to harm you, for example trying to
> poison you or kill you? How do you explain this?*

iii. Delusions of reference

These are false beliefs held by the subject that other people, events or objects have a particular and unusual meaning specifically for him. For example, he may be convinced that the casual glances of passers-by signify their knowledge that he is homosexual, or that the tone of voice of a television newsreader is intended to convey a message especially for him. When the individual realises that the feelings he experiences originate within himself, they are known as ideas (as opposed to delusions) of reference.

Delusions/ideas of reference

> *Q: Do people ever do or say things which (seem to) have a special meaning for you?*
> * *Q: Do you see any reference to yourself on TV or in the papers?*

iv. Grandiose delusions

The subject believes that he possesses exceptional powers or talents, or that he is a person of great importance, sometimes with a special purpose or mission in life. These delusions are most frequently encountered in manic states, but they can also occur in schizophrenia and organic disorders.

> * *Q: Is there anything special about you?*
> * *Q: What is your opinion of yourself compared to other people? (better, worse, the same?)*
> * *Q: Do you have special abilities or powers? Is there a special purpose or mission to your life?*

v. Delusions of jealousy

These are usually based upon the subject's false belief concerning the supposed infidelity of his spouse or partner, with highly dubious or improbable evidence being offered in support of his allegations. They are more frequently encountered in men, especially those who drink heavily, and may lead to violent and homicidal acts (*see* p. 398: Othello syndrome).

> * *Q: Do you have any reason to be jealous of anybody?*
> *Q: Do you trust your partner, or do you have any reason to believe that your partner is deceiving you?*

vi. Erotic delusions

Abnormal ideas of this kind are more common in females, and usually involve a false belief of being loved or admired by someone who in reality is remote and inaccessible, such as a person of high standing or public renown. The object of desire may be relentlessly pursued despite his clear lack of interest in, or overt rejection of, his admirer (*see* p. 398: de Clérambault's syndrome).

vii. Nihilistic delusions

The individual believes that certain things, such as the world, his loved ones, his career, parts of his body or indeed his entire self, no longer exist. These delusions are most commonly encountered in severe depressive illnesses (*see* p. 399: Cotard's syndrome).

viii. Delusions of guilt and worthlessness

In delusions of guilt, the subject often believes that he has committed a wicked act or performed some moral transgression, which in reality is trivial or non-existent, but for which he feels he ought to be punished. In some cases this may lead to a suicide attempt. Delusions of worthlessness may result in an individual rejecting help or treatment because he believes he does not deserve it, or that he is beneath contempt. Both are most frequently encountered in the setting of a depressive illness.

> *Q: Do you feel you have committed a crime, or sinned greatly, or deserve punishment?*

ix. Hypochondriacal delusions

These are false convictions of ill-health, which are held despite reassurance from doctors or other professionals that they are groundless. The individual may believe that he is suffering from a terminal illness, or describes distressing symptoms which are without substance, such as obstruction of the throat or rotting of the bowels.

5. Perceptual Abnormalities

Abnormal perceptual experiences involve sensory distortions and sensory deceptions.

(a) SENSORY DISTORTIONS

Sensory distortions are due to perceived alterations in either the intensity, quality or spatial form of the stimulus. For example, colours might appear more vivid, sounds louder or softer, and objects can seem larger (macropsia) or smaller (micropsia). Distortions may result from organic states (such as those induced by drugs, metabolic changes or infection), intense anxiety or heightened emotion.

(b) SENSORY DECEPTIONS

Sensory deceptions involve either illusions, true hallucinations or pseudo-hallucinations.

i. Illusions

Illusions are misinterpretations of external sensory stimuli to produce a false perception. For example, the howling of the wind may be mistaken for a cry of distress, or the shadow of a tree in poor light is incorrectly perceived as being the figure of a man. Illusions can occur in functional and organic conditions, as well as in individuals who are not mentally disordered, such as people suffering from extreme fatigue.

ii. True hallucinations

These differ from illusions in that they are false perceptions which arise in the absence of any external stimulus. They are experienced as being situated in the outside world (as opposed to being 'in the mind'), and therefore have the same substance, clarity and permanence as real perceptions. They can occur in all sensory modalities and cannot be produced or dismissed at will, the subject having no insight into their true nature. Hallucinations may be perceived as originating in the external environment, or emanating from within the subject's own body.

When eliciting an experience which appears to be hallucinatory, it is important to determine not only its source (external or internal space), but also the content, timing, frequency and effect on the patient. For example, in the case of auditory hallucinations the following questions should be asked:

* *Q: I should like to ask you a routine question which we ask of everybody. Do you ever seem to hear noises or voices when there is no one about, and nothing else to explain it?*
* *Q: Are these voices (or noises) in your mind or can you hear them through your ears?*
* *Q: How do you explain the voice(s)?*
* *Q: What does (do) the voice(s) say?*
* *Q: Do you hear several voices talking about you?*
* *Q: Do you hear your name being called? Do they speak directly to you?*
* *Q: Do they refer to you as 'he' ('she')?*
* *Q: Do they seem to comment on what you are thinking or reading or doing?*
  Q: How often do you hear the voices/sounds? Is there any particular time of day or situation when they occur?

Hypnagogic hallucinations are experienced just as the subject is falling asleep, and hypnopompic hallucinations at the time of awakening. They are frequently auditory, and both types can occur in the absence of mental illness.

The most commonly encountered hallucinations are auditory and may take the form of voices, music, singing or noises. They can occur in the context of functional illnesses, such as schizophrenia or affective disorders (*see* Chapters 5 and 8), as well as in certain organic states, i.e. delirium, dementia, temporal lobe epilepsy, alcohol or drug abuse.

The presence of visual hallucinations should always raise the possibility of an organic disorder, especially alcohol withdrawal and other delirious states. Olfactory, gustatory and tactile hallucinations are less common, but may occur in a variety of functional and organic disorders.

> *Q: Have you seen/smelt/tasted/felt anything that puzzled or frightened you and that others were not aware of?*

iii. Pseudohallucinations

This is a confusing and ambiguous term because it is used in two distinct ways. On the one hand, it is applied to a form of mental imagery, in which perceptual experiences, although vivid, tend to be fleeting and lack the substance and clarity of normal perceptions or true hallucinations. Even so, they cannot be produced or dismissed at will. A further distinction from true hallucinations is that they are experienced in subjective space, sometimes referred to as the 'mind's ear' or 'mind's eye'. The second use of the term is to describe hallucinations which the subject recognises as having no place in the external world. An example of the latter is in the case of phenomena which sometimes occur in the acute stages of bereavement, when the deceased's voice may be heard or their form seen by the spouse or other close relative (*see* Chapter 7). Pseudohallucinations (in either sense of the term) do not necessarily signify mental disorder, although they can occur in several psychiatric conditions.

6. Cognitive State

Cognition is the faculty of knowing and perceiving. The cognitive state examination tests **orientation**, **concentration/attention**, **memory** and **general knowledge**, the latter being a guide to the level of intelligence. Where there is clear evidence of impairment, more specific tests of brain function may be carried out (*see later*).

Consciousness is defined as the state of awareness of the self and the environment, and may be obviously impaired during examination, as evidenced by drowsiness or sleepiness. However, several levels of consciousness exist along the continuum between full awareness and coma, and this may not be apparent unless specifically tested for, sometimes on more than one occasion. When consciousness is impaired, one or more aspects of cognitive function are affected. It is important to look for fluctuations in the level of consciousness during the interview, and to determine from other observers if variations occur throughout the day. There are no signs which are specific for minor impairment (clouding) of consciousness, and its detection rests upon clinical judgement based on the following indicators:

(a) evidence of drowsiness or reduced awareness of the environment
(b) fluctuations in the level of consciousness during examination or reported at other times. These may only be apparent at night-time or when the patient is fatigued
(c) evidence of dullness, inactivity or uncertain behaviour in the absence of drowsiness
(d) impairment of orientation, (see following pages). Lack of orientation for time is the most sensitive indicator, followed by place and then person in more severe cases
(e) poor concentration resulting in disruption of the train of thought or conversation. Attention is focused on subjective stimuli rather than external events
(f) impairment of registration and short-term memory recall; long-term memory may also be affected.

Altered states of consciousness are discussed further in Chapter 9.

i. ORIENTATION

Orientation should be determined for time, place and person. Disorientation is most commonly found in organic disorders.

> Q: What is the time/day/date/month/year?
> Q: What is this place you are in now?
> Q: What is your name? Who am I? Who is this person (e.g. pointing to a nurse)?

ii. CONCENTRATION AND ATTENTION

These may be impaired in functional illnesses (such as mania or depression) and in organic states. Apparent memory defects, particularly those seen in depressive illnesses, are usually due to poor concentration since both functions are interrelated.

In addition to an overall impression of distractability, concentration and attention may be specifically tested for by asking:

> *Q: Please give me the months of the year/days of the week in reverse order.*

or by the serial 7s test:

> *Q: Please subtract 7 from 100, and then continue to take 7 away from the remainder (i.e. 100 . . . 93 . . . 86 . . .)*

In both tests, the time taken and number of mistakes made should be recorded.

iii. MEMORY AND GENERAL KNOWLEDGE

Specific tests should only be interpreted in conjunction with an overall impression of memory function gained from the subject, and from information given by others. Nervousness during the interview or alteration in mood can dramatically affect performance, so that it might be necessary to see the individual on more than one occasion to verify the consistency of any apparent defects.

Tests of **immediate memory** include the ability to register new information and recall it straight away, such as repeating a series of four or five digits forwards and backwards. Since this also tests concentration to some extent, any impairment in the latter may result in defective recall.

Short-term (or recent) memory can be judged by assessing the subject's capacity for new learning. He is given a name and address and asked to repeat it following an interval of 5 minutes, to see how well it has been retained. In addition, memory for recent events may be determined by testing the individual's recollection of current news items, television programmes or personal happenings that can be verified, such as the details of meals or ward outings.

Long-term (or remote) memory is more difficult to test, since personal information given cannot always be easily validated (e.g. when the subject married or when children were born). Consequently, it is useful to ask about items of common general knowledge, such as the years World War II began and ended, or the name of the prime minister at that time. Inconsistencies in the sequence in which events are described should be noted, as well as recording selective impairment of memory for particular incidents or periods of time, such as before and after accidents.

Memory testing should also note the quality of the patient's answers as well as their content. **Confabulation** (a falsification of memory), and **perseveration** (the inappropriate repetition of a previous answer or act) are both suggestive of a dementing process (*see* Chapter 9).

Short-term (recent) memory

> *Q: I'm going to give you a name and address and when I've finished please repeat it. (This is to check that registration has been adequate.) Try and remember it, because I shall ask you again in 5 minutes' time.*

The name and address should be seven items, e.g. John Holbrooke, 5 Croft Avenue, Windsor, Berkshire. (The number of attempts before the information is fully registered should be noted, as well as any errors on recall.)

> *Q: Have you read anything interesting in the papers/seen anything on television recently? Tell me about it.*

Long-term (remote) memory and general knowledge.

> *Q: Who was prime minister throughout most of World War II?*
> *Q: What is the Queen's name/names of her children?*
> *Q: Can you name five cities in England?*

It is also useful to ask *verifiable* personal details, such as birth dates or anniversaries. The interviewer should allow for cultural differences and poor intellect when interpreting answers. The level of intelligence can be estimated from the educational history, work record, interests and general knowledge of the individual, but it may be determined more accurately by **psychometric testing** (*see* Chapter 18).

In patients suspected of having an organic brain disorder, further cognitive assessment may be necessary to help determine the location and extent of the cerebral lesion. These include tests for language and arithmetical functions, apraxia and agnosia.

iv. TESTS FOR LANGUAGE AND ARITHMETICAL FUNCTIONS

Impairment of the expression and comprehension of language is referred to respectively as **expressive** and **receptive dysphasia**. These can be tested for during the interview by assessing the subject's ability to converse normally and to understand questions put to him in written or verbal form. **Nominal dysphasia** is impairment of the ability to name specific objects when asked to do so. **Dysgraphia** and **dyscalculia** refer to impairment of the abilities to write and to solve mathematical problems.

v. TESTS FOR APRAXIA

Apraxia may be defined as the inability to carry out purposeful actions, in the absence of any significant motor or sensory dysfunction. It occurs in association with lesions of the parietal lobe, and can be tested for in several ways.

In **constructional apraxia** the subject is unable to copy or construct simple geometric figures, while **motor apraxia** is an inability to perform simple acts when asked to do so. The individual with **dressing apraxia** is incapable of putting on or removing garments such as a jacket or cardigan.

> *Q: Show me how a soldier salutes.*
> *Q: Copy this drawing for me (house, clock face, square, circle)*
> *Q: Please take your cardigan off and put it on again.*

vi. TESTS FOR AGNOSIA

Agnosia is defined as 'perception stripped of meaning', and occurs in association with parietal lobe dysfunction. The defect cannot be explained by sensory impairment, mental deterioration or disorders of consciousness and attention. It can present as an inability to recognise objects visually (**visual agnosia**) or by touch (**astereognosis**), as well as familiar faces (**prosopagnosia**), colours, sounds (**auditory agnosia**) and certain parts of the body (e.g. **finger agnosia**).

> *Q: (Pointing to a familiar object such as a chair or table) What is that, and what is it used for?*

7. Insight

Insight refers to the level of accurate understanding that an individual has as to the nature of his condition, its causation and his need for treatment. Consequently, insight may be described as being either intact, partial or absent.

> * *Q: Do you think there is anything the matter with you?*
> * *Q: What do you think it is?*
> * *Q: Could it be a nervous condition?*
> * *Q: What do you think the cause is?*
> * *Q: Why did you need to come to hospital?*
> *Q: Do you think you need treatment?*

8. Physical Examination

Every patient should be physically examined to determine whether presenting psychological symptoms are in any way attributable to organic illness. It is also important to assess the overall state of the individual's physical health, and where appropriate, further investigations such as haematological, biochemical or radiological procedures may be required.

SUMMARY

The Psychiatric History

1. **General information**: name and address, age and sex, marital status, occupation, country of origin, religion, patient's status (in- or outpatient, informal or detained).
2. **Presenting complaint/reason for referral**: brief verbatim account, including its effect on the subject's life.
3. **History of presenting condition**: duration, nature and chronological order of symptoms, possible precipitants, aggravating and relieving factors (including any treatment received), related disturbances of bodily function — sleep, appetite, weight, energy, libido.
4. **Family history**: personal details of parents and siblings, home atmosphere, record of any psychiatric or physical disorder in other family members.
5. **Past psychiatric history**: for each previous episode of mental disorder record the name of hospital where treated, date and duration of care, diagnosis, precipitants, treatment and outcome.
6. **Past medical history**: record any significant physical illnesses, accidents, operations or other hospital admissions; note drugs prescribed (past and present).
7. **Personal history**: a. **Early development and childhood** — problems during pregnancy and birth, developmental milestones and any evidence of delay, periods of separation from care givers, domestic stability and level of contentment, psychological and physical health. b. **Schooling** — ages of starting and finishing at each school, qualifications gained, any periods of prolonged absence (note reasons), relationships with peers and teachers, level of enjoyment, antisocial behaviour. c. **Employment** — details of present and previous jobs, periods of unemployment. d. **Psychosexual and marital history** — menstrual and sexual history, dates of current/previous marriage(s), details of spouse/partner and children, periods of separation, details of recent sexual activity.
8. **Social history**: details of accommodation and financial circumstances, leisure interests and hobbies, social relationships, tobacco, alcohol and illicit drug use (level of consumption/abuse/dependency), brief profile of daily activity; forensic history.
9. **Premorbid personality**: character, predominant mood, attitudes, self-image (an independent account should always be obtained).
10. **Additional history from other informant(s)**: independent source.

The Mental State Examination

1. **Appearance and behaviour:** bodily proportions and posture, dress and level of self-care, facial characteristics, overall state of health, social behaviour (rapport, manner, eye contact, degree of cooperativeness), apparent level of consciousness, level of motor activity and any associated disorders of movement.
2. **Mood:** subjective account of prevailing mood, objective emotional expression, appropriateness, constancy and reactivity of affect.
3. **Speech:** pattern, quantity and rate.
4. **Thought content:** obsessive-compulsive phenomena, phobias, depersonalisation/derealisation, suicidal thoughts, ideas of hopelessness/worthlessness, abnormal ideas and beliefs (delusions).
5. **Perceptual abnormalities:** sensory distortions and sensory deceptions: illusions, true hallucinations, pseudohallucinations.
6. **Cognitive state:** level of consciousness, orientation for time, place and person; concentration and attention, memory — immediate, short-term, long-term; general knowledge and estimated level of intelligence, further tests of language and arithmetical function, tests of visuospatial function (apraxia and agnosia).
7. **Insight:** level of understanding as to the nature of the condition, its causation and the need for treatment.
8. **Physical examination.**

REFERENCES AND FURTHER READING

Gelder, M., Gath, D., Mayou, R. (1983). Interviewing, clinical examination and record keeping. In *Oxford Textbook of Psychiatry*, pp. 32–66. Oxford: Oxford University Press.

Institute of Psychiatry (1987). *Notes on Eliciting and Recording Clinical Information*. Oxford: Oxford University Press.

Wing, J. K., Cooper, J. E., Sartorius, N. (1974). *The Measurement and Classification of Psychiatric Symptoms*. Cambridge: Cambridge University Press.

3 PERSONALITY DISORDERS

Personality is a difficult term to define, but is generally held to refer to those aspects of a person's behaviour, thinking and emotional reactions which are enduring and predictable throughout a wide range of circumstances and life situations. Features of personality would therefore include an individual's persisting attitudes, values, feelings and intellectual capabilities.

PERSONALITY DEVELOPMENT

The influence of heredity on the developing personality is indicated by the findings of twin studies, which have shown a greater concordance of certain personality traits among monozygotic compared to dizygotic twin pairs. Furthermore, differences in temperament between infants can be identified shortly after birth (e.g. fractiousness or placidity), many of which persist into childhood and even later life.

Normal personality development is dependent on normal brain maturation and functioning, so that any adverse intrauterine, perinatal or postnatal influences which cause damage to the central nervous system may lead to the development of a disordered personality (*see* p. 349). Psychodynamic factors, including the effects of early interpersonal relationships between child and caregivers, also need to be considered, and these are discussed further in Chapter 13.

The effects of emotional deprivation or a disturbed family life on personality development are difficult to establish. Although some children reared in this manner do have abnormal personalities as adults, this is not always the case. The role of learning is also important, and may have a significant effect in modifying aspects of innate temperament. A child who is naturally placid might learn to become more aggressive if this is the manner in which his parents habitually interact. Consequently, it would seem that the personality is shaped as a result of the interplay between biological and environmental factors, as well as through opportunities for social interaction. There is no evidence to support the previously held view that an association exists between personality type and body build.

PERSONALITY AND ILLNESS

Personality has an important bearing on people's responses to physical illness (*see* Chapter 15), and also their susceptibility to develop certain types of psychiatric disorder. For example, someone who leads a totally ordered and controlled existence is more likely to become anxious or depressed when faced with change or uncertainty, than a person who thrives on challenges and novel situations. Similarly, the clinical features of a mental disorder may be greatly influenced by aspects of the personality. For instance, persecutory delusions may be a prominent feature of a depressive illness in someone with a suspicious and untrusting nature.

Although an association between certain personality types and specific psychiatric conditions evidently exists (e.g. obsessional personalities are prone to develop depressive illnesses and obsessional neuroses), others do not seem to confer any susceptibility to mental illness. Consequently, schizoid personalities are no more liable than other types to develop schizophrenia (although it was once considered that they were), nor are hysterical (histrionic) personalities aetiologically linked with hysterical neurosis.

THE ASSESSMENT OF PERSONALITY

Behaviour and patterns of social interaction can vary from one situation to another and be influenced by different environmental conditions. For example, a man, who is normally aggressive or controlling within his peer group, may initially appear calm and subdued in the presence of authority figures, or feel daunted by the attendance of staff members at a ward meeting. Consequently, it is impossible to make an objective assessment of personality on the basis of one interview. Furthermore, the behaviour of patients may be a reflection of mental illness rather than underlying personality, or an admixture of both. Therefore, any interpretation of current behaviour must be made in the light of past modes of functioning, supplemented wherever possible by information from an independent source.

Personality inventories are psychological tests which have been developed to assist the clinician in the assessment of personality disorders. They attempt to discriminate between normal and abnormal personalities using standardised questions about attitudes and emotional reactions, as well as physical and psychological symptoms. Although theoretically useful, their clinical application is limited by problems of validating responses in the presence of mental illness. In addition, because the tests are self-administered, subjects have a tendency to answer questions in a way which reflects their wish to be seen in a favourable light, thereby leading to further inaccuracies.

NORMAL AND ABNORMAL PERSONALITY

Because personality is commonly understood as one of the ways of differentiating between people, the concept of **normality** is difficult to establish. This is further complicated by the fact that certain ideas, emotional reactions and behaviour appear to be universal, while others are culture-bound or limited still further to specific groups or individuals. Bearing these factors in mind, any attempt to define **abnormal personality** will have obvious limitations. ICD 9 defines personality disorder as 'deeply ingrained, maladaptive patterns of behaviour, generally recognisable by the time of adolescence or earlier, and continuing throughout most of adult life, although often becoming less obvious in middle or old age. The personality is abnormal either in the balance of its components, their quality and expression, or in its total aspect. Because of this deviation or psychopathy, the patient suffers or others have to suffer, and there is an adverse effect upon the individual or on society.' (In this definition, the term 'psychopathy' is used to denote *all* abnormal personalities. However, later in this chapter, it is used more specifically to describe a personality in which antisocial behaviour is a prominent feature.)

Consequently, the concept of **personality disorder** embraces a number of elements, namely:

1. the characteristics of the personality, which is distorted by an exaggeration or imbalance of its constituent traits
2. the behaviour of the individual, which is identified as being maladaptive from an early age
3. the presence of suffering, either of the self, others or society.

Difficulties sometimes arise when trying to determine whether **deviant behaviour** results from a personality disorder or mental illness, which may have important implications with regard to treatment (*see later*). Certain personality disorders lead to abnormal behaviour only when the person is subjected to some form of stress, while in others, it can occur in the absence of any clear precipitant. In general, recent behavioural changes in an individual who previously functioned normally are more likely to be the result of mental illness, whereas if the current abnormal behaviour has been present from an early age, it is probably attributable to a personality disorder. The limitations to making such a distinction are evident where illness has persisted for many years (as may occur in chronic schizophrenia), when long-term abnormal behaviour results from mental retardation, or where no independent history of earlier behaviour is available. Diagnostically, it is possible for mental illness and personality disorder to coexist (*see* p. 8).

The presence of **suffering** is perhaps most easily determined when behavioural patterns are clearly maladaptive. For example, some individuals are consistently aggressive towards others without apparent reason, while the abnormally suspicious personality may suffer by constantly doubting the intentions of others. The highly obsessional individual might be unable to complete tasks because of unrealistic attention to detail, and as a result, persistently experiences a sense of failure by setting himself impossible standards of perfection.

The **classification** of personality disorders is largely descriptive, and is based upon the identification of specific clusters of observable phenomena (**personality traits**), which are then assigned to a diagnostic category. In practice, such a system is fraught with difficulties because:

1. the combination with which traits appear in any diagnostic category is highly variable
2. clinically, considerable overlap occurs between the different proposed entities
3. nearly all the traits which constitute abnormal personalities can sometimes be identified to a lesser degree in personalities considered to be normal
4. the criteria for deciding whether a personality is abnormal (by virtue of the balance of its components, their quality and expression, or in its total aspect) are often vague and ill-defined.

ICD 10 is likely to differentiate between personality disorders, personality trait accentuation and personality change. **Personality disorder** and **personality trait accentuation** are distinguished from one another by their severity and their pervasiveness. While the latter involves a relatively moderate aggravation of a single trait, or of a few interrelated traits, with little or no impairment in social functioning, personality disorders proper are characterised by marked abnormalities of the total aspect of the person and cause serious personal distress or social dysfunction. Both differ from personality change in the timing and the mode of their emergence. Personality trait accentuation and personality disorders are developmental conditions which appear in childhood or adolescence, are not secondary to other mental disorders or brain disease, and continue into adulthood. In contrast, **personality change** is acquired, usually during adult life, following severe or prolonged stresses, extreme environmental deprivation, serious psychiatric disorders, or brain disease or injury.

SPECIFIC PERSONALITY DISORDERS

Some of the personality disorders which are listed in both ICD 9 and DSM III-R, and the traits which they are identified by, are shown in Table 3.1. Not all of the traits are present in every case, and some disordered personalities may have favourable aspects as well as the detrimental characteristics mentioned. Although many of the terms listed are widely

Table 3.1 Personality Disorders

Type	Features
Obsessional (anankastic)	Rigid and inflexible personality, bigotry, meanness, obstinacy, excessive perfectionism and cleanliness, indecisiveness and pedantry (some obsessional traits may be viewed favourably by others, i.e. dependability, precision, punctuality, high moral standards)
Histrionic (hysterical)	Egocentricity, insincerity, vanity, emotional shallowness, tendency to dramatise situations, sexual immaturity and frigidity, craving for excitement, flirtatiousness, attention-seeking, manipulative and dependent behaviour, capacity for self-deception and inconsistency (favourable traits in normal personalities may include liveliness, social attractiveness and theatrical ability)
Paranoid	Suspiciousness and mistrust of others, over-sensitivity to setbacks or criticism, absence of tenderness and sentimentality, tendency towards jealousy and aggressiveness, excessive ideas of self-importance and self-reference, argumentativeness
Schizoid	Introspectiveness, aloofness, detachment from socialising, lack of emotional warmth, tendency to solitary existence, self-absorbed with inner fantasy world (such traits may be advantageous in those who need to live or work in isolated environments)
Affective	Disorders of mood control *persisting throughout life:* 1. **depressive personality** — tendency to gloominess and pessimism, unwarranted worrying, constant misery and diminished capacity for enjoyment 2. **hyperthymic personality** — persistent optimism and cheerfulness (irrespective of the circumstances), rashness and lack of judgement 3. **cyclothymic personality** — tendency to alternate between depressive and hyperthymic forms (this may be a precursor to bipolar affective disorder)
Explosive	Tendency to outbursts of anger or violence, poor emotional control, absence of any other antisocial behaviour
Asthenic (dependent)	Passive tendencies, compliant with the wishes of others, lack of assertiveness, lack of vitality, avoidance of responsibility, tendency to manipulate others into caring for them

continued overleaf

Table 3.1 *Continued*

Type	Features
Borderline	Feelings of emptiness and boredom, impulsive or unpredictable behaviour, poor sense of identity, instability of mood, tendency to self-mutilation, unstable and intense relationships, poor control over anger and aggression, intolerance of being alone
Narcissistic	Increased sense of self-importance, desire for constant attention, rich fantasy life, anger or indifference in response to criticism, selfishness, disregard for others, egocentricity

used clinically, it is often preferable to give a brief description of the personality rather than to use a diagnostic label which may be misleading.

ICD 10 is likely to provide diagnostic guidelines for the following personality disorders: paranoid, schizoid, dyssocial, impulsive, histrionic, anankastic, anxious, dependent, other and unspecified forms.

An important concept from both the psychiatric and legal viewpoint is the psychopathic or antisocial personality disorder (see below). Once again, it must be reiterated that what is being discussed is an imprecise clinical entity, the characteristics of which are highly variable. Consequently, there is considerable danger in labelling someone a 'psychopath', with all the pejorative connotations that this entails, without qualifying those aspects of the personality or manifest behaviour which led to such a diagnosis being made.

PSYCHOPATHIC PERSONALITY DISORDER (antisocial personality disorder or sociopathy) (This will probably be classified as 'dyssocial personality disorder' in ICD 10.)

Development of the Concept

Throughout the nineteenth century, it was recognised that there was a group of people who shared the common features of a lack of moral values and a tendency to outbursts of violence, occurring in the absence of intellectual impairment, delusions or hallucinations. Various terms were used to describe such behaviour by physicians in Europe and America — 'manie sans delire' (Pinel, 1801), 'moral derangement' (Rush, 1812) and 'moral insanity' (Prichard, 1835).

In 1891, Koch used the term **psychopathic inferiority** to describe similarly abnormal behaviour occurring in the absence of major mental illness or intellectual impairment. Kraepelin (1907) introduced the term

psychopathic personality to expand this concept and emphasised that the behaviour of such individuals caused suffering to others. Schneider (1923) postulated that there was an additional group of personality disordered people who only caused suffering to themselves. A further classification was introduced in 1939 by Henderson, who described three kinds of psychopathic personality: the **aggressive** type (violent, with a tendency to self-harm); the **inadequate** type (unstable, passive, hypochondriacal and dishonest); and the **creative** type (self-minded and ruthless, yet often gifted and imaginative).

The term **sociopathy** became popular in the USA in the 1960s, and reflects the impact that psychopathic personalities have on society through their antisocial behaviour (DSM III-R now favours the term **antisocial personality**). In the UK, **psychopathic disorder** is defined in the Mental Health Act as one of the forms of mental disorder for which compulsory admission and detention in hospital may be necessary (*see* Chapter 24). Scott (1960) attempted to outline the common elements contained in the various definitions of psychopathic disorder, these being:

1. an exclusion of psychotic illness or subnormality (mental retardation) *? isn't this a pers disorder definition ?*
2. the disorder is persistent from an early age
3. behaviour is described as abnormally aggressive, antisocial, seriously irresponsible or inadequate
4. society is impelled to deal with such individuals.

Clinical Features

Those who accept the concept of a psychopathic personality identify a number of features which are said to be characteristic of the disorder, although the combination in which they occur will vary. They include:

1. a lack of remorse or feeling for others
2. impulsive behaviour and poor tolerance of stress
3. an inability to learn from experience
4. a tendency towards violent and aggressive behaviour
5. irresponsibility and a disregard for social obligations
6. a poor understanding of personal motivation.

The antecedents of psychopathic personality may be evident from early childhood or adolescence. There is often a history of conduct disorder, hyperactivity, truanting or suspension from school, and a general failure to respond to disciplinary measures. Delinquent behaviour, persistent lying and fighting are other common features at this time.

In adult life, interpersonal relationships tend to be superficial, unstable and short-lived. Sexual activity begins at an early age and sometimes develops into promiscuous behaviour. Marriages are often volatile and unsuccessful, and there may be a history of violence, repeated separations or divorce. The individual's work record tends to be poor, and is marked by frequent job changes, dismissals, impulsive walkouts, absenteeism and an inability to get along with colleagues or accept orders from superiors. Some psychopaths resort to petty criminal acts which are characteristically performed on impulse, so that the forensic record can be extensive. A history of alcohol or drug abuse is often elicited, and bouts of anxiety or depression may be associated with suicidal threats or gestures. By their mid-30s, many psychopathic personalities show some degree of maturation, in that their antisocial behaviour becomes less overt, although interpersonal relationships often remain chaotic.

Aetiology

A **genetic influence** has been suggested by twin and adoption studies (*see* Chapter 1), although the difference in concordance rates between monozygotic and dizygotic twin pairs is not as clear cut as with other psychiatric disorders in which genetic factors are implicated. Electro-encephalographic (**EEG**) studies have shown some minor abnormalities in the traces of those individuals diagnosed as having psychopathic personalities. The pattern produced resembles that found in children, which has led to the proposal that the disorder may be associated with 'immaturity' of the cerebral cortex. Another theory advocates that psychopaths are born with '**underactive autonomic nervous systems**', and that their 'sensation-seeking' behaviour is an attempt to compensate for this underactivity.

A number of **environmental factors** in infancy and early childhood have been implicated in the development of psychopathic personality disorder. These include prolonged maternal deprivation, family discord and a history of parental antisocial behaviour or alcohol abuse. **Psychoanalytical theory** relates psychopathy to the underdevelopment of the superego (*see* Chapter 13), while **learning theory** focuses on maladaptive conditioning and modelling in childhood.

Management

Since personality encompasses the concept of enduring traits of human behaviour, some psychiatrists hold the view that disorders of personality are untreatable. In the case of psychopathy, attempts at treatment often yield disappointing results, and any changes which occur in behaviour are usually minimal. **Drugs** have a limited role in the management of psychopathic personality disorder, and are only occasionally indicated to relieve stress or symptoms of anxiety. Dynamic **psychotherapy** is of little help in such cases, although the subject may benefit from a supportive relationship in which firm boundaries are established to define the limits of acceptable behaviour through the use of a contract (*see* Chapter 13). **Behavioural techniques** and **counselling** can be employed to help the individual avoid stressful situations and cope with feelings of frustration when these arise. Drug or alcohol-related problems should be dealt with by appropriate means (*see* Chapter 11).

Short-term hospital admission may occasionally be indicated in times of crisis, but prolonged inpatient care is inappropriate in a conventional psychiatric unit. In some cases, admission to a **therapeutic community** can be of benefit. These specialised units have developed treatment programmes in which modification of behaviour is attempted by peer pressure. This is applied through the process of living together in a democratic community that makes and implements its own rules and disciplines. In this way, the individual is encouraged to assume responsibility for his own actions and to develop increased means of self-control over his behaviour. Those with psychopathic personalities who are extremely dangerous or violent may need to be treated in an interim secure unit or Special Hospital (*see* p. 410).

SUMMARY

1. **Personality** refers to those aspects of a person's behaviour, thinking and emotional reactions which are enduring and predictable throughout a wide range of circumstances and life situations. Its **development** appears to be contingent upon the interplay between biological, environmental and social factors.

2. Because personality is used as a way of differentiating between people, the concept of **normality** is difficult to establish. The concept of **personality disorder** embraces a number of elements: (a) the characteristics of the personality, which is distorted by an exaggeration or imbalance of its constituent traits; (b) the behaviour of the individual, which is identified as being maladaptive from an early age; (c) the presence of suffering, either of the self, others or society. Abnormal behaviour may reflect an underlying personality disorder or the presence of mental illness, so that an independent history of earlier conduct is essential when attempting to differentiate between them.

3. The **classification** of personality disorders is largely descriptive, and is based upon the identification of specific clusters of observable phenomena, which are then assigned to a diagnostic category. The concept of a **psychopathic** or **antisocial personality disorder** is important from both the psychiatric and legal viewpoint. Clinical features are said to include a lack of remorse or feeling for others, impulsive and aggressive behaviour, poor tolerance of stress, an inability to learn from experience, lack of responsibility and poor insight. Antisocial behaviour is usually identifiable

from an early age extending through to adulthood, when difficulties with interpersonal relationships and work are often evident. A history of recidivism, alcohol or drug abuse may also be elicited. Although several aetiological theories exist, the causation of the disorder remains unclear, and its existence as a discrete entity continues to be disputed. Many psychiatrists consider psychopathy to be untreatable, although in some cases, admission to a therapeutic community may be of benefit.

REFERENCES AND FURTHER READING

Hamilton, J. R. (1987). The management of psychopathic offenders. *British Journal of Hospital Medicine;* **38**: 245–50.

Henderson, D. (1939). *Psychopathic States*. New York: W.W. Norton.

Koch, J. L. A. (1891) *The Psychopathic Inferiorities*. Ravensburg: Dorn.

Kraepelin, E. (1907) *Clinical Psychiatry* (trans. A. R. Diefendorf). New York: Macmillan.

Kurland, H. D., Yeager, C. T., Arthur, R. J. (1963). Psychophysiological aspects of severe behaviour disorders. *Archives of General Psychiatry;* **8**: 599-604.

Pinel, P. (1801) *Traité Medico-Philosophique sur l'Alientation Mentale, ou la Manie*. Paris: Richard Caille et Ravier.

Prichard, J. C. (1835) *A Treatise on Insanity and Other Disorders Affecting the Mind*. London: Sherwood, Gilbert and Piper.

Rush, B. (1812) *Medical Enquiries and Observations Upon the Diseases of the Mind*. Philadelphia.

Rutter, M. (1987). Temperament, personality and personality disorder. *British Journal of Psychiatry*; **150**: 443–58.

Schneider, K. (1923). *Psychopathic Personalities* (translation of 9th edn. (1950)). Vienna: F. Deuticke.

Scott, P. (1960). The treatment of psychopaths. *British Medical Journal;* **i**: 1641–46.

4

THE NEUROSES

The term **neurosis** was first used in the eighteenth century to describe disorders of the nervous system for which no physical cause could be found. **Freud** later used the term **psychoneurosis** to apply to three specific syndromes; anxiety hysteria (now referred to as phobic anxiety), obsessive-compulsive neurosis and hysteria. He attributed the development of these conditions to unconscious conflicts arising within the mind, between needs, wishes and innate drives, and the forces which control their fulfilment (*see* Chapter 13). He differentiated them from anxiety neurosis, which was considered to have a biological causation, although in the course of time the term 'neurosis' came to refer to all of these conditions. In considering the causation of the psychoneuroses, Freud was of the opinion that the aetiological factors were the same as those concerned in personality development. This concept has persisted, and is reflected in current psychoanalytical theories concerning the association between neurosis and personality disorder (*see* Chapter 13).

The modern use of the terms **neurosis** and **neurotic** is confusing because one or the other is applied in a number of different ways as:

1. a general term to mean minor mental illness
2. a pejorative term to describe 'highly strung' or anxious individuals (a 'neurotic' old woman)
3. a description of certain 'mental processes' that are a means of responding to and coping with stress, which are sometimes maladaptive (neurotic defence mechanisms, *see* p. 263)
4. a description of specific symptoms, such as anxiety, depression, obsessional thoughts and physical symptoms (with no organic basis) which may be a common reaction to stress in everyday life (**neurotic symptoms**)
5. a descriptive term for a group of disorders (**the neuroses**), in which psychological reactions to stress are grossly exaggerated — anxiety states, phobic disorders, obsessive-compulsive neurosis, hysteria, depressive neurosis, hypochondriasis and the depersonalisation syndrome.

The problems surrounding the concept of the neuroses as 'illnesses' have been discussed elsewhere (see p. 9). However, if neurotic symptoms are viewed as maladaptive reactions to stress, it can be argued that the so-called neuroses are merely a reflection of an underlying disorder of personality, and should be considered as such, rather than as discrete entities or illnesses.

Many people present to general practitioners displaying an admixture of mild or transient neurotic symptoms (such as anxiety, sadness, tiredness or excessive concern about bodily functions), which usually resolve spontaneously or following simple reassurance. It is only when the symptoms become more severe or persistent, that the subject is likely to be considered as suffering from a 'neurosis'. Difficulties also arise when attempting to reliably differentiate the neuroses into specific categories on the basis of symptom content. In textbooks, the conditions are named after the predominant symptom, e.g. anxiety neurosis or obsessional neurosis. In practice, the clinical picture may be much less clear, so that symptoms of anxiety or depression can be just as prominent as obsessional phenomena in a person with a diagnosis of obsessional neurosis.

All classification systems are based upon grouping together disorders with common features, on the basis of aetiology, pathological changes or symptomatology. With regard to the neuroses, most definitions make use of negative rather than positive criteria, so that it is easier to explain what a neurosis is not, rather than what it is. Criteria include:

1. an absence of any demonstrable organic cause (such as tumour, epilepsy or infection) to account for symptoms
2. no loss of contact with external reality (compare with psychosis)
3. an absence of any gross abnormality or disorganisation of the personality
4. behaviour which may be greatly affected, but usually remaining within socially acceptable limits.

Aetiology

From the above, it will be apparent that the causation of the neuroses is not clearly understood. A predisposition to developing a neurosis may be **genetically** determined, and also reflected by abnormalities of **personality**. From a psychosocial viewpoint, 'normal' functioning requires a balance to exist between the stress factors of everyday life and the coping mechanisms which counteract them. When this equilibrium becomes disturbed, a neurosis might result. The capacity to deal with stress is governed by personality (some aspects of which may be inherited), physical health, past experience and supportive relationships. Theoretically, the more severe the abnormality of personality, the less severe the stress needs to be to cause a neurosis. **Stress factors** which may act as precipitants include adverse conditions of living and work, life events and interpersonal conflicts.

Several other hypotheses have been advanced to account for the development of neurotic symptoms. **Psychoanalytical theory** proposes that neuroses in adult life are a resurfacing of conflicts which were not resolved in childhood (*see* Chapter 13). **Learning theory** views neurotic symptoms as learned behaviour attempting to reduce anxiety, which is perceived as an innate drive. Finally, social models of causation stress the importance of the **environment** and the personal significance which the individual attaches to circumstances surrounding the development of neurotic symptoms.

In conclusion, it can be seen that the factors involved in the development of neurotic symptoms are complex. Although the concept of neuroses as discrete entities is controversial, the terms used to describe them remain in widespread clinical use, and are likely to persist for the foreseeable future. Consequently, it is important for the student to have an understanding of their use in psychiatric practice. On the following pages, several of the neurotic disorders are described in accordance with their classification in ICD 9. Although the authors accept that the value of diagnostic labels for neuroses is limited and somewhat artificial, it does provide a basis for explaining some of the ideas of causation associated with specific neurotic symptoms, as well as the methods used in treating them.

The concept of neurosis is not likely to be retained as a 'major organising principle' in ICD 10. With the exception of 'neurotic depression', the disorders described in this chapter will probably be included in one overall group known as 'neurotic, stress-related and somatoform disorders'.

ANXIETY STATES

Anxiety may be defined as an emotional state with the subjectively experienced quality of fear, and is usually a normal phenomenon which occurs in response to stress. Small amounts benefit functioning by increasing efficiency, alertness and concentration. However, when anxiety increases so that it is out of proportion to a provoking stimulus, it becomes a hindrance and is said to be 'pathological'. A threat may be recognised as the cause of some anxiety states, but this is not always the case, since attacks can also arise spontaneously. Where the fear leads to avoidance of the provoking stimulus, it is referred to as **phobic anxiety** (*see* Phobic disorders p. 58).

Clinical Features

Anxiety states may be **generalised** and persistent or occur in the form of unpredictable **panic attacks**.

The clinical features can be grouped into:

1. **psychological symptoms** which include fear and a sense of foreboding, difficulty in concentrating, feelings of irritability and intolerance of noise
2. symptoms due to **motor tension**, including headache (caused by muscle tension in the scalp and neck), chest pain (due to intercostal muscle spasm), backache and limb stiffness
3. symptoms caused by **autonomic overactivity**, resulting in breathlessness, palpitations, diarrhoea and vomiting, abdominal cramps, dry mouth, sweating, restlessness, tremor and frequency of micturition
4. symptoms related to **sleep disturbance** — characteristically, the anxious subject has difficulty in getting off to sleep (as opposed to waking early); vivid dreams and nightmares are common and the patient wakes intermittently
5. **physical signs** of anxiety which include a tense and worried facial expression, tremulousness, visible evidence of perspiration, tachycardia, overbreathing and fidgeting or overactivity.

A 27-year-old secretary attended her general practitioner complaining of feeling perpetually tired, tense and anxious. She described herself as 'always having been a worrier', but matters had noticeably deteriorated in the past 3 months. She was now unable to sleep properly, as the day's problems kept turning over in her mind, and although she maintained an active social life and the capacity to enjoy herself, she worried constantly about her appearance and what others thought of her. Her appetite and weight had remained constant and she denied feeling depressed. Her doctor prescribed an anxiolytic drug (*see below*) and suggested referral to a psychiatrist which the woman declined to accept.

A 47-year-old business executive began to experience panic attacks which occurred three or four times a week after several of his colleagues were made redundant. He was unable to predict their onset, and on one occasion, he awoke in a distressed state in the middle of the night. In between these episodes he felt well and calm. During the attacks he experienced a sense of impending doom, accompanied by hyperventilation, a feeling of tightness in the chest, palpitations and profuse sweating, which lasted for about 20 minutes. Afterwards, he felt tired and 'drained of energy'. Treatment consisted of relaxation training (*see below*) and psychotherapy sessions, during which he was able to explore his fears about the future. Over the course of the next few months, the attacks subsided in frequency and severity.

Epidemiology

Onset is frequently during early adulthood, although some people experience symptoms for the first time in middle age. Estimates vary widely, but approximately 3% of the general population are affected at any one time, with females outnumbering males.

Aetiology

Three main theories of causation exist:

1. **Genetic theory** — anxiety states tend to 'run in families'. Those who suffer in this way may have genetically determined anxious predispositions. Current life stresses can then cause the development of an anxiety state.
2. **Attachment theory** — suggests that anxiety results from a reactivation in later life of feelings of insecurity experienced in childhood and infancy due to inadequate 'attachment' to a stable parent figure.
3. **Psychoanalytical theory** — proposes that anxiety in adult life is a resurfacing of 'psychological conflicts' which were not resolved in childhood (*see* Chapter 13).

Management

This can be considered in terms of psychological, physical and social treatments.

1. PSYCHOLOGICAL TREATMENTS

Simple support through talking and listening is of fundamental importance. In addition, intrapersonal difficulties may be helped by **dynamic psychotherapy**, during which conflicts can be explored (*see* Chapter 13).

Behaviour therapy is employed through **relaxation techniques**. The subject learns to recognise and relieve muscular tension, and to control irregularities of breathing. By becoming 'physically relaxed', mental relaxation follows as a matter of course (*see also* Chapter 13).

2. PHYSICAL TREATMENTS

Benzodiazepines (such as diazepam and lorazepam) are 'minor tranquillisers' which became very popular for treating anxiety states as they are effective, safe in overdose and were thought to be non-addictive. It is now recognised that dependency *does* occur, and withdrawal symptoms (feeling tense, tremulous, sweaty and panicky) are common when the drugs are stopped. Consequently, if their use is considered to be really necessary, they should only be prescribed in short courses and at low dosage (*see* Chapter 12).

Buspirone (BuSpar), is a recently introduced anxiolytic which is structurally unrelated to the benzodiazepines, and has a number of important clinical differences (see Chapter 12).

Beta-blockers (such as propranolol) are useful in the treatment of anxiety states where physical symptoms are prominent and distressing (e.g. flushing, sweating and palpitations). These drugs are non-addictive, but are contraindicated in certain medical conditions such as asthma, heart failure and diabetes.

Antidepressants, including monoamine reuptake inhibitor (MARI) and monoamine oxidase inhibitor (MAOI) drugs, are also used (*see* Chapter 12). Those with sedative properties, such as amitriptyline, reduce anxiety and help relieve insomnia. However, tolerance eventually develops to these effects. MAOIs also have anxiolytic activity, but their potentially dangerous interaction with certain foodstuffs and other drugs limit their usefulness.

In those few cases where anxiety remains very severe and incapacitating and responds to no other form of treatment, **psychosurgery** may be considered as a last resort (*see* p. 99).

3. SOCIAL MANAGEMENT

This should include a general appraisal of current crises and difficulties which may have precipitated or aggravated the condition. For example, social intervention might involve rehousing if the patient is living in crowded or unsuitable accommodation. Marital or family work to resolve interpersonal conflicts can be helpful in conjunction with other forms of treatment.

Prognosis

The outcome in anxiety states is variable. In general, the longer symptoms have persisted, the worse the prognosis.

PHOBIC DISORDERS

Normal fears are common among children and some adults. A mild fear of heights, darkness, rodents or spiders is considered to be within normal limits in our culture, provided it does not interfere with the individual's ability to carry on his everyday life. If the fears become more intense and handicapping they are known as phobias.

A **phobia** is said to exist when:

1. a fear is out of proportion to the demands of the situation
2. the fear cannot be reasoned or explained away
3. it is beyond voluntary control
4. the fear leads to avoidance of the provoking stimulus.

Clinically, there are three main groups of phobias: **agoraphobia, social phobias** and **simple phobias** (sometimes referred to as monosymptomatic phobias).

Epidemiology

Phobias are relatively uncommon, affecting about six per 1000 of the population, although only one-third of these are seriously disabling. Two-thirds of agoraphobic patients and those with social phobias are female. Simple phobias are equally common in men and women, except for those involving animals, where women once again predominate.

Aetiology

The cause of phobic disorders is not clearly understood, although both agoraphobia and social phobias may develop in the context of emotional or social difficulties. Simple phobias may be remnants of childhood fears, some of which are learned by imitation and others by conditioning. Why some of these persist into adulthood is not known. Because so many people are afraid of the same things, it has been suggested that some fears are 'prepared'. This concept regards phobias as a persistence of behaviour which was adaptive or useful long ago. For example, avoidance of animals was once of survival value. However, there is no clear evidence that a tendency to develop phobias is inherited.

Agoraphobia

The literal meaning of this term is 'a fear of the market place'. It is used clinically in a wider context to include individuals who become anxious or afraid in crowds, when they travel on public transport or in lifts, and when they go shopping or leave the safety of their own homes. The fear is often heightened in places which cannot be easily left, such as a crowded room. Most sufferers develop symptoms for the first time between the ages of 15 and 35 years. The illness often has a fluctuating course, with periods of exacerbation and remission continuing for many years.

Clinical features develop as follows:

1. initially, there is a fear of certain situations such as crowds, travelling on public transport or being in enclosed spaces. This leads to:
2. anxiety-related symptoms as to what may happen under these circumstances (ideas of fainting, vomiting or losing control). This results in:
3. avoidance behaviour which might take the form of becoming house-bound, only venturing out when accompanied or avoiding travel on public transport. Others may reduce anxiety by turning to drugs or alcohol as a way of coping.

Other non-phobic symptoms may also be present, such as depression.

A 54-year-old married woman became unable to leave the house on her own shortly after her daughter, an only child, married and left home. Her husband had to accompany her on weekend shopping trips, which were always made in the car, since she was also afraid of travelling on public transport. During the week, her daughter and a neighbour carried out errands for her. She was referred for treatment when she admitted to her general practitioner that bruises on her face were the result of a fall at home caused by having too much to drink. She was consuming a bottle of sherry during the daytime in an attempt to overcome her feelings of despair regarding her inability to leave the house alone.

A successful programme of exposure therapy (*see later*) enabled her to travel unaccompanied, and led to a dramatic reduction of her alcohol intake. To minimise the risk of relapse, she accepted an offer of psychotherapy, and during these sessions was able to come to terms with her feelings of loss and anxiety concerning her daughter leaving home. One year after the completion of treatment she remained symptom-free.

Social Phobias

Social phobias are persistent and irrational fears of situations in which an individual may be observed by others (e.g. restaurants or cinemas) and subsequently behave in an embarrassing or humiliating way (such as vomiting or fainting in public). As a result, the patient feels it necessary to avoid such situations.

A 26-year-old accountant had felt uneasy for many years in small social gatherings, such as dinner parties and eating out in restaurants. Following his engagement, his feelings of uneasiness intensified, so that on one occasion, when invited to dinner by his future in-laws, he became extremely nauseous, vomited a number of times and spent the rest of the evening in the toilet. From this time onward, he avoided visiting places where he felt he might be observed by others. Despite combined therapy involving anxiolytic medication and graded exposure (*see below*), his symptoms only partially resolved, and tended to recur when he was under stress.

Simple Phobias

Simple (monosymptomatic) phobias are persistent and irrational fears of particular objects, events or circumstances, other than those described in agoraphobia and social phobias. These include fears of spiders, dogs, heights and darkness, and lead to an overwhelming desire to avoid them.

A 44-year-old police officer had a fear of hypodermic needles which had been present for as long as he could remember, so that he avoided all situations where he might require an injection or be exposed to needles. Shortly after joining the police force, he was asked to donate blood in an emergency, and so great was his fear that he falsely declared that he had a venereal disease in order to be excused. He saw his phobia as a character weakness, and managed to conceal it from his family and colleagues for many years, until he was involved in a car accident and refused to allow his wounds to be sutured. Following this, he was persuaded to seek psychiatric help, and was successfully treated by a programme of graded exposure to needles (*see below*).

Management

The management of phobic disorders should begin with a general assessment of the condition, followed by specific therapeutic measures.

GENERAL ASSESSMENT

An assessment is necessary to determine whether the anxiety experienced by the subject relates to a specific stimulus or is more generalised. As a rule, behaviour therapy is more likely to succeed in the former case, but there are other reasons why treatment may fail. Assessment should also determine whether:

1. the subject has employed dangerous coping strategies to deal with his fears, such as abusing alcohol or drugs
2. the subject's family has been in collusion, such as children accompanying an agoraphobic mother on outings to avoid going to school
3. secondary gain factors are perpetuating the phobic symptoms. For example, a husband who has to accompany his wife on every trip from the home may also be reducing her insecurity about their relationship, in that while he is with her, he cannot be with someone else
4. phobic symptoms are part of another clinical syndrome, such as depression. In this case, recognition of the primary disorder is important, since its successful treatment may also resolve the phobic symptoms.

SPECIFIC THERAPEUTIC MEASURES

The mainstay of treating phobic disorders is through the behavioural treatment of **exposure**. This is based on the principle of encouraging the subject to re-enter situations which provoke anxiety and to remain in them until the fear subsides.

Graded exposure is an approach whereby the subject is progressively exposed to the feared situation one step at a time. The therapist must first gain the subject's trust, and explain that avoiding situations acts to maintain the phobia. A **hierarchy of anxiety-provoking stimuli** is then constructed in steps of increasing difficulty. In the case of an agoraphobic patient with a fear of leaving the house to go out shopping alone, the stages might involve the following:

1. walking to the gate at the end of the front path
2. walking to the bus stop at the end of the road, perhaps at first with a companion, and then alone
3. boarding a bus to go to the shops
4. entering a quiet shop to purchase one article
5. buying groceries at a supermarket unaccompanied and then returning home.

Many more steps than outlined above may be necessary. The subject should be urged to take an active part in his own treatment and does not need to be accompanied by the therapist during exposure. However, praise for completing each step of the hierarchy is an important element in encouraging further exposure.

The individual is able to proceed up the hierarchy when anxiety for the preceding stage has become minimal. It is helpful if each attempt at 'exposure' is recorded in a diary, so that both subject and therapist can monitor progress. If at any stage the level of anxiety becomes unbearable and the patient contemplates escaping, control may be regained by **relaxation training** (*see* Chapter 13).

Flooding involves exposing the patient to the feared object or situation without using a graded approach. Thus, a patient with a fear of shopping might be taken to a crowded supermarket and helped to remain there until all fear has dissipated. Flooding is effective provided each session is of sufficient duration (ideally 1–2 hours long), and the patient stays in contact with the stimulus until all fear has gone. However, there is no evidence that this technique produces better results than graded exposure, and some authorities consider that the distressingly high levels of arousal that can be produced limit its usefulness as a form of therapy.

Systematic desensitisation, a form of graded exposure in fantasy, is still occasionally used as a preparatory step to treat phobias that cannot be easily dealt with *in vivo* (e.g. a fear of flying). The subject is encouraged to form a mental picture of the phobic situation, proceeding through increasingly stressful stages (e.g. going to the airport, walking to the plane, etc.). The ensuing anxiety is then dealt with by relaxation techniques. It is not a very effective procedure, and may take many weeks for any noticeable improvement to occur.

Drugs have a place in the treatment of phobic disorders, but are most effective when used in conjunction with behaviour therapy. Some patients find the prospect of exposure too frightening, and consequently are unable to enter therapy. In these cases, **benzodiazepines** are sometimes used in the early stages of treatment before an exposure session, although they should be discontinued as soon as possible. **MAOI** antidepressants also reduce anxiety in phobic patients, but the effect takes several weeks to develop. When depressive symptoms coexist, **MARI** antidepressants, which include tricyclic compounds, may be useful.

Prognosis

The outcome in phobic disorders is variable, so that some patients never recover completely. There may be periods of remission alternating with episodes of relapse for months or years.

OBSESSIVE-COMPULSIVE NEUROSIS

Obsessions are recurrent ideas, thoughts, images or impulses which enter the mind and are persistent, intrusive and unwelcome. Although they are recognised as a product of his own mind, the individual regards them as absurd and alien to his personality. Attempts are usually made to ignore or resist them.

Obsessional **thoughts** have a variety of themes, frequently of an unpleasant or blasphemous nature. When they result in continuous pondering, they are known as **ruminations.** Obsessional **images** are frequently vivid and often morbid or violent, such as repeatedly seeing the scene of an accident or the tombstone of a loved one. Obsessional **impulses** may have a similar content, such as persistent urges to stab children. Obsessional **doubts** concerning actions that have not been completed may lead to rituals involving checking and counting. Obsessional **ideas** or fears of contamination can result in compulsive washing. Obsessional symptoms also sometimes occur in early dementia, schizophrenia, anorexia nervosa and depressive illness.

A 28-year-old married man complained that mental images of male genitalia formed in his mind whenever he talked to other men. He found the experience extremely distressing, since he had no conscious homosexual inclinations. When he attempted to resist the images, this merely served to intensify them, and he eventually sought help from his general practitioner. Initial treatment with medication was unsuccessful, and he was referred to a clinical psychologist for further help.

Compulsions or **rituals** are obsessional motor acts which, although voluntary, are performed with reluctance, since they too are regarded as absurd and alien to the personality. The act is therefore carried out with a sense of compulsion coupled with a desire to resist. If resistance is attempted, anxiety mounts and can only be reduced by yielding. In severe cases, symptoms can be very distressing and crippling in their effect on the person's life. Patients may spend hours on end preoccupied with their obsessions or performing rituals, so that they are unable to work, relax or socialise.

A 57-year-old single woman developed a compulsion for washing and grooming her dog, which started after she noticed the animal was scratching. Although she accepted the assurance of her vet that the animal was not infested, she was unable to overcome the idea that he might be 'contaminated' or resist the urge to clean him. As a result, she bathed him four to five times a day, followed by long sessions of grooming, so that she had little time for anything else. Acknowledging the absurdity of her behaviour and the danger to the dog's health, she attempted to overcome her problem by entrusting his care to a friend.

Soon afterwards, however, she developed obsessional ideas that the living room carpet might contain dog fleas, and consequently felt compelled to conduct a minute examination of the pile which lasted for several hours. She was only able to alleviate her feelings of anxiety by repeatedly shampooing it. At this point, her distress and exhaustion led her to seek help.

Aetiology

Seventy per cent of those who develop obsessional neurosis have a premorbid **obsessional personality**, features of which include meanness, rigidity of character, orderliness, excessive cleanliness and a fondness for collecting things (*see* Chapter 3). At present, there is little evidence to suggest that obsessional neurosis is genetically determined.

The **psychoanalytical view** of causation sees these phenomena as a defence against cruel or aggressive impulses. By filling the mind with obsessional thoughts, other ideas are unable to enter consciousness (*see* Chapter 13).

Epidemiology

The condition is uncommon, occurring in approximately five per 1000 of the general population. Males and females are affected equally, with the onset in most cases before the age of 35.

Management

Compulsions (motor acts) are easier to treat than obsessions. In both cases, **behaviour therapy** is the cornerstone of management (*see* Chapter 13).

Compulsive acts may be helped by **response prevention** (*see* page 277). In this form of behaviour therapy, the subject is instructed to desist from carrying out the unwanted behaviour. Except in very severe cases, constant supervision does not appear to be necessary, so that merely telling the patient to refrain serves as an adequate control. This leads to an increase in anxiety, which eventually abates along with the compulsive behaviour if the subject is able to desist from performing his rituals (c.f. exposure). Certain acts, such as compulsive hand-washing, are often associated with a fear of contamination. Under these circumstances, it may be helpful for the subject to 'practise restraint' by deliberately soiling his hands (such as rummaging through a wastebin) and then resisting the urge to clean them. This treatment will need to be carried out several times before the patient is able to cope with the resultant anxiety.

Obsessions may respond to **thought stopping** (*see* p. 278). The patient is encouraged to relax and then ruminate, so that the obsessional thought is uppermost in his mind. At this point, the therapist shouts 'Stop!' and the patient attempts to cease ruminating. Additional reinforcement can be obtained by a mildly painful stimulus experienced at the same time, such as the subject pulling on a rubber band attached to his wrist. Eventually, he learns to internalise control by shouting 'Stop!' to himself whenever the obsession occurs, and by associating pain with his ruminations.

Clomipramine, an antidepressant drug, is claimed to have specific 'anti-obsessional' properties, but its effectiveness is probably limited to patients with clear-cut depressive symptoms. **Psychosurgery** is indicated as a last resort in severe cases of chronic, unremitting, incapacitating illness which have failed to respond to other methods of treatment (*see* p. 99).

Prognosis

Two-thirds of all cases show some improvement with treatment. Patients with severe symptoms, persistent life stresses and premorbid obsessional personalities have the worst prognosis. The course of the illness may be constant, or fluctuate with periods of exacerbation and remission.

HYSTERIA

Hysteria is derived from the Greek word for womb — *hustera*. The ancient Greeks believed that the uterus was capable of wandering throughout the body, and by pressing on other organs, could produce a malfunction in them. The notion that hysteria was a disorder of the mind was first introduced over 200 years ago, although the idea that it was a condition exclusive to women persisted for much longer. In the nineteenth century, Charcot, a French neurologist, demonstrated that hysterical disorders could be produced (and relieved) in susceptible individuals by hypnosis and suggestion (*see* Chapter 13).

The terms **hysteria** and **hysterical** have been applied widely and imprecisely in medical and general usage, so that there is little universal agreement as to their meaning. For example, they are used to describe a personality type (*see* p. 47), a state of severe distress as seen in a tantrum, and physical symptoms for which examination findings and laboratory tests reveal no cause.

The term 'hysteria' is unlikely to be included in ICD 10, and conditions of this type will probably be classified as dissociative disorders of memory, awareness, identity, movement and sensation.

Aetiology

Hysterical neurosis is a term applied to a condition in which signs and symptoms of disease occur in the absence of physical pathology. Furthermore:

1. it arises in response to **stress** and confers some **advantage** to the individual
2. in contrast to malingering, symptoms are not created deliberately, but instead are constructed **unconsciously** around the person's own notion of the disorder which may be gained from past experience, personal knowledge or by observing the behaviour of others
3. symptoms are not attributable to overactivity of the autonomic nervous system.

The concept of hysteria is difficult to understand, as the idea that symptoms are 'constructed' (albeit unconsciously) gives the impression that the subject is wilfully manufacturing his condition for some ulterior motive. In fact, this is not the case, and the individual is no more or less aware of the mechanism of causation of his symptoms than is someone with organic illness. Although a cheerful acceptance of disability is sometimes seen in hysterical neurosis (**la belle indifference**), other patients can be profoundly distressed by their dysfunction.

Hysterical symptoms confer advantage through primary or secondary gain. In **primary gain**, anxiety over a psychological conflict is excluded from consciousness. For example, a soldier preparing for battle may be unable to acknowledge his underlying fear of injury or death, and might therefore resolve his dilemma by unconsciously developing a paralysed limb. In this condition, he is unable to fight and yet is not seen by himself or others as a coward. **Secondary gain** consists of the practical advantages which can be achieved by using the symptoms, such as the increased attention of others or the abrogation of responsibilities. In the above case, this might include hospitalisation and the care and concern of the nursing staff. It is not exclusive to hysterical disorders, and is sometimes seen in patients with organic illness.

Clinical studies have demonstrated that a high percentage of patients diagnosed as suffering from hysterical neurosis subsequently develop physical or psychiatric illness which could have accounted for the original symptoms. Therefore, it must initially remain a provisional diagnosis, particularly to avoid the risk of any new evidence of organic disease being ignored. Because hysteria is provoked by stress, if none is found, nor any element of gain determined, the diagnosis must be in doubt.

Clinical Features

Symptoms in hysteria can cover the entire spectrum of physical and mental illness. The accuracy of symptom reproduction tends to be influenced by the level of knowledge the person has about the condition, but even so, there are usually clear differences between features of an hysterical disorder and those of an organic illness. For example, someone with hysterical blindness may consistently avoid bumping into objects and people, while the pattern of hysterical anaesthesia in a limb does not correspond to anatomical innervation. Furthermore, symptoms can often be exacerbated or diminished by suggestion on the part of the examiner, although this phenomenon is sometimes observed in organic disorders.

Clinical features may be classified as **dissociative states** or **conversion symptoms**.

DISSOCIATIVE STATES

These are sudden but temporary alterations in the normally integrated functions of consciousness (and sometimes motor behaviour). They include:

1. **Hysterical amnesia**: an abrupt memory loss for a specific and often traumatic episode, although more commonly, the individual complains that he knows nothing of his earlier life. This contrasts with his ability to use learned information from the past that does not have personal or emotional significance, such as using a knife and fork or dressing himself.

2. **Fugue state**: hysterical amnesia accompanied by wandering. The sufferer may end up many miles from home, with no recollection of how or why he got there. Fugues can also occur in depressive illness and certain organic states.
3. **Somnambulism** or sleep-walking is often regarded as a dissociative state.
4. **Multiple personality**: a rare condition in which the individual may have several different personalities, none of which has any apparent knowledge of the others.

A 31-year-old woman was brought by the police to a casualty department late one night, having been found wandering along the hard shoulder of a motorway with no shoes on. She carried no means of identification and was unable to remember her name, address or other personal details; nor could she account for her recent behaviour. She appeared physically well, and was otherwise able to converse lucidly and rationally, demonstrating that she was fully orientated in time and place. On examination, there was no obvious evidence that she abused drugs or alcohol.

The woman was admitted to hospital overnight and was identified the next day by her husband, who had reported her to the police as a missing person. It later transpired that on the morning of her disappearance, she had received a letter from a credit card company threatening legal action unless she rapidly settled a large debt, which had remained outstanding for several months. An hysterical fugue state was diagnosed, and following arrangement of a bank loan by her husband to settle the debt, her amnesia rapidly resolved.

CONVERSION SYMPTOMS

These symptoms were so named by Freud, because he saw them as resulting from psychological energy which had been 'converted' into physical symptoms, thereby providing relief from some intolerable stress and avoiding conflict. They are often suggestive of neurological disease and include seizures, paralysis, ataxia, anaesthesia, mutism (aphonia), pain, blindness and deafness.

A 34-year-old married woman developed a sudden paralysis of both legs, for which no organic cause could be demonstrated. Her relatives reported that 10 days previously, her younger sister had suffered a transection of the spinal cord following a car accident, which had rendered her paralysed from the neck down.

The two were very close and the patient had always been protective towards her younger sister. During several interviews, it became apparent that she experienced intense guilt surrounding the accident. Consequently, the development of 'conversion symptoms' served to resolve her conflict in which she felt that she (rather than her sister) should have been injured. Over the course of several weeks, during which time she received regular psychotherapy, her symptoms gradually resolved.

Briquet's syndrome or somatisation disorder (DSM III-R) was first defined by a group of American physicians (St Louis hysteria). It is characterised by the development of multiple, persistent physical complaints, for which there is no demonstrable organic basis. The condition is thought to be confined to women, who most commonly describe cardiac, respiratory and menstrual problems. The onset is said to be before the age of 30 and the disorder is thought to run a life-long, fluctuating course. There is considerable debate regarding its validity as a specific clinical entity, and some authorities would argue that people who present in this way demonstrate many of the characteristics described in certain personality disorders.

Epidemiology

The prevalence of hysteria is difficult to determine, and although now generally uncommon in Europe and North America, it is more evident in underdeveloped societies. Women probably outnumber men, and it seldom appears for the first time after the age of 40. Hysterical symptoms sometimes affect groups of people *en masse* (epidemic hysteria), especially when they share some common stress, such as schoolchildren prior to an examination.

Management

This must always begin with a thorough physical examination, followed by investigations to exclude organic illnesses such as temporal lobe epilepsy, cerebral tumour and dementia. Patients who are under stress often feel inhibited or unable to discuss their problems, so that **psychotherapy** may be helpful. Attention should be directed towards the factors which are thought to have precipitated the condition. **Abreaction** by hypnosis or by intravenous administration of a sedating drug is a method of lowering arousal and enabling the subject to talk about his difficulties (*see* Chapter 13). Finally, an explanation as to the nature of the symptoms, and simple reassurance that they will subside is often helpful.

Prognosis

The outcome in most cases is good, with a rapid and complete recovery. However, when symptoms persist for more than one year, they are likely to remain intractable.

DEPRESSIVE NEUROSIS

Some less severe forms of depression frequently fulfil the criteria for neurotic disorders, in that they have no organic basis, they result from stress factors acting on a predisposed personality, and sufferers do not lose touch with external reality. Anxiety and other neurotic symptoms are also sometimes present. Therefore, minor depressions are sometimes classified among the neuroses.

The concept of depressive neurosis is unlikely to be retained in ICD 10. An episode of depression which fulfils the criteria outlined above will probably be classified under the affective disorders as a mild depressive episode (*see* p. 86). Diagnostic guidelines will include mild or absent biological symptoms of depression, evidence that the disorder causes both distress and interference with ordinary activities and lasts for a minimum of two weeks.

The issue as to whether there is just one type of depression differing only in severity, or two types which differ in regard to aetiology, symptoms and management, has not been resolved. The subject is discussed more fully in Chapter 5.

HYPOCHONDRIASIS

This condition derives its name from the ancient belief that it was associated with physical disorders of organs below the costal margin, hence 'hypo-chondriasis'.
Hypochondriasis may be defined as:

1. an excessive concern with one's health in general, or
2. an unrealistic interpretation of physical signs or sensations as being abnormal, leading to a preoccupation with the fear of having a serious disease.

The unrealistic fear persists despite medical reassurance and causes impairment in social or occupational functioning. Hypochondriacal symptoms are most often seen as a feature of a **depressive illness.** Hypochondriasis occurs more frequently among men, the lower social classes, the elderly and those closely associated with disease (such as medical students).

Treatment initially involves a search to exclude organic pathology. If part of a depressive illness, hypochondriacal symptoms may fade as the depression resolves. Simple support and reassurance are important, while avoiding a detailed discussion of the symptoms with the patient.

DEPERSONALISATION SYNDROME

The symptom of **depersonalisation** is an experience whereby the subject feels 'as if' he is no longer real, which has an associated unpleasant quality. It is *not* a delusional belief, because the person is aware of the nature of the change he experiences. When the feeling of unreality relates to the subject's environment ('as if' the world around him is not real), the term **derealisation** is used. Derealisation can occur alone or together with depersonalisation. Feelings of being outside oneself, inability to experience strong emotion, or changes in the perception of body or limb size are also sometimes included as part of the so-called **depersonalisation syndrome**.

Depersonalisation and derealisation may occur as features of other psychiatric disorders, such as anxiety, depression and schizophrenia, or in normal people under stress. Treatment is of the underlying condition, although in most cases the symptoms are short-lived and self-limiting.

A 34-year-old woman suffering from an anxiety state described the symptoms of depersonalisation in the following way: 'My voice seems as if it's unreal, and when I look at my hands and legs, I ask "Is this me?" I know it must be, it just seems unpleasantly strange.'

A 38-year-old woman complained of having lost the capacity to experience emotion. She described the symptoms of depersonalisation and derealisation as 'I feel as if my spirit has left my body. I see the world around me, but I don't feel as if I'm part of it anymore'.

SUMMARY

1. The term **neurosis** is applied in a number of different ways, especially to describe a group of disorders (the neuroses) in which psychological reactions to stress are grossly exaggerated. Furthermore, there is no evidence of organic brain disorder, sufferers do not lose touch with external reality, behaviour usually remains within socially acceptable limits and the personality is not grossly abnormal or disorganised. There is considerable debate surrounding the concept of neuroses as illnesses, and it is often difficult to differentiate them reliably into specific categories on the basis of symptom content.
2. The neuroses include anxiety states, phobic disorders, obsessive-compulsive neurosis, hysteria, depressive neurosis, hypochondriasis and the depersonalisation syndrome. Their causation remains unclear, although neurotic symptoms in adult life may result from an interaction between genetic, psychological and environmental factors.
3. **Anxiety** is an emotional state with a subjectively experienced quality of

fear. When it increases so that it is out of proportion to a provoking stimulus, it becomes a hindrance and is said to be 'pathological'. Anxiety states may be generalised and persistent or occur in the form of unpredictable panic attacks. Three per cent of the population are affected, with onset frequently in early adulthood. Clinical features include psychological symptoms, symptoms due to motor tension, autonomic overactivity and sleep disturbance, as well as physical signs of anxiety. There is some evidence of a genetic predisposition, interacting with environmental factors to precipitate the disorder. Treatment includes the use of psychotherapeutic and behavioural techniques, benzodiazepines, beta-blocker and antidepressant drugs, as well as social measures. Prognosis is variable.

4. A **phobia** is a fear which is out of proportion to the demands of the situation, so that it cannot be reasoned or explained away. It is beyond voluntary control and leads to avoidance of the provoking stimulus. Clinically, there are three main groups — agoraphobia, social phobias and simple phobias — but they remain relatively uncommon and their causation is not clearly understood. Agoraphobia literally means a 'fear of the market place', although it is clinically used in a wider context to include those who become anxious or afraid in a variety of settings, such as in crowds or travelling on public transport. Social phobias are persistent and irrational fears of situations in which an individual may be observed by others, and subsequently behave in an embarrassing or humiliating way, such as vomiting or fainting in public. Simple (monosymptomatic) phobias are persistent and irrational fears of particular objects, events or situations (such as spiders, dogs, heights and darkness), which lead to an overwhelming desire to avoid them. The management of phobic disorders usually involves the assessment of provoking and perpetuating factors, followed by exposure treatment. Outcome is variable.

5. **Obsessions** are recurrent ideas, thoughts, images or impulses which enter the mind and are persistent, intrusive and unwelcome. Although they are recognised as a product of his own mind, the individual regards them as absurd and alien to his personality. Attempts are sometimes made to ignore or resist them. **Compulsions** (or rituals) are obsessional motor acts which, although voluntary, are performed with reluctance, since they too are regarded as absurd and alien to the personality. The act is therefore performed with a sense of compulsion, coupled with a desire to resist. These conditions are uncommon and 70% of those affected have a premorbid obsessional personality. Behaviour therapy is the cornerstone of management, utilising response prevention to treat rituals and thought stopping to control obsessional phenomena. Clomipramine is sometimes useful, although intractable cases may require psychosurgery as a last resort. Two-thirds of all cases of obsessive-compulsive neurosis show some improvement with treatment.

6. **Hysteria** is a term sometimes applied to signs and symptoms of disease

which occur in the absence of demonstrable physical pathology, and in response to some stressor. Symptoms usually differ significantly from those of organic illness, and are constructed unconsciously around the person's own notion of the disorder gained from past experience, personal knowledge or by observing the behaviour of others. They are not attributable to overactivity of the autonomic nervous system, and confer some advantage or gain to the individual. Hysterical dissociative states are sudden but temporary alterations in the normally integrated functions of consciousness (and sometimes motor behaviour). They include hysterical amnesia, fugue states and multiple personality. Hysterical conversion symptoms are derived from Freud's concept of mental energy being 'converted' into physical symptoms, thereby providing relief from some intolerable stress. They are often suggestive of neurological disease and include paralysis, anaesthesia, blindness, deafness, muteness and seizures. The management of hysteria should begin with a thorough physical examination, followed by investigations to exclude organic illness. Abreaction and psychotherapeutic measures may be helpful, and in most cases the prognosis is good.

7. **Depressive neurosis** describes less severe forms of depression which fulfil the criteria for neurotic disorders. **Hypochondriasis** involves excessive concern with one's health in general, or an unrealistic interpretation of physical signs or sensations as being abnormal. This can lead to a preoccupation with the fear of having a serious disease, and most commonly forms part of a depressive illness. **Depersonalisation syndrome** includes the symptoms of depersonalisation and derealisation, in which the individual feels as if he or the world around him is unreal.

REFERENCES AND FURTHER READING

Gelder, M. G. (1986). Neurosis: another tough old word. *British Medical Journal*; **292**: 972–73.

Kenyon, F. E. (1976). Hypochondriacal states. *British Journal of Psychiatry*; **129**: 1–14.

Lloyd, G. G. (1986). Hysteria: a case for conservation? *British Medical Journal*; **293**: 1255–56.

Marks, I., Horder, J. (1987). Phobias and their management. *British Medical Journal*; **295**: 589–91.

Sedman, G. (1970). Theories of depersonalisation: a reappraisal. *British Journal of Psychiatry*; **117**: 1–14.

Slater, E. T. O., Glithero, E. (1965). A follow-up of patients diagnosed as suffering from hysteria. *Journal of Psychosomatic Research*; **9**: 9–13.

Stern, R. S., Cobb, J. P. (1978). Phenomenology of obsessive-compulsive disorder. *British Journal of Psychiatry*; **132**: 233–40.

Tyrer, P. (1979). Anxiety states. In *Recent Advances in Clinical Psychiatry 3* (Granville-Grossman, K. L., ed.) pp. 161–83. Edinburgh: Churchill Livingstone.

5

THE AFFECTIVE DISORDERS

The mood of an individual can change many times throughout the day in response to events and circumstances. Such fluctuations are usually short-lived, and because most are appropriate and understandable in the context of situations which provoke them, they are considered normal.

The **affective disorders** are concerned with abnormalities of affect or mood, especially those involving **depression** and **elation**. Their recognition is important, because untreated they can cause prolonged suffering, which may in turn lead to serious disruption of the person's life and the risk of suicide.

In these disorders, mood changes are sustained over a period of time, although this alone does not necessarily signify that an individual is suffering from an affective illness. For example, sadness and feelings of depression following the loss of a loved one may last for months or even longer, and in most societies would be considered normal. To allow for this wide variation in emotional response, mood is sometimes defined as being abnormal if:

1. the mood changes are more severe or last longer than would normally be expected
2. the event which caused the change in mood appears insufficient to explain the duration or severity of the symptoms.

Consequently, distinguishing normal from abnormal mood changes can sometimes be extremely difficult, and the diagnosis of affective disorders may rely upon accompanying changes in:

1. **bodily functions** (such as alterations in sleep pattern)
2. **psychomotor function** (the speed at which people think and move)
3. the **content of thoughts**.

In certain cases, depressive illnesses and mania are classified as **functional psychoses** (*see* p. 9), along with schizophrenia. Milder forms of depression are sometimes classified as **neuroses** (*see later*).

74

DEPRESSIVE ILLNESS

The term **depression** is used both generally and by doctors to describe:

1. an isolated symptom
2. a normal reaction to adverse circumstances
3. a disturbance of mood lasting a day or two
4. a disturbance of mood sustained for weeks or months
5. a collection of signs and symptoms which constitute an illness.

The principal feature of a **depressive illness** is a **sustained lowering of mood**, from which the sufferer cannot be distracted. In its most severe form, the subject is unable to enjoy anything in life (**anhedonia**), and as a consequence the world seems dull, grey and joyless. The feeling is often said to have a unique quality, and is described as being quite different, for example, from that experienced following bereavement. In addition to important abnormalities of thought, perception and cognitive function that may be present (*see later*), a number of physical symptoms and changes can occur which are referred to as the **biological features of depression**. These include:

1. alteration in sleep pattern
2. diurnal variation of mood
3. changes in weight, appetite and bowel habit
4. variation in level of activity
5. reduction of sexual energy.

Sleep Pattern

Sleep is disturbed, the subject characteristically awakening at 3 or 4 a.m. and unable to sleep anymore (**early morning wakening**).

Diurnal Mood Variation

The morning may be experienced as the most difficult time of the day, when mood is at its lowest and mental and physical activity are almost impossible to initiate (**diurnal variation of mood**). As the day progresses, matters usually improve, so that by evening the subject feels relatively normal.

Appetite, Weight and Bowel Habit

Poor appetite is common and **weight loss** may be dramatic. In severe cases, 5–10 kg (10–20 lb) can be lost in a matter of weeks. Patients may cease to eat and drink completely, so that their management becomes a medical as well as a psychiatric emergency. Bowel function is frequently altered, with **constipation** a common complaint.

Level of Activity

Patients sometimes take to their beds or sit for hours in a chair with expressionless faces, hardly talking or moving and showing little interest in their surroundings (**psychomotor retardation**). Alternatively, the individual may display signs of extreme **agitation**. Under these circumstances, he is unable to sit still, frequently pacing up and down or wringing his hands and constantly asking for (but deriving little) reassurance from others.

Reduction of Sexual Energy

Loss of libido and impotence are often early features of a depressive illness, and women may cease to menstruate.

Abnormalities of Thought Content

Ideas of **guilt, self-deprecation** and **worthlessness** can occur, which in extreme cases may become **delusional** in intensity. For example, sufferers sometimes believe they are responsible for all the ills of the world, or are convinced that they will be punished for some terrible crime. Delusional ideas might also be expressed about the physical state of their bodies (**hypochondriacal delusions**). Severely depressed patients may believe that their intestines have rotted away or that their blood vessels are filled with poison. In extreme cases, they might be convinced that they are already dead or that the world no longer exists, citing these beliefs as a reason for not eating or drinking. Abnormal convictions of this kind which refer to non-existence of the self, others or the world are termed **nihilistic delusions**. Thinking is often preoccupied with **ideas of suicide**, death and dying. If asked, such patients may describe the future as 'black' or 'hopeless' and see no chance that matters can improve. Suicide is therefore an ever-present risk (*see* Chapter 6).

Perceptual Abnormalities

Sometimes, the sufferer experiences **auditory hallucinations** and is troubled by voices talking to him. Their content is frequently deprecatory, saying things such as 'You're no good' or 'You deserve to suffer'. Occasionally they are imperative, commanding the individual to harm or even kill himself. Other hallucinations can involve the experiences of unpleasant smells or tastes.

Cognitive Function

Loss of interest in formerly pleasurable pastimes and pursuits is made worse by **difficulty in concentration**, so that activities (such as watching television or reading a book) are rapidly abandoned after a few short minutes. Memory is seemingly affected because poor concentration prevents new information being registered properly. In elderly depressed patients, this can give the impression of a dementing illness (**depressive pseudodementia**, *see* p. 166).

A 54-year-old married company director visited his general practitioner complaining of poor sleep, difficulty in concentrating at work and lack of energy for the previous 2 months. On physical examination, his doctor could find no abnormality, and a full blood count and erythrocyte sedimentation rate (ESR) were both normal. He was prescribed some sleeping tablets, advised to ease up at work and asked to return in a fortnight.

Two weeks later, his wife requested a home visit as she was concerned about her husband who had been off work for several days. He was eating very little, appeared to have lost weight, and was complaining that his bowels were 'blocked up'. He no longer bothered to dress or shave during the day, and although he went off to sleep at a normal time, she would find him pacing the bedroom in the early hours. He was preoccupied with non-existent financial worries, and talked repeatedly about being 'better off dead'. Concerned about the deterioration in his mental state and the possible risk of suicide, the doctor suggested admission to the local psychiatric unit, which the patient was persuaded to accept.

In hospital, he was observed to awaken every morning at about 5 a.m., although he would stay in bed, until coaxed out to breakfast by the nursing staff. He ate very little and lost a further 3 kg in weight during the first week of his admission. His conversation was preoccupied with the state of his health, in particular his bowels, and he repeatedly talked about 'doing away with myself' because he felt he was a burden to everyone and a total failure. He could not be distracted from his misery and interacted very little with the other patients. He also reported hearing voices talking to him whilst he was in the lavatory, saying 'you're useless' and 'why not kill yourself?'

Because of the sustained disturbance in mood, physical changes, abnormalities of thought content and auditory hallucinations, he was diagnosed as suffering from a severe depressive illness.

MANIA AND HYPOMANIA

Full-blown **mania** is an uncommon occurrence, usually because help is sought and treatment instigated before the extreme phase of the condition is reached. **Hypomania** is said to exist while the illness is developing. It is therefore similar to, but not as severe as, a manic episode.

In ICD 10, hypomania is likely to be used to denote a persistent, mild degree of elation of mood and increased energy and activity, without delusions and hallucinations.

The 'core' feature of mania and hypomania is a **persistent elevation of mood** or increased sense of well-being, associated with mental and physical **overactivity**. Sometimes, **irritability** (without evidence of euphoria) predominates. Although the mood is mainly cheerful, it may be frequently punctuated by periods of depression or anger which can last from a few minutes to several hours. During these episodes, suicide attempts are a real risk, and outbursts of aggression or violence may occur if the individual's needs or wishes are not immediately met.

In the early stages of the illness, the euphoric mood is said to have an 'infectious quality', so that people in the company of manic or hypomanic individuals find it difficult not to laugh or smile at their antics. However, those who know the person well recognise that their behaviour is excessive.

Manic patients typically have an **abundance of energy** which manifests itself in terms of speech, thought and action. Talk is characteristically loud and rapid (**pressure of speech**), and sometimes contains **rhymes, jokes** or **puns**. During conversation, the patient may suddenly burst into song or emphasise his words with expansive theatrical gestures. As the condition progresses, speech can become unintelligible, not only due to excessive speed, but also because connections between thoughts and words become increasingly disjointed (**flight of ideas**, *see* case history below). When asked, the patient may describe his thoughts as **racing**. A **decreased need for sleep** is often associated with phrenetic planning and activity, resulting in physical exhaustion. Although numerous tasks might be undertaken simultaneously, few (if any) are completed. Manic patients are highly **distractable** with poor powers of concentration. A line of conversation may suddenly switch to commenting on the decor of the room or some extraneous noise.

The subject's appraisal of himself often alters too, varying from an increase in self-esteem to markedly **grandiose ideas or delusions.** In the belief that he is a person of great importance with special powers or talents, he may undertake spectacular ventures, such as attempting to meet personally with politicians and royalty, or hiring an auditorium to display musical talents which in reality are limited or non-existent. At a more mundane level, advice might be offered on matters which are totally beyond the realm of his knowledge. **A loss of financial constraint** can result in the purchase of unusual or unnecessary items, while money may be given away to casual acquaintances, so that serious debts are sometimes incurred.

The appearance of manic patients is occasionally indicative of their condition, with bright and garish clothes being worn, and females displaying excessive amounts of poorly applied make-up. Social activity usually increases (often inappropriately), such as renewing old acquaintances by telephoning them in the middle of the night! **Disinhibited behaviour** is common, especially in terms of heightened or inappropriate sexual activity. **Hallucinations**, when experienced, are frequently understandable in the context of the altered mood state. For example, one woman reported hearing the voice of Jesus telling her to lead her fellow patients to salvation, as she was now endowed with the power to heal all sickness.

A 34-year-old married school teacher had suffered from recurrent bouts of mania for 3 years. He had been taking lithium (*see* management p. 102) for the past 12 months, which had effectively controlled his mood swings, but at the end of the summer term he decided to stop taking his medication against medical advice, as he felt certain that he was now cured.

Six weeks later, his wife telephoned the hospital and reported that her husband had become increasingly irritable and moody. He had taken to staying up late at night and playing his records loudly, which had twice resulted in the neighbours calling the police. She was now particularly worried, because that morning, a salesman had called to arrange the installation of an expensive sauna and solarium that her husband had ordered for their semi-detached house. When she later confronted him about their inability to afford such a luxury, he became abusive and aggressive, and stormed out of the house.

He had been seen by his general practitioner several times, but all requests for him to visit the hospital or take his medication had been refused. Consequently, his psychiatrist agreed to see him at home. On arrival, he found the patient sitting in the living room, surrounded by masses of school work taken home for marking in the holidays. He had told his wife that he was perfecting a method of marking ten essays simultaneously, to prove to his colleagues that he was 'the most innovative member of staff'. When asked by the doctor what he was doing, he replied 'I'm trying to mark ten pieces of work, not pieces of eight. I'm not Long John Silver or a bloody parrot you know, or would you? What are you a doctor or a vet? Niet! I'm a Russian — rushin' around here, rushin' around there. I bet you're here for the Communist Party; bring a bottle did you?'

Apart from exhibiting 'flight of ideas', his speech was rapid and it was virtually impossible to interrupt him. He refused admission to hospital, and in view of his general condition and behaviour, he was compulsorily detained. On admission, he was given an intramuscular injection of chlorpromazine and slept for 12 hours. On awakening, he agreed to take medication orally.

Untreated mania is a potentially serious condition, because lack of sleep and sustained overactivity can lead to physical exhaustion and on occasion, death. Before this stage is reached, both the patient and others are at risk of serious accident or financial ruin through lack of judgement and reckless behaviour. Even with treatment, some patients will swing rapidly into a depressive illness. The risk of suicide is high, and it is estimated that 15% of those who suffer from manic and depressive illnesses will eventually take their own lives (a 30-fold increase compared with the general population).

Although brief episodes of depression are common in manic illnesses, they are rarely sustained. However, when the patient describes a predominantly depressed mood and thought content in the setting of manic behaviour, this is known as a **mixed affective state**. Occasionally, manic patients present as mute and motionless (so-called **'manic stupor'**).

In the elderly, the diagnosis of mania may be easily missed because elation of mood is often absent and overactivity not prominent. Patients frequently present with irritability and mildly disinhibited or aggressive behaviour.

The ICD 9 classification of mania currently used in the UK does not specify how long symptoms need to be present in order to make the diagnosis. ICD 10 is likely to introduce diagnostic guidelines for manic episodes which include symptoms that are severe enough to be handicapping and last for at least one week. The mood change should be accompanied by increased energy and several symptoms frequently found in mania, such as pressure of speech, decreased need for sleep and grandiosity.

The descriptions that have been given of depressive and manic illnesses demonstrate the typical features of these disorders (Table 5.1). However, in practice the diagnosis is not always easy, and some of the difficulties involved will be considered in the next section.

CLASSIFICATION

Affective disorders have been classified in many ways, which is confusing since no particular method has gained general acceptance. Axes of classification are based upon:

1. the underlying cause
2. differences in the clinical features
3. whether the patient experiences recurrent bouts of depression alone, or a combination of depression and mania
4. whether or not contact with reality is maintained
5. the severity of the illness.

As a consequence, a multitude of descriptive terms have arisen, including psychotic, endogenous, reactive, neurotic, manic-depressive,

Table 5.1 Summary of the typical features of depressive and manic illnesses

	Depressive illness	Mania/Hypomania
Mood	Lowered	Elevated and/or irritable
Behaviour	Retardation/agitation, loss of interest	Overactive, reckless, distractable and disinhibited
Speech	Reduced quantity and rate	Increased quantity and rate (pressure of speech), rhymes and puns
Perceptual abnormalities	Hallucinations (mood-congruent)	Hallucinations (mood-congruent)
Thoughts	Ideas or delusions of guilt, self-harm, worthlessness, nihilism	Grandiose ideas or delusions, racing thoughts and flight of ideas
Sleep	Disturbed with early morning wakening	Reduced need for sleep
Appetite	Reduced	Variable
Weight	Frequently decreased	Variable
Sexual activity	Decreased	Increased

bipolar and unipolar. Some of them are used inconsistently, conveying different ideas from those originally intended. Why then is any form of classification necessary? In practical terms, it is recognised that different types of affective disorder vary in their management and outcome. A clearly defined system of classification aids management by giving an indication of the most appropriate form of treatment and the likely course of the illness. The following section reviews the various classifications which are in common use, and gives a brief account of how they evolved. Some of them are confusing because the discrete clinical entities described rarely exist in practice, and considerable overlap between different types is often encountered.

Classification 1: unipolar and bipolar affective disorders

Those who experience depressive illnesses alone are described as suffering from a **unipolar affective disorder.** There should be a history of at least three separate episodes of depression, with complete recovery in between, and no evidence of mania.

ICD 10 is likely to introduce the categories of **depressive episode** (see p. 86) and **recurrent depressive disorder** (which in either case may be mild or severe). The diagnosis of recurrent depressive disorder should only be made if the subject has had at least two episodes fulfilling the descriptions given for a mild or severe depressive episode, (see p. 86) and without any history of a manic episode. At least two of the episodes should have lasted for a minimum of two weeks, and the two should be separated by at least six months of normal mood in order to be confident that they are indeed distinct.

Those who experience both manic and depressive illnesses are described as suffering from a **bipolar affective disorder**. There should be a history of at least one episode of mania and one episode of depression. Repeated episodes of mania without depression are also classified as bipolar. This is because most authorities agree that patients with recurrent mania will eventually develop a depressive illness at some time in their life.

The term manic-depressive illness does *not* have precisely the same meaning as bipolar affective disorder. The former is an outdated term and best avoided.

The diagnosis of mania is usually made easily and presents few problems. There may, however, be great difficulty in diagnosing hypomania, which at its mildest is hard to distinguish from a lively or active personality.

ICD 10 is likely to introduce the following categories for bipolar affective disorder:
1. **Bipolar affective disorder, currently manic** – the subject is currently manic, symptoms should have lasted for at least one week and be severe enough to produce a definite impairment of function. There should be a history of at least one other affective episode, manic or depressive, in the past.
2. **Bipolar affective disorder, currently depressed** – the current depressive episode should be severe enough to be handicapping and should have lasted for at least two weeks. There is at least one well authenticated manic episode in the past.
3. **Bipolar affective disorder, currently mixed** – the subject has had at least one well authenticated manic episode in the past and currently exhibits either a mixture or a rapid alternation of manic and depressive symptoms.
4. **Bipolar affective disorder, currently in remission**.

Classification 2: primary and secondary affective disorders

A **secondary affective disorder** is one which is either:

1. preceded by another psychological illness or
2. associated with a physical illness.

In contrast, a **primary affective disorder** has no such identifiable causative link. The importance of this classification relates to management, in that treatment of the underlying condition usually results in resolution of the secondary affective disorder. Psychological and physical illnesses which are associated with affective disorders are considered in the section on aetiology (*see* p. 92).

Classification 3: endogenous/ psychotic versus reactive/ neurotic depression

In some people who present with depressive symptoms, affective changes may not be as severe as in a depressive illness. Furthermore, mood can fluctuate, so that the individual complains of his depression coming over him 'in waves', rather than the loss of ability to enjoy life being complete. Consequently, he can usually be distracted from his misery, albeit for a short time. Feelings of despair are often worse in the evenings (rather than the mornings), and although bodily functions are commonly affected, they are not consistent with the characteristic biological changes found in a depressive illness. For example, weight may be gained rather than lost, particularly if appetite increases to compensate for feelings of distress. Sleep is not always disturbed, but when it is, the subject frequently complains of difficulty in getting to sleep (early insomnia) or waking intermittently, rather than early morning wakening. In some cases, sleep can be excessive (hypersomnia).

Feelings of anxiety are commonly present, but ideas of guilt and self-blame are unusual, the individual tending to blame others for his predicament. Nevertheless, people presenting with this clinical picture may be so distressed that they have difficulty in coping with the demands of life, and will sometimes express suicidal ideas which may even be acted upon.

Where the onset of these symptoms follows on from, or is attributed to an event such as the end of a relationship or the loss of a job, the condition is sometimes known as a **reactive depression**. Those who use this nomenclature would refer to a depressive illness as an **endogenous depression**, since it ostensibly comes 'out of the blue' and is attributed to internal causes. Many psychiatrists consider this division unsatisfactory because there is considerable evidence that life events are influential in nearly all cases of depression. Although symptom patterns are said to be clearly distinguishable between the two types, in clinical practice this is not always so.

Further confusion arises in that the terms **psychotic** and **neurotic depression** are sometimes respectively applied to the descriptions given for endogenous and reactive forms of the illness. A more appropriate use of the expression 'psychotic' is reserved for those cases of depression where insight is lost and delusions and/or hallucinations are present.

Although the terms endogenous/psychotic and reactive/neurotic are commonly applied in clinical practice, there are a number of objections to their continued use. Not all psychiatrists accept that there are different types of depression, and many believe that these terms simply represent varying degrees of severity of a single condition. In addition, it is fairly common to encounter patients who exhibit cardinal features of both types. This lends weight to the argument that depressive illness can be depicted on a continuous spectrum, with endogenous/psychotic features at one extreme and reactive/neurotic features at the other, so that the vast majority of sufferers fall somewhere in between (*see* Fig. 5.1).

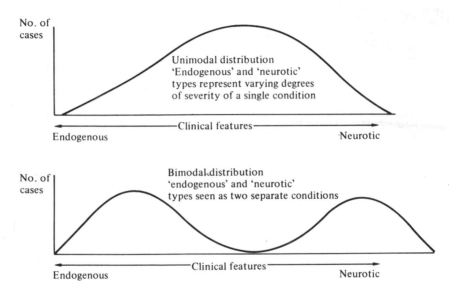

Fig. 5.1 Unimodal and bimodal models of depression

American psychiatrists have attempted to reduce ambiguity by replacing the terms endogenous/psychotic and reactive/neurotic with **major depressive episode** (melancholia) and **dysthymic disorder** (dysthymia) as defined in DSM III-R (*see* p. 10). Rather than relying on vague criteria, the difference between the two is determined quantitatively according to the duration and number of symptoms elicited from a supplied list. However, the debate continues as to whether the disparity between endogenous/psychotic and reactive/neurotic depression is qualitative (comprising two different illnesses) or quantitative (one illness varying in degree of severity). Because differences do exist in terms of response to treatment, it is probably worthwhile preserving the concept of a distinction, irrespective of the labels used. A summary of the differences between the various types of depression discussed in this section is given in Table 5.2.

Table 5.2 Summary of differences between various 'types' of depression

Terminology used	Depressive illness (out of the blue)	external cause
	Endogenous depression	Reactive depression
	Major depressive episode (melancholia)	Dysthymic disorder
	Psychotic depression	Neurotic depression
Mood	Diurnal variation worse in a.m.	Diurnal variation not present, or worse in p.m.
	Persistently lowered	May fluctuate
	Total loss of enjoyment	Can be distracted from misery
Sleep	Early morning wakening	Difficulty in getting to sleep, intermittent wakening or hypersomnia
Appetite and weight	Poor appetite, weight loss may be considerable in a matter of weeks	Appetite often normal and may gain weight
Suicidal thoughts	Frequently present	Sometimes present
Guilt	Often present, blame themselves for real or imagined misdemeanours	Infrequent, usually blame others for their predicament
Delusions and hallucinations	May be present in severe cases	If present, not due to depressive symptoms
Psychomotor activity	May be grossly retarded in movement and thought	Gross retardation very unusual
Anxiety symptoms	May be present	Commonly present
Attitude to the future	Seen as very bleak and hopeless	Occasionally seen as bleak and hopeless
Sexual activity and libido	Reduced or absent	May be reduced or normal

ICD 10 is likely to introduce the terms 'severe depressive episode' and 'mild depressive episode' as respective synonyms for 'endogenous' and 'neurotic' types of depression.

ICD 10 is likely to introduce the categories of **severe depressive episode** and **mild depressive episode**. In both forms, the subject suffers from lowering of mood, reduction of energy and decrease in activity. In the severe form, there are accompanying 'biological' or 'endogenomorphic' symptoms and loss of self-esteem. Ideas of worthlessness, guilt, sin and imminent disaster may become delusional, with auditory hallucinations congruent with the depressed mood. In particularly severe cases, there is an increased danger of successful suicide, and motor and psychic retardation may progress to stupor. The depressive episode should be severe enough to cause both distress and interference with ordinary activities, and should last for a minimum of two weeks. A mild depressive episode is one which lacks the distinguishing and more severe features of a severe depressive episode. The subject may still suffer considerable distress and interference with ordinary activities, but biological symptoms are mild or absent. Motor and psychic retardation, delusions and hallucinations are also absent. As with a severe depressive episode, symptoms should last for a minimum of two weeks.

EPIDEMIOLOGY

Because of disagreement over definitions and classification, the epidemiology of the affective disorders is difficult to determine. In addition to problems with differentiating between normal unhappiness and depressive illness, varying methods used to collect data add to the confusion. However, despite these factors, certain trends can be identified (Table 5.3).

AETIOLOGY

No single theory has emerged as to the principal cause of affective disorders. As a result, a number of different 'models' of causation have been proposed.

1. Genetic Theories

The results of **family**, **twin** and **adoption studies** (*see* p. 7) demonstrate that genetic influences are stronger in bipolar than unipolar disorders. Overall, it is probably a **tendency** to develop affective illness that is inherited, and other factors are required to precipitate the conditions which are recognised as mania or depression.

2. Biochemical Theories

These have been advanced to explain the actions of drugs used in the management of affective disorders. In the early 1950s, it was noted that

Table 5.3 Epidemiology of bipolar and unipolar affective disorders

	Bipolar	Unipolar
Mean age of onset of first illness	Approximately 30 years	No consistent figure can be determined from research findings
Approximate incidence	20/100 000/year	200–400/100 000/year (some studies report much higher figures)
Lifetime expectancy*	1%	10–20%
Sex ratio	M:F = 1: 1.3	M:F = 1:2
Social class	Upper > lower	No distinction
Risk to first-degree relatives	Increased risk of unipolar and bipolar disorders	Increased risk of unipolar disorders only

* Percentage of population expected to develop the illness during their lifetime.

reserpine, a drug commonly used at that time to treat high blood pressure, frequently produced severe depression. It was later shown that reserpine lowered the levels of certain neurotransmitters within the central nervous system. The **monoamine theory** proposes that a deficiency of the biogenic amines **noradrenaline** and **serotonin (5-hydroxytryptamine)**, causes depression, while an excess results in mania. Consequently, it is accepted that antidepressant drugs probably exert their effect by increasing the level of these monoamines through inhibition of their natural breakdown.

However, this theory does not account for all known facts. For example, some patients with depressive illness do not respond to antidepressants, and although an increase in monoamine levels occurs immediately, clinical improvement can be delayed for up to 4 weeks in those who do respond. Despite these drawbacks, it does provide a useful model for the development of further compounds to treat affective disorders.

Other biochemical theories that have been proposed implicate alterations in sodium and water metabolism, but their significance is not clearly understood.

3. Endocrine Theories

A chemical or hormonal change which could be measured to make or support a clinical diagnosis of depression would, of course, be of considerable benefit. Although the level of the hormone **cortisol** is known to be raised in some patients with depressive illness, this finding alone has little diagnostic value as levels are also elevated in subjects under stress. However, measuring cortisol levels in response to an injection of dexamethasone may be of some help in confirming the diagnosis of depression. When the synthetic hormone dexamethasone is injected, the normal response is for the production of cortisol by the body to be reduced for some hours; i.e. dexamethasone suppresses plasma cortisol levels. However, when dexamethasone is given to depressed patients with raised cortisol levels, a significant number (approximately two-thirds) fail to undergo suppression. This is known as a positive **dexamethasone suppression test**.

4. Environmental Theories

Environmental factors probably exert their effect in conjunction with genetic and other influences in the development of affective illness.

THE ROLE OF LIFE EVENTS

Feelings of sadness and unhappiness which follow traumatic or unpleasant experiences are part of everyday life. It is therefore understandable that adverse **life events** of this kind should have been studied to investigate any connection that exists between them and the onset of affective illness. The **context** of the life event is also important. For example, the death of an only child of middle-aged parents may have an entirely different connotation to the loss of a new-born infant of a young couple with several other children.

Because many depressed patients desperately search for a cause of their unhappiness, they may falsely attribute responsibility for their condition to a particular event when reviewing the recent past. Thus, a man who has lost his job may pinpoint this as the cause of his depression. In fact, he may well have been sacked because he was already depressed, which caused him to become inefficient and led to his dismissal. Far greater significance could be attributed to the event if its occurrence was **independent** (such as the loss of a job through redundancy), and could not therefore result from illness.

Most studies agree that depressed people report more adverse life events in the period before the onset of their illness than do normal controls over the same time span. The interval covered varies from a few weeks to several months. However, looking at the population as a whole, most life events are not followed by affective illness. In considering why some individuals are more susceptible than others to develop depression,

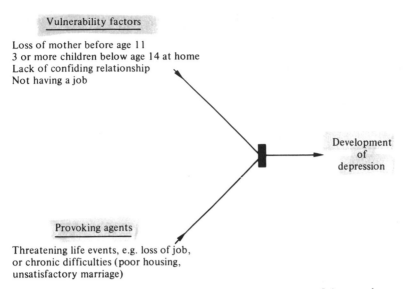

Vulnerability factors

Loss of mother before age 11
3 or more children below age 14 at home
Lack of confiding relationship
Not having a job

Development
of
depression

Provoking agents

Threatening life events, e.g. loss of job,
or chronic difficulties (poor housing,
unsatisfactory marriage)

Fig. 5.2 The role of social factors in the development of depression
based on a study of working-class London women

a study was conducted of depressed women in London. A number of
vulnerability factors were identified which did not bring about depression
themselves, but required the additional presence of **provoking agents**,
these being threatening life events or chronic difficulties (such as poor
housing or an unsatisfactory marriage). The vulnerability factors identified
were:

1. having lost one's mother before the age of 11
2. three or more children under the age of 14 at home
3. lack of a confiding relationship with another adult
4. not having a job.

Although it would not be valid to implicate these factors in the
development of all cases of depression, the findings do nevertheless
provide a useful basis for understanding the role of environmental
influences in the causation and perpetuation of affective disorders
(Fig. 5.2).

Stressful life events also appear to play a role in the onset of manic
illnesses, although less research has been conducted in examining this
association than with depression.

EARLY LOSS

Sigmund Freud felt that depression in later life was a re-awakening of loss
which occurred in childhood. The death of a parent early on seems to have

some bearing on the development of depressive illness, although the degree of influence of such an event remains in doubt.

5. Psychological Theories

ANALYTICAL THEORIES

Freud interpreted the self-accusations made by some depressed patients as relating to feelings about some loss in their lives. Loss and rejection naturally evoke feelings of anger which are directed towards the lost 'object'. Those who become depressed are said to do so because they turn this anger inwards (introjection), thereby punishing themselves (*see* Chapter 13).

COGNITIVE THEORY OF DEPRESSION

The traditional association between mood and thinking is that a lowering of the former results in morbid thoughts of despair, which in turn may lead to suicidal ideas and actions.

The cognitive theory of depression (developed by Beck) views the matter differently, in proposing that the lowered mood which occurs in depressed patients **results** from 'automatic' thoughts. These take the form of 'negative ideas' in which the person sees himself, the world around him and the future unfavourably. This pattern of thinking has probably become established over many years, and the subject may be unaware that he is engaging in such activity.

When faced with a problem, the self-defeating content of the depressed person's thoughts distorts the evidence to produce a gloomy picture, so that events are interpreted in a negative way without considering alternatives. For example, 'The fact that the girl at last night's party wouldn't dance with me proves that I am unattractive to women.' This theory of causation has recently been utilised to treat depression by **cognitive therapy** (*see* p. 279).

LEARNED HELPLESSNESS

This theory is based upon the observation of behavioural changes in animals that are subjected to unpleasant stimuli (such as electric shocks), which they cannot take steps to avoid or control. Under these conditions the animals become hypoactive and passive, eat very little and lose weight, demonstrating comparable features to depression in humans. The theory of learned helplessness proposes that depressive disorders in man occur as a result of an acceptance by the subject that his actions will have no effect in altering the course of events. To date, there is little experimental evidence to support the hypothesis.

6. Miscellaneous Causes of Affective Illness

Depression (and rarely mania) can occur in association with the following:

1. physical illnesses (*see* Chapter 15)
2. other psychiatric disorders
3. the administration of certain drugs
4. surgical procedures and trauma
5. childbirth (*see* Chapter 20).

Details are shown in Table 5.4.

THE MANAGEMENT OF DEPRESSION

Management will depend to some extent upon the presenting features of the illness, as well as the therapist's view of its causation. In clinical practice, it is useful to consider each case of depression individually and, ideally, an **eclectic approach** should be adopted using aspects of different therapies to suit the needs of the patient, while concentrating on those which appear to give the best response.

The **severity of the illness** is the main factor in determining whether a patient should be treated at home or in hospital. The majority of cases are mild, and can be managed successfully in outpatients or by the general practitioner (*see* p. 101). More severe cases may require admission to hospital, particularly if there is a serious risk of suicide or the person is unable to cope with his usual responsibilities. (The management of the suicidal patient is considered in Chapter 6.) Severely retarded patients, especially those who live alone, might well die from dehydration or lack of food if left to themselves.

In addition to nursing and medical care, hospital provides a supportive, non-stressful environment which allows time away from the psychosocial difficulties that may have caused or exacerbated the illness.

Management is best considered in terms of:

1. **physical treatments**: including drug therapy, electroconvulsive therapy (ECT) and (rarely) psychosurgery
2. **psychological treatments**: involving psychotherapeutic and cognitive techniques
3. **social aspects of treatment**: utilising community support and rehabilitation.

Table 5.4 Miscellaneous causes of affective disorders

	Depression	Mania or depression
Physical disorders		
(a) Endocrine	Addison's disease Hypothyroidism Hypopituitarism Parathyroid disorders	Cushing's syndrome Thyrotoxicosis
(b) Metabolic	Electrolyte disturbance Renal failure Acute porphyria	Hepatic failure
(c) Haematological	Anaemias (B_{12}, folate, iron) Leukaemias	
(d) Neurological	Parkinson's disease Cerebrovascular accident Cerebral lupus *Huntington's?*	Multiple sclerosis Temporal lobe epilepsy Space-occupying lesions Acute and chronic organic reactions
(e) Infections	Influenza Infectious mononucleosis	Encephalitis Syphilis (general paresis) Viral hepatitis, AIDS
(f) Neoplasia	Primary or metastatic malignancy	
(g) Trauma and surgery		Depression common post-operatively and following head injury
Psychiatric disorders	Anxiety states, phobias, schizophrenia, obsessive-compulsive neurosis, anorexia/bulimia nervosa	

Drugs — Many drugs have been implicated in precipitating affective disorders, but in most cases the mode of causation is unclear

	Reserpine, methyldopa, barbiturates, alcohol, isoniazid, oral contraceptives, digoxin, sulphonamides, immunosuppressants	Steroids, L-dopa, antidepressants (mania only), amphetamines

Although each will be considered separately, this is purely for descriptive purposes, as all aspects of treatment are complementary to one another.

1. Physical Treatments

(a) DRUG THERAPY

Once a diagnosis of depression has been made, the decision to use drugs depends upon a number of factors. Mild depressive symptoms which are a response to environmental stress and crises tend to resolve spontaneously or with simple treatment, such as sympathy, reassurance and advice on problem-solving. Under these circumstances drugs are rarely necessary.

Where mild symptoms persist for months, or the patient is more severely ill, there are strong indications for the use of antidepressants. A persistent lowering of mood from which the patient cannot be distracted, together with 'biological' features (early morning wakening, diurnal mood variation and loss of weight or appetite), suggest that a good response to drug treatment can be expected.

Monoamine Reuptake Inhibitors (MARIs)

These drugs inhibit the degradation of biogenic amines, by preventing their reuptake at the synaptic cleft. They are usually first choice in the drug treatment of depression and include the **tricyclic antidepressants**. Their effectiveness has been well proven over the past 25 years, their unwanted effects and contraindications are clearly understood, and they are relatively inexpensive to prescribe. The mode of action of MARIs relates to the 'amine hypothesis' of depression (*see* p. 87).

A large number of tricyclic compounds are available, and in terms of their efficacy there is little to choose between them. The choice of drug is largely determined by the range of side-effects and how these are tolerated by the patient. Further details of these compounds are given in Chapter 12.

The use of MARI drugs is not without problems. The onset of their antidepressant action is relatively slow and variable, 2 – 4 weeks elapsing before any noticeable improvement in mood occurs. However, unwanted actions can develop after the first dose. Consequently, a 'lag period' is created, during which the individual may experience unpleasant drug-related symptoms, but no therapeutic benefit. This is one of the reasons why patients stop taking their medication before it has had time to work. However, some of the other actions of these drugs are therapeutically useful. For example, compounds which are sedating (such as amitriptyline) may help to induce sleep and relieve feelings of tension where anxiety or agitation are prominent features of a depressive illness.

Because MARIs have a long half-life, they are therapeutically effective if given once a day. They should only be given in divided doses to reduce troublesome side-effects. The more times a patient has to remember to take his medication, the less likely he is so to do. Treatment should continue for at least 6 months following the resolution of symptoms, to minimise the risk of relapse.

Since their antidepressant effect takes 2–4 weeks to develop, MARIs should be taken for at least 5–6 weeks before a course of treatment is said to be unsuccessful. Providing the patient has definitely been taking the drug at an adequate dosage, there is little to be gained by trying another compound from this group, and other treatments should then be considered.

MARI antidepressants are highly dangerous in overdose, and this must be borne in mind when they are prescribed to depressed patients who may harbour suicidal ideas. The risk can be minimised by assessing the patient at frequent intervals, only giving medication to cover the period until he is seen again, and by entrusting the handling of the tablets to a relative or friend. Tricyclic antidepressants should also be prescribed with caution in the elderly, because a normal therapeutic dose for a young adult may prove to be toxic in an older person, and side-effects can be especially troublesome. Treating the depressive phase of a bipolar illness with MARI antidepressants can sometimes produce a rapid swing into mania.

Monoamine oxidase inhibitors (MAOIs)

As their name suggests, MAOIs act by inhibiting **monoamine oxidase** enzymes, which are responsible for the intracellular breakdown of monoamines within the central nervous system. Consequently, the levels of the neurotransmitters noradrenaline and 5-hydroxytryptamine are elevated, which is thought to account for the drugs' antidepressant actions.

MAOIs have been shown to be less effective in the management of depressive illness than MARI antidepressants, and are therefore rarely used as a first line treatment. They also have the potential to interact dangerously with certain drugs and foodstuffs. However, they do have a place in the management of 'resistant' depression and in illnesses where a large component of anxiety exists. MAOIs are discussed more fully in Chapter 12.

The new antidepressants

Because of the many problems with both tricyclic antidepressants and MAOIs in terms of their troublesome unwanted effects, and toxicity in overdose, newer antidepressants have been developed in an attempt to overcome these difficulties.

Most of the new drugs inhibit monoamine reuptake, but a few are believed to work in different ways to produce mood elevation. Many of them do not produce the same side-effects as tricyclics and MAOIs, but a number of new problems have arisen with their administration which are equally troublesome. In some cases, this has led to their withdrawal from use (*see* Chapter 12).

(b) ELECTROCONVULSIVE THERAPY (ECT)

This is a physical treatment which involves the passage of an electric current through the brain in order to induce a fit.

Historical development

The use of electricity to cure illness dates back to ancient times, when the electric torpedo fish was found to relieve headaches if applied to the scalp. By the eighteenth century, numerous accounts existed of physicians using electrical current to cure grief reactions, depression and anxiety states. Throughout the nineteenth and early part of the twentieth century, doctors continued to experiment with this method of treating mental disorders.

During the 1920s, it was a commonly held belief that schizophrenia and epilepsy could not coexist in the same individual. Although this assumption is now known to be false, it nevertheless provided the basis for the use of ECT as a therapeutic procedure, initially in schizophrenia and later in depression. In 1933, Meduna, a Hungarian physician, began using intramuscular injections of camphor to induce fits in schizophrenic patients, on the assumption that the occurrence of a seizure by artificial means would cause the condition to remit. The method was unreliable in producing convulsions, but Meduna's work inspired two Italian research workers, Cerletti and Bini, to extend their animal experiments on the electrical induction of fits to human subjects. In 1938, they treated their first subject, a mute vagrant found wandering in a Rome railway station. He was given an electrical stimulus to the head, following which he improved rapidly without apparent ill effect. There is, however, some doubt as to what was wrong with him!

By the 1940s, the use of ECT for the treatment of schizophrenia had become widespread. However, the failure of many patients to improve, coupled with the observation that an elevation in mood frequently occurred following a convulsion, resulted in a gradual shift of its use away from schizophrenia towards treating depression.

Initially, ECT was administered without a general anaesthetic. Although the patient immediately became unconscious following the passage of current, severe injuries often resulted from fractures of the spine or long bones, due to the powerful muscle contractions occurring at the time of the seizure. In the early 1950s, **modified ECT** was gradually introduced, and this is now standard practice. A short-acting general anaesthetic and muscle relaxant are given prior to inducing the fit, in order to prevent such complications and to make the treatment less distressing for the patient.

Indications for use and mode of action

The use of ECT is an emotive subject, partly because the prospect of passing electricity through the brain is for many people abhorrent. In addition, there is a risk of fatality, although this is negligible and is mainly associated with the administration of the anaesthetic, rather than the procedure itself. For these reasons, ECT is not usually considered as a first-line treatment for depression, despite the fact that antidepressant drugs (and indeed the untreated illness) are themselves associated with significant rates of mortality.

As a general rule, a favourable response to ECT is more likely where **biological features of depression** predominate. Other particular indications include:

(i) the presence of depressive delusions, such as false convictions of guilt, worthlessness, illness and financial ruin
(ii) serious risk to life through refusal to eat or drink, self-neglect or active suicidal intent
(iii) psychomotor retardation or depressive stupor
(iv) failure to respond to, or comply with, drug treatment
(v) a contraindication to using antidepressant drugs because of intolerable side-effects or poor physical health of the patient.

How ECT works is not clearly understood, but it has been postulated that it increases the sensitivity of post-synaptic monoamine receptors in the brain. In addition to the management of depression, it can also be sometimes used to treat **manic illnesses** which have failed to respond to neuroleptics or lithium, and schizophrenic illnesses in which **catatonic features** are prominent. In other forms of schizophrenia, ECT has been shown to be less effective than neuroleptic drugs.

Procedure

ECT is usually administered in the morning, and the patient has nothing to eat or drink from midnight onwards. The subject lies on a bed or couch in the treatment area and is put to sleep with a short-acting general anaesthetic. The anaesthetist also administers a muscle relaxant to prevent the severe spasms which would otherwise occur when the seizure is induced.

Unilateral   Bilateral

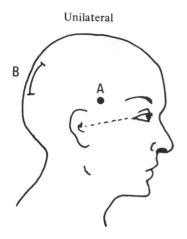
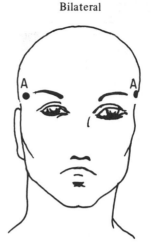

Point A is 4 cm above the mid-point
between the angle of the orbit and
the external auditory meatus. Point   Point A on both sides is the same as
B should be a minimum of 12 cm from   for unilateral placement.
from Point A, without crossing the
midline.

Fig. 5.3 Position of the electrodes in unilateral and bilateral ECT

The psychiatrist in attendance then places two small electrodes on the scalp, which may be applied **unilaterally** or **bilaterally** (Fig. 5.3), having first moistened the underlying skin with a saline solution to ensure good electrical contact. (Unilateral placement of the electrodes is nearly always on the right side of the head in people who are right-handed, i.e. overlying the non-dominant hemisphere. Determining laterality with left-handed subjects is more complicated.)

An electric current of very low voltage is passed between the electrodes for a few seconds to induce a fit. Because of the suppressing effect of the muscle relaxant, all that may be evident is a slight twitching of the toes or a flickering of the eyelids for anything up to one minute, although more powerful contractions of the limbs are sometimes observed. If no fit is seen following the passage of the current, it is normal practice to repeat the procedure once more. After a few minutes, the patient recovers consciousness, and within 30–45 minutes is able to return to the ward. The advantages and disadvantages of unilateral and bilateral ECT are summarised in Table 5.5.

On balance, the advantages of unilateral ECT outweigh the disadvantages, and it seems to be the treatment of choice in most cases. However, where speed of action is essential (e.g. in cases of high suicide risk and other life-threatening situations), bilateral ECT is preferable.

Table 5.5 The advantages and disadvantages of bilateral and unilateral ECT

	Bilateral	Unilateral
No. of treatments needed	6–8 treatments usually required for resolution of symptoms. Initial improvement frequently more rapid than with unilateral	May require one or two additional treatments compared with bilateral ECT
Seizure	Bilateral seizure usually occurs	Seizure may occur in only one hemisphere or not at all
Side-effects	More likely to be confused immediately after treatment and complain of headache. Amnesia may be severe but is reversible	Headache, confusion and amnesia absent or less severe than with bilateral treatment

Precautions and contraindications to ECT

ECT should never be administered to a patient with **raised intracranial pressure**. Other than this, each case must be individually evaluated by judging the risk of giving the treatment against that of withholding it. Patients who have a cerebral tumour or aneurysm, or who give a recent history of heart attack, stroke or other cardiorespiratory problems which create an anaesthetic risk, should be assessed very carefully before the decision is taken to give ECT. Where appropriate, it is permissible to give the treatment during pregnancy, to patients with epilepsy, in cases of senile dementia with depressive symptoms, and in those fitted with a cardiac pacemaker. In individuals with bipolar affective illness, treatment with ECT may precipitate mania.

Medicolegal aspects

An explanation of the procedure, its benefits and dangers must be given by the doctor, following which the patient is required to give **written consent** before ECT is administered. Where this is refused or the individual is too ill to give permission, provisions exist within the Mental Health Act 1983 to treat the patient without his consent if ECT is considered essential (this is discussed further in Chapter 24).

(c) PSYCHOSURGERY

Psychosurgery is the destruction of normal or abnormal brain tissue in order to bring about changes in behaviour or emotions. Today, its use is restricted to a very small number of patients each year (*see below*).

Various techniques have been used on human subjects for over 100 years, and originated from observations of the docile behaviour which was induced in monkeys following removal of parts of their frontal lobes.

In the 1930s and 1940s, the **standard prefrontal leucotomy** was the most widely used procedure, performed on thousands of patients with unremitting symptoms of schizophrenia, chronic agitation and depression. It involved severing nerve pathways between the frontal lobe and the rest of the brain by inserting a specially curved blade known as a leucotome through burr holes in the skull. By the 1950s, this treatment had fallen into disrepute because of poor results and the high incidence of side-effects such as **epilepsy, incontinence** and **unwanted personality changes** (apathy, disinhibition and intellectual impairment). There was also a significant mortality rate, and consequently, the introduction of safer and effective drug treatments signalled the end of the widespread use of this technique.

Psychosurgery is currently restricted to intractable cases of depression (as well as chronic anxiety and obsessional neurosis), in which symptoms are seriously disabling, have persisted unabated for at least 2 years and have failed to respond to other forms of treatment. Modern techniques are highly specialised and utilise sophisticated procedures. Selected areas of the brain are identified through precise stereotactic methods and then destroyed by the use of radioisotopes, freezing, ultrasound or electro-coagulation. Side-effects are minimal, the mortality rate is negligible, and with careful patient selection some improvement can be expected in most cases.

Psychosurgery is a controversial procedure because it involves the irreversible destruction of 'normal' brain tissue and its mode of action is unknown. Consequently, the Mental Health Act 1983 requires the informed consent of the patient *and* the concurring second opinion by representatives of the Mental Health Act Commission before any procedure is performed (*see* Chapter 24).

2. Psychological Treatments

Psychological treatments for depression can be considered in terms of supportive and dynamic psychotherapy and cognitive therapy.

Supportive psychotherapy (*see* Chapter 13) is given to most patients in some form, and sometimes is the mainstay of treatment. It aims to minimise disabling symptoms by encouraging the expression of feelings, demonstrating empathy with the individual's problems, and offering support and advice where appropriate.

Dynamic psychotherapy (*see* Chapter 13) is aimed at helping certain patients to develop an understanding of the nature of their problems. It may be especially useful where inter- or intrapersonal difficulties are a prominent feature of the clinical picture. A degree of psychological awareness is required, in which the individual must be responsive to interpretations of behaviour and feelings, and be prepared to challenge long-standing attitudes and ideas. Severe illnesses, particularly where gross retardation or depressive delusions are present, are not amenable to this form of therapy. Older depressed patients may be unwilling or unable to review distant events in relation to present feelings.

Cognitive therapy (*see* Chapter 13) is a relatively new form of treatment which has been shown to be effective in milder cases of depression, sharing similar limitations to those of dynamic psychotherapy. It involves a relearning of responses to situations, so that ways of thinking which lead to depressive feelings are avoided. Positive attitudes are encouraged by exploring alternative possibilities. For example, 'my girlfriend didn't phone last night. . .' might be because she was late home from work or felt unwell, rather than. . . 'because she doesn't love me'. In practice, encouraging patients to generate 'alternative assumptions', and believe them, is a complex process requiring a considerable amount of time.

3. Social Aspects of Treatment

Many patients have social problems involving difficulties with accommodation, financial matters and relationships, which may have precipitated or serve to perpetuate their depressive symptoms. Consequently, specific treatments (such as drugs) often require some form of concurrent **social intervention** to be effective. For example, a woman living in severely overcrowded conditions, who displays features of depressed mood, early morning wakening and weight loss, might well benefit from a course of antidepressants. However, improvement is unlikely to occur or be sustained unless consideration is given to her accommodation problems. Assistance of this kind can be provided by the psychiatric social worker, who is able to liaise with **community services** such as the housing department, employment agencies, self-help groups and social security authorities.

As soon as the more severe physical and psychological symptoms have resolved, a carefully prescribed and monitored **occupational therapy programme** forms an integral part of general management. Work and domestic assessment is followed by retraining in areas where skills have been diminished through lack of motivation or loss of confidence (*see* Chapter 14). Various activities such as **art, pottery** and **drama** can be used to increase self-esteem by developing an individual's creativity, as well as serving to encourage social interaction with other patients and staff.

DEPRESSION IN GENERAL PRACTICE

The majority of patients who complain of depressive symptoms are seen and treated by their general practitioners. Minor depressive episodes in response to stress and social dysfunction form a significant part of the family doctor's workload, although most people improve spontaneously or with appropriate counselling. More persistent cases of depression often arise in association with some form of chronic social pathology (such as marital breakdown or alcohol abuse). Because many of these disorders are environmentally determined, increasing social support and teaching patients better coping strategies are probably the most effective ways of bringing about sustained improvement, rather than solely prescribing drugs.

Studies have shown that antidepressants are widely used in the primary care setting, although family doctors tend to prescribe these drugs in lower dosages and for shorter periods of time than hospital psychiatrists. Compliance with medication in general practice is very poor, and one study showed that 40% of patients prescribed antidepressant drugs had stopped taking them after a fortnight, which increased to 60% within 3 weeks. In nearly every case, the doctor did not know of the decision, and yet ironically, the reason most frequently given for discontinuation was that the patient felt better.

Patients do seem to improve more quickly if their doctor is aware that they have psychiatric symptoms. Physical complaints are often a prominent feature of minor depressive disorders seen in general practice, and can readily lead to the true nature of the diagnosis being missed (*see* Chapter 13). Certain characteristics have been identified in general practitioners who are good psychiatric 'case detectors'. These include an empathic style (*see* p. 275), using non-directive and open-ended questions, being sensitive to verbal and non-verbal cues, and not reading the case notes during the consultation!

When dealing with a case of depression, it is useful for the general practitioner to consider its severity (mild, moderate, severe), the presence of any special features (agitation, suicidal thoughts, delusions), possible precipitating or perpetuating factors, as well as any previous episodes of mania or depression.

THE MANAGEMENT OF MANIA

Most patients with hypomania or mania will eventually require **hospitalisation**. Even in the early stages of the illness, judgement may be impaired, and when associated with reckless and disinhibited behaviour, can lead to adverse consequences for the patient and his family. Lack of insight, combined with a subjective sense of well-being, commonly results in the patient refusing medication, so that effective outpatient treatment is impossible. Admission to hospital not only provides a safe and secure environment, but ensures regular compliance with drugs until recovery. Where admission is refused, **compulsory detention** may be necessary (*see* Chapter 24).

On admission to hospital, a urine sample should be obtained as soon as possible to exclude the presence of illicit drugs which may have precipitated or aggravated the illness. Many patients have been overactive for days or weeks prior to hospitalisation, having had little sleep and paying scant attention to their diet and fluid intake. **Skilled nursing care** is the cornerstone of management, not only in consideration of the patient's physical condition, but also in terms of gaining the individual's trust at a time when he is largely out of control. The experienced nurse knows how to deal with frequent irritable and aggressive outbursts, using a minimum of confrontation and physical restraint, and avoiding provocation. This can be achieved by providing some boundaries to the patient's behaviour, but at the same time sharing their sense of fun when this is appropriate and harmless. Channelling the individual's excessive energy towards safer activities is also important.

Treatment of the Acute Illness

Lithium is a specific antimanic drug (*see* Chapter 12), but large doses are needed to control the acute illness and its onset of action takes approximately 5–10 days. Therefore, a neuroleptic drug, such as **chlorpromazine** (which has sedative properties), is usually administered concurrently to control symptoms until lithium becomes effective. Alternatively, **haloperidol** is sometimes used, and may be preferable in cases where hypotension is likely to be particularly dangerous (such as in dehydrated patients). However, it should be prescribed with care when combined with lithium, as a potentially life-threatening disorder has been attributed to this drug combination.

Lithium can only be given in oral form, and where the patient is very disturbed or refuses to take it, initial management will rely solely on neuroleptic drugs (sometimes given intramuscularly) until improvement occurs. Once symptoms abate, neuroleptic medication can be rapidly tailed off, and lithium levels adjusted to maintain control and minimise side-effects. In the acute illness, the use of lithium alone is confined to mild cases.

In those patients who fail to respond to medication, and especially where their behaviour constitutes a serious risk to themselves or others, **ECT** may be given. One or two treatments can effect rapid resolution in an otherwise resistant illness.

Follow-up and Maintenance Therapy

Once the acute symptoms have settled, a decision is required regarding maintenance therapy. Patients who have recurrent manic or hypomanic episodes (either alone or in association with depressive illness) may benefit from **continuous lithium treatment** (*see* Chapter 12). However, because lithium is a drug with a narrow therapeutic range and a number of potential long-term side-effects (especially those involving the kidney and thyroid gland), therapy of this kind requires constant monitoring. Therefore, for the duration of treatment, which may be for life, the patient must attend for regular blood tests to ensure a therapeutic dose is being taken, and to detect impending toxicity. Some patients find these requirements unacceptable, while others default because they become certain that they are cured and no longer need medication.

An alternative to this approach is to use **depot neuroleptic drugs,** particularly in those patients with poor compliance or where there are contraindications to lithium therapy. However, the risk of tardive dyskinesia militates against this being used as a first-line treatment. More recently, the anticonvulsant drug **carbamazepine** has been shown to be useful in the prophylaxis of bipolar affective disorders, particularly where rapid mood swings occur ('rapid cyclers').

PROGNOSIS OF AFFECTIVE DISORDERS

The duration of illness in most cases is less than 6 months, although the condition tends to recur. In one study conducted over a 15-year period, only 5% of subjects had a depressive illness which was not followed by further episodes of mania or depression. The corresponding figure for single attacks of mania or hypomania was less than 1%. The time interval between successive episodes is variable, but tends to shorten with increasing age.

The risk of relapse in depressive illnesses which have responded to MARI (tricyclic) antidepressants can be reduced by continuing the drug for at least 6 months from the time of clinical recovery. Lithium taken continuously has been shown to be effective in reducing the number of manic and depressive episodes in bipolar patients, although it does not prevent their recurrence totally. The effectiveness of lithium in the prophylaxis of unipolar affective disorders is less apparent.

SUMMARY

1. **Affective disorders** are characterised by sustained abnormalities of 'affect' or mood, either depression or elation. They may be accompanied

by alterations in bodily function, thought content, perception and behaviour.

2. **Depressive illness**: this characteristically involves a persistent lowering of mood, which in its most severe form leads to an inability to enjoy anything in life (anhedonia). Associated biological features of depression include early morning wakening, diurnal mood variation, poor appetite, weight loss, constipation, loss of libido, psychomotor retardation or agitation. Abnormal depressive thoughts can involve ideas or delusions of guilt, worthlessness, ill health, nihilism, hopelessness and suicide. Occasionally, in a severe illness, the sufferer experiences unpleasant and deprecatory auditory hallucinations. Loss of interest and poor concentration are other common features of depression.

3. **Mania and hypomania**: the core feature of these disorders is a persistent elevation of mood or increased sense of well-being, associated with overactivity and a reduced need for sleep, although irritability without euphoria can predominate. Speech is frequently increased in both quantity and rate (pressure of speech), and this may be associated with racing thoughts and flight of ideas. Rhyming and punning may also occur. The individual tends to be distractable and disinhibited, and might entertain grandiose ideas or delusions. Hypomania is similar to, but not as severe as, full-blown mania.

4. **Classification** of affective disorders: several different systems exist, but only some are useful in determining treatment and prognosis. Classifications currently in use include unipolar/bipolar affective disorders, endogenous/reactive and psychotic/neurotic depression, primary and secondary affective disorders, as well as major depressive episode and dysthymic disorder (as defined in DSM III-R).

5. The **epidemiology** of affective disorders is difficult to determine accurately, although certain trends can be identified. Unipolar disorders are more common than bipolar disorders. Women outnumber men 2:1 in unipolar disorders, whereas sex distribution is approximately equal in bipolar illnesses.

6. **Aetiology**: a number of different models of causation have been proposed, although no single theory predominates. A genetic influence has been demonstrated by family, twin and adoption studies. The monoamine theory proposes that depression is probably due to a deficiency of biogenic amines at certain strategic sites in the brain, while mania is thought to result from a relative excess of these neurotransmitters. Endocrine changes which are observed in affective disorders, such as raised cortisol levels, may result from non-specific stress. Environmental determinants, which include life events and vulnerability factors, probably exert their effect in conjunction with genetic and other influences to cause affective illness. Analytical theories view depression as internalised anger following some kind of loss. The cognitive model suggests that depressed mood is secondary to persistent negative thoughts about the self, the

world and the future. The theory of learned helplessness proposes that depression arises because of acceptance by the subject that his actions will not alter the course of events. Physical illnesses, other psychiatric disorders, drugs, trauma and childbirth have all been implicated in the causation of affective disorder.

7. **Management of depression**: the majority of cases are mild and are effectively dealt with by the general practitioner. More severe or persistent cases may require hospital admission. Physical treatments include antidepressant drugs (MARIs and MAOIs), ECT and (rarely) psychosurgery. MARI drugs are most effective when biological features predominate, but 2–4 weeks can elapse before a therapeutic effect is evident. They should be continued for at least 6 months following recovery to minimise the risk of relapse. Where no response occurs, ECT should be considered, especially in cases where depressive delusions or psychomotor retardation are present, and the risk of suicide is high. Supportive psychotherapy is an important element of treatment in all cases of depression, although dynamic therapy is most effective when inter- and intrapersonal difficulties are prominent. Cognitive therapy is only appropriate in mild cases of depression. Social intervention may involve attention to problems surrounding accommodation, financial matters and life-style. Liaison with community services is often necessary. Occupational therapy forms an integral part of the rehabilitation of depressed patients. Most cases of depression seen by general practitioners probably respond better to psychosocial intervention than to drug treatment.

8. **Management of mania**: hospitalisation is usually required, and drug treatments together with skilled nursing care are the cornerstone of management. Neuroleptics are usually prescribed initially for the acute stages of the illness together with lithium, the latter also being used for long-term prophylaxis. ECT is sometimes effective in resistant cases.

9. **Prognosis**: the duration of affective illness in most cases is less than 6 months, although the condition tends to recur.

REFERENCES AND FURTHER READING

Angst, J., Baastrup, P., Grof, P., Poldinger, W., Weis, P. (1973). The course of monopolar depression and bipolar psychosis. *Psychiatry, Neurology and Neurosurgery*; **76**: 489–500.

Beck, A. T., Rush, A. J., Shaw, B. F., Emery, G. (1979). *Cognitive Therapy of Depression*. New York: Guilford Press.

Blacker, C. V. R., Clare, A. W. (1987). Depressive disorder in primary care. *British Journal of Psychiatry*; **150**: 737–51.

Brown, G. W., Harris, T. (1978). *Social Origins of Depression*. London: Tavistock Publications.

Cerletti, U., Bini, L. (1938). Un nuovo metodo di shokterapia; l'elettroshock. *Bulletin Academia Medica di Roma*; **64**: 136-38.

Cookson, J. C. (1985). Drug treatment of bipolar depression and mania. *British Journal of Hospital Medicine*; **34**: 172–75.

Coppen, A. (1967). The biochemistry of affective disorders. *British Journal of Psychiatry*; **113**: 1237–64.

Kendell, R. E. (1976). The classification of depressions: a view of contemporary confusion. *British Journal of Psychiatry*; **129**: 15–28.

Mindham, R. H. S., Howland, C., Shepherd, M.(1973). An evaluation of continuation therapy with tricyclic antidepressants in depressive illness. *Psychological Medicine*; **3**: 5–17.

Paykel, E. S. (1978). Contribution of life events to causation of psychiatric illness. *Psychological Medicine*; **8**: 245-53.

Paykel, E. S., ed. (1982). *Handbook of Affective Disorders*. Edinburgh: Churchill Livingstone.

Pippard, J., Ellam, L. (1981). *Electroconvulsive Treatment in Great Britain*. Royal College of Psychiatrists, Ashford: Headley Brothers Ltd.

Schou, M. (1986). Lithium treatment. *British Journal of Psychiatry*; **149**: 541–47.

6

SUICIDE AND NON-FATAL DELIBERATE SELF-HARM

Every year in the UK several thousand people take their own lives. Significantly, many of those who kill themselves have recently consulted their doctor or told others of their plans. Although not all of these deaths are preventable, a proportion could perhaps be averted, and it is therefore important for doctors and other health care workers to be aware of the signs and risk factors which indicate that someone is likely to attempt or commit suicide.

SUICIDE

Suicide may be defined as an intentional, self-inflicted, life-threatening act which results in death.

Epidemiology

Approximately **4500** people commit suicide each year in the UK. A falling suicide rate in the 1960s and early 1970s was attributed to several factors, including the removal of coal gas from the domestic supply, a reduction in the number of barbiturates prescribed, and a general improvement in psychiatric services. However, since then, the rate appears to be rising once again, although the reasons for this remain unclear. Across all age groups, male suicides outnumber female, although the gap is diminishing, particularly among the elderly. The suicide rate increases with age, being very rare in childhood and reaching a peak in the mid-60s for women and a decade later for men. There is an increased risk among the divorced, widowed or single, and those in social classes I and V. More suicides occur in the spring than at other times of the year, with a higher incidence among those living in urban as opposed to rural areas.

Methods Used

Drug overdosage (most commonly with antidepressants and analgesics) accounts for approximately half of all suicides. The remainder result from more **violent methods** which include hanging, drowning, wounding, shooting, gassing, jumping from buildings or in front of moving vehicles or trains.

Aetiology

Several **psychiatric disorders** are associated with an increased risk of suicide, particularly affective illnesses, alcohol and drug abuse, early dementia, schizophrenia, anorexia nervosa and some personality disorders. An increased rate is also found among epileptics, as well as those who suffer **physical illnesses** which cause severe pain or handicap. Suicide sometimes follows **bereavement** and other **losses** such as retirement, divorce or unemployment, and is also associated with **social isolation**. Approximately 50% of those who kill themselves have made an attempt on their lives in the past.

The Assessment and Management of the Suicidal Patient

A person who says he intends to take his own life, or has thoughts of so doing, must be taken seriously. Enquiring about suicidal feelings does not increase the likelihood of them being acted upon, and indeed, many people derive comfort from the knowledge that their plight is understood, and often welcome the opportunity to share the burden of their despair.

A carefully taken **history** should determine the frequency and intensity of suicidal thoughts and whether the subject has considered how he intends to take his life, or if he has made active plans to do so. Ideas of hopelessness and despair for the future need to be enquired about, since their presence greatly increases the likelihood of a suicidal person killing himself. Similarly, it is important to know if there are reasons that prevent him from taking his life, such as religious beliefs or a fear of causing suffering to relatives. The subject should be asked about any current social or interpersonal problems and the state of his physical health, as well as details of past psychiatric illnesses and previous suicide attempts. **Mental state examination** will need to include a careful assessment of mood, thought content and cognitive function. Persecutory ideas or delusions sometimes lead to suicidal acts, and occasionally such patients talk of harming relatives or friends (extended suicide), whom they believe are also suffering. Factors to be taken into account when assessing the degree of suicidal risk are shown in Table 6.1.

When the risk is gauged to be high, it is advisable to admit the person to **hospital** in order to minimise the likelihood of self-harm, and to allow time to deal with any underlying psychological, physical or social precipitants. Occasionally, suicidal patients who refuse informal admission may need to be compulsorily detained.

Supervision on the ward should be as unobtrusive as possible, even

Table 6.1   Assessment of the suicidal patient — factors associated with an increased risk

---

Social status
1. Male, aged over 40
2. Unemployed or retired
3. Divorced, widowed, separated
4. Immigrant status
5. Living in a deprived urban area

Current problems
1. Suffering from affective disorder, early dementia, schizophrenia, alcohol or drug abuse, epilepsy, anorexia nervosa
2. Suffering from a chronically disabling or painful physical illness (especially the elderly)
3. Recent loss, e.g. bereavement, divorce, retirement, redundancy
4. Living alone or in isolation, lack of social support

Family history
Affective illness, suicide, alcohol dependence

Personal history
1. Psychiatric illness especially affective disorder, alcohol abuse
2. Previous suicide attempts

Personality
Psychopathic personality disorder, with impulsive or aggressive tendencies

Mental state
1. A clear statement of suicidal intent
2. Suicidal thoughts (especially if these involve plans or have resulted in preparation for the act)
3. Feelings of hopelessness, worthlessness or despair
4. Significant lowering of mood associated with weight loss and insomnia
5. Persecutory delusions
6. Auditory hallucinations or delusions of control which instruct or compel the subject to take his life

---

when a special nurse is assigned to observe the patient, although all staff must be alerted to the risk of suicide. A significant number of suicidal patients who enter hospital will already be taking psychotropic medication, but this may have been prescribed inappropriately or in less than adequate dosage. If psychiatric illness is present, it should be actively treated, and in the case of depression, the use of **antidepressants** or **ECT** will need to be considered (*see* Chapter 5). Those in whom depressive symptoms and suicidal feelings arise as a consequence of alcohol or drug abuse may rapidly improve within a short time of becoming abstinent.

Talking with suicidal patients and encouraging them to discuss their problems is of great importance, and may help to instil a sense of hope for the future, even though they currently see none. As the crisis passes, and the subject is once again able to accept that his life has some purpose, active **social intervention** needs to aim at decreasing isolation and dealing with any other problems, such as accommodation or financial difficulties, which may be present. Following discharge, regular **follow-up** by the hospital or primary health care team should be arranged. An ongoing therapeutic relationship is not only important to provide support, but also to ensure that management plans are implemented, and that a resurgence of any symptoms of mental illness is rapidly detected.

Not everyone who expresses suicidal thoughts or intentions will need admission to hospital. Some people, in the face of a sudden crisis, rapidly feel unable to cope with the situation, and respond by expressing ideas of self-harm as the only means of solving their problem. Under such circumstances, regular **counselling** by the family doctor or on an outpatient basis may be sufficient to provide the individual with the support he needs until the crisis is over. In addition, practical steps to resolving the predicament can be explored, and the subject helped to learn more constructive ways of dealing with future problems.

In cases where the person is not admitted to hospital, it is frequently advisable, as an added precaution, to give a telephone number where help can be reached at relatively short notice both day and night (such as the acute admission ward). The knowledge that assistance is available if needed, and the ability to speak with someone at a time of crisis, may help to reduce the risk of self-harm. Whenever it is difficult to evaluate the suicidal risk or the dependability of the person's social support network, it is always safest to arrange admission until more information is available.

NON-FATAL DELIBERATE SELF-HARM (DSH)

Deliberate self-harm (sometimes referred to as **parasuicide**) can be defined as an intentional, self-inflicted, non-fatal act effected by physical means, drug overdosage or poisoning. It is done in the knowledge that it is potentially harmful, and in the case of drug overdosage, that the amount taken was excessive. Although the majority of those who commit acts of this type do so without the intention of killing themselves, the suicide rate for this group in the following 12 months is **100 times** greater than for the general population. Consequently, each act of DSH needs careful assessment, however trivial the intent may seem.

Epidemiology

It is difficult to determine accurately the number of incidents of non-fatal DSH, but current estimates in England and Wales suggest that the total is in the order of **several hundred thousand** cases per year, and seems to be increasing, especially among the young. Unlike suicide, females predominate over males by a ratio of 2:1 across all age groups, the highest rate occurring in those aged between 15 and 24 years. An increased risk is associated with being divorced or single, of low or middle social class, and living in poor urban areas.

Methods Used

Drug overdosage accounts for over 90% of all cases in the UK, analgesic (aspirin and paracetamol) and psychotropic compounds (benzodiazepines and antidepressants) being the most common types of medication used. **Self-mutilation** is involved in the remainder, and usually entails superficial lacerations to the wrists or forearms. Rarely, deeper wounds are inflicted to the neck or abdomen, or other violent forms of self-injury are perpetrated, such as shooting, hanging or jumping in front of trains. These methods usually indicate a high degree of suicidal intent.

Aetiology

Most individuals who deliberately harm themselves (but survive) do so in response to **stress** and often display minor depressive symptoms. In others, aspects of a **personality disorder** may be evident, characterised by impulsivity, immaturity and aggressive tendencies. Nearly half of all acts of DSH are carried out while under the influence of **alcohol**. Major psychiatric illness is much less common than in those who commit suicide.

Adverse **social factors** are common precipitants of non-fatal DSH. These include distressing life events (such as marital breakdown or the end of a relationship), unemployment, poor housing, financial problems, ill health and social isolation.

The **motives** in cases of DSH are often complex or vague, and not always revealed by the subject. Although many initially claim they wished to die, most acts are performed impulsively, as a 'cry for help' or to escape from an intolerable situation. Further reasons given include an attempt to manipulate or punish others, and to test the benevolence of fate by 'dicing with death'. Studies have indicated that within 24 hours of the act, only 10% of individuals regret not dying and continue to demonstrate serious suicidal intent.

Assessment Following an Act of Deliberate Self-Harm

The assessment interview should take place in an environment where privacy is ensured (not in the corridor of the casualty department or at the bedside in an open ward), and at a time when the person has recovered from any toxic effects related to overdose or poisoning. It is important to obtain an independent account from relatives or friends of events leading up to the act, and to ask nursing and other staff about the patient's behaviour since admission. The circumstances surrounding the act are often a more accurate indicator of suicidal intent than the individual's stated aims. Some people who genuinely wished to kill themselves may deny their true intentions, while others (such as those who are attention-seeking or embarrassed about their behaviour), may falsely claim that they wanted to die.

The **aims of assessment** are to:

1. establish the degree of suicidal intent at the time of the act and at present
2. establish the risk of further acts of non-fatal DSH or subsequent suicide
3. diagnose any underlying physical or psychiatric disorder and decide upon treatment
4. determine the nature of any personal or social problems which may have precipitated the act, i.e. difficulties with relationships, housing, employment, finances and sexual identity
5. identify the extent of the individual's coping resources and support system, and decide upon the most appropriate form of help
6. decide upon further arrangements for the patient — should he be discharged home, referred to outpatients or admitted to hospital?

Suicidal intent at the time of the act is indicated by:

1. evidence of premeditation, e.g. saving up tablets
2. taking precautions to avoid discovery
3. failing to alert potential helpers after the act
4. carrying out the act in isolation
5. performing 'final acts' in expectation of death, such as leaving a suicide note or writing a will
6. the method used — particularly violent and aggressive acts which allow little chance of survival i.e. shooting, jumping onto railway lines or from buildings, throat-cutting and hanging. However, even when an apparently trivial overdose is taken, intent can still be high, as patients have varying ideas as to what constitutes a 'lethal' amount of drug.

Persistent suicidal intent following an act of DSH is indicated by the continuing expression of suicidal wishes or plans, regret at failing to die and hopelessness for the future (*see* Table 6.1 regarding the **risk of subsequent suicide**).

About one in five of those who commit an act of DSH will make a repeated attempt within the next 12 months, and approximately 2% will **succeed** in killing themselves. The **risk of further acts of DSH** is increased if there is a past history of similar attempts or of treatment for psychiatric disorder. Other risk factors include abuse of drugs or alcohol, being widowed, divorced or separated, evidence of a psychopathic personality disorder or a criminal record, and being unemployed or of low social class.

Management

Since the majority of people who commit an act of DSH have no intention of killing themselves, and are not suffering from any major psychiatric disorder, most can be discharged home following assessment. Where evidence of mental illness is found, or the patient presents a significant suicidal risk, admission to hospital is usually necessary, and management should proceed as outlined on p. 108. In the majority of cases, intervention is concerned with **improving coping skills** and **resolving any personal or social problems** that led up to the act. Many of the difficulties which are encountered can be dealt with by the general practitioner or by enlisting the help of other agencies, such as social services. Occasionally, outpatient counselling may be of benefit if, for example, there is evidence of marital or relationship difficulties, or intrapersonal problems are encountered which require further evaluation.

PREVENTION OF SUICIDE AND DELIBERATE SELF-HARM

There is no clear evidence that psychiatric intervention following acts of deliberate self-harm has been effective in reducing the rate of further attempts. **Primary prevention** has been aimed at improving ways of detecting the potential victim of suicide, increasing the help available to those faced with social and emotional problems, and limiting the availability of prescribed drugs which are frequently used in suicide attempts. A general practitioner with an average-sized list will, as a rule, have one case of suicide among his patients every 5 years. Consequently, the large number of people with psychosocial difficulties seen each day by family doctors means that effective screening of this group is impractical. Furthermore, careful control of repeat prescriptions and avoiding the excessive dispensing of drugs may be of some benefit, but does not prevent the use of medication bought 'over the counter' or prescribed for someone else. The **Samaritan organisation** provides a 'round the clock' nationwide telephone service manned by volunteers, which offers support and advice to people at a time of crisis. Evaluation of their effectiveness has been limited by the guarantee of anonymity to those who enlist their help. However, many people seen after an act of DSH say they knew of the existence of the Samaritans beforehand.

Table 6.2 Summary of suicide and non-fatal DSH in the UK

	Non-fatal DSH	Suicide
Age	Commonest in young age groups	More common in late middle age and the elderly
Sex	F>M	M>F
Marital status	Highest rates in divorced and single	Highest rates in divorced, single and widowed
Employment	Associated with unemployment	Associated with unemployment and retirement
Social class	Commonest in social class V	Commonest in social classes I and V
Urban/rural	Urban>rural, inner cities	Urban>rural
Evidence of mental illness	Major mental illness in 10%	Major mental illness in 90% (depression and alcohol)
Physical health	Usually healthy	May be evidence of terminal or disabling illness, associated with intractable pain or physical handicap
Method used	Drug overdosage in 93% of cases	Drug overdosage in about 50% of cases, violent methods used in remainder
Incidence	Not known, probably >30 times suicide rate	9–10/100 000/year, rising again
Season	No seasonal variation	Commonest April–June
Personality	Evidence of psychopathy	No specific type

SUMMARY

1. Approximately 4500 people commit **suicide** each year in the UK. Drug overdosage accounts for one-half of such deaths, the remainder dying by more violent means. Associated risk factors include being male, divorced or widowed, middle-aged or elderly, unemployed or retired, suffering a recent loss or living in social isolation. Certain psychiatric disorders, notably depression and alcohol dependence, carry an increased risk of suicide, along with physical conditions which cause severe pain or handicap. A past history of suicide attempts and expressed ideas of hopelessness are also important factors. In cases where the risk of suicide is judged to be significant, admission to hospital should be arranged. Any

underlying psychiatric or physical disorder needs to be treated, and steps taken to resolve personal or social problems that have been identified. Follow-up and community support are important once the patient has been discharged from hospital.

2. Several hundred thousand acts of **non-fatal deliberate self-harm** are thought to be carried out each year. Such behaviour is most prevalent among the young (especially females), drug overdosage being the method usually employed. The act frequently follows some stressful event, although the motives expressed are often vague and complex. Associated factors include unemployment, divorce and relationship problems, social isolation or deprivation, ill-health, personality disorder and alcohol abuse. Major psychiatric illness is uncommon.

3. Assessment following an act of DSH should aim to establish the degree of current suicidal intent and that at the time of the act, and to evaluate the risk of further attempts or of subsequent suicide. Management is directed towards treating any underlying physical or psychiatric disorder, improving coping skills and attempting to resolve the personal or social problems that led up to the act. **Preventive measures** seem to have had a limited effect in reducing the number of suicides and cases of non-fatal DSH, both of which appear to be on the increase.

REFERENCES AND FURTHER READING

Bancroft, J. H. J., Hawton, K., Simkin, S., Kingston, B., Cumming, C., Whitwell, D. (1979). The reasons people give for taking overdoses: a further inquiry. *British Journal of Medical Psychology*; **52**: 353–65.

Barraclough, B. M., Bunch, J., Nelson, B., Sainsbury, P. (1974). A hundred cases of suicide: clinical aspects. *British Journal of Psychiatry*; **125**: 355–73.

Department of Health and Social Security (1984). *The Management of Deliberate Self-Harm*. London: DHSS (Health notice HN (84) 25).

Hawton, K. (1987). Assessment of suicide risk. *British Journal of Psychiatry*; **150**: 145–53.

Kessel, N. (1985). Patients who take overdoses. *British Medical Journal*; **290**: 1297–98.

Kreitman, N., ed. (1977). *Parasuicide*. Chichester: Wiley.

Platt, S. (1986). Parasuicide and unemployment. *British Journal of Psychiatry*; **149**: 401–5.

7 BEREAVEMENT

The term **bereavement** is probably derived from the Saxon word **reave**, meaning to rob, which graphically describes the feeling many people experience following a loss. The expression of grief which ensues is part of a process of realisation and gradual relearning, a way of coming to terms internally with what is an established reality in the outside world. Although bereavement is most frequently associated with the death of a loved one, grief is often experienced following other losses (some of which may be symbolic), such as retirement, divorce, moving house or undergoing an operation.

The response to loss in terms of its duration, mode of expression and outcome is extremely variable, so that the concept of 'normal grief' has obvious limitations, and in part is determined by personal as well as cultural values. For example, an elderly couple may mourn the death of an only child for the rest of their lives, which many people would consider an understandable and 'normal' response. By contrast, actively grieving for a pet 2 years after its death would probably be regarded as abnormal by most standards.

Although some losses ultimately have a favourable outcome by promoting maturity, emotional strength and a sense of responsibility in the bereaved, others may result in the development of psychiatric illness. Consequently, it is important to recognise responses which are indicative of abnormal or 'morbid grief', as well as identifying predisposing factors in those thought to be at risk of its development (*see later*).

THE PROCESS OF NORMAL GRIEF

Initially, there may be a period of **shock** and **denial** prior to the expression of grief. Subsequently, episodes of acute distress known as **pangs of grief** are experienced, during which **anxiety** symptoms are often severe, and **yearning** or crying out is accompanied by an urge to **search** for the departed, to the exclusion of other activities. This impulse is usually counteracted by a conscious acknowledgement of the absurdity and futility of such behaviour, so that a compromise is reached. The cry is stifled, and the urge to search is sometimes replaced by **motor restlessness** and fervent mental activity in which events leading up to the loss are repeatedly reviewed, as if attempting to discover what went wrong and somehow remedy matters. Although the bereaved sometimes report seeing or hearing the dead person, insight into the nature of these phenomena (**illusions or pseudohallucinations**) is nearly always retained.

Sometimes, discomfort is so great that **defence mechanisms** are unconsciously employed to avoid, deny or delay the expression of grief (*see* p. 263). **Denial** results in the bereaved continuing to function as if nothing had happened, with perhaps the only evidence of arousal being signs of autonomic overactivity. **Anger** directed at the deceased — 'If only he'd taken more care of himself' — at the self — 'If only I'd looked after him better' — or at the doctor — 'It's your fault for not treating him soon enough' — is another means of coping with overwhelming grief. Sometimes, a sense of shame and perplexity arises in response to the irrationality of such feelings, and this may lead to the development of **guilt** and **depression**.

A 22-year-old West Indian man severely injured his right hand in an industrial accident, following which his thumb and index finger needed to be amputated. In the immediate postoperative period he was generally pleasant and cooperative, although the nursing staff were perturbed about his apparent lack of concern for his injuries, and his inappropriately cheerful manner. He refused to see the prosthetics technician, and when visited by a union representative concerning the possibility of a claim for compensation, he could see no point in discussing the details of the accident with him. He resisted all efforts to persuade him to see a psychiatrist, and the next day took his own discharge against medical advice. One week later, he was admitted to casualty having taken an overdose of sleeping tablets.

Between episodes of acute distress, a **chronic disturbance** is evident, in which a persistent sense of helplessness and hopelessness is experienced, so that the bereaved feels lost and dejected, without any sense of purpose or direction. **Functional changes**, such as anorexia, weight loss and sleep disturbance are common, and vulnerability to illness is increased due to changes in the body's physiological defences. During the period of adjustment following bereavement, interest is temporarily lost in the outside world and **disengagement** occurs. Social contacts are shunned, apart from perhaps a few intimate friends or relatives, and new or threatening experiences are avoided, safety being ensured by staying close to home.

The **manner** in which grief is expressed differs from one culture to another. In some, it is highly ritualised and an occasion for communal mourning, in which public displays of emotion are actively encouraged. As a result, there is considerable social pressure to force people into overt mourning. In other societies where a 'stiff upper lip' attitude is endorsed, grieving remains a private matter. When deprived of social support, the bereaved sometimes turn to doctors for help, and derive comfort from the medical profession by adopting the **sick role**.

With the passage of time, **recovery** is heralded by pangs of grief becoming less frequent, less intense and of shorter duration. Appetite gradually returns and overeating may occur, while the resurgence of sexual feelings (at a time when their expression seems inappropriate) may produce a sense of guilt. Eventually, the individual begins a process of **re-engagement** with the outside world, during which he gradually accepts the reality of his changed circumstances, renews former acquaintances and interests, and is able to develop new relationships. The length of time from loss to recovery varies from person to person, and although memories and feelings persist, they come to be viewed in a different perspective. **Anniversaries** are times when pangs of grief can temporarily recur.

Other Responses Which Occur Following Loss

In addition to the expression of grief, an alteration in the physical health of the bereaved can occur following loss. Studies have demonstrated an increased death rate from **heart disease** among widowers in the first 6 months following bereavement, when compared with age-matched controls. Other conditions such as **asthma**, **rheumatoid arthritis** and **ulcerative colitis** may deteriorate during this period, although paradoxical improvement is sometimes noted. It is possible that in these cases, the illness might have represented an emotional outlet which had been blocked while the deceased was alive. An association between the development of cancer and bereavement has also been proposed, although no conclusive link has yet been established.

Marked **behavioural changes** are sometimes seen, and may reflect the emergence of personality traits which were previously repressed. For example, a son might resort to gambling or drinking after his father's death, whereas before he led a staid existence. The development of **psychiatric disorder** following bereavement can be an exacerbation of a pre-existing state, or alternatively, arise *de novo*, symptomatically covering the entire spectrum of functional disorders. Chronic grief (*see below*) may merge imperceptibly into a **depressive illness**, and the distinction between the two can sometimes be very difficult. However, it is important not to 'medicalise' normal grief routinely by automatically prescribing psychotropic drugs, since they may delay the grieving process, and in the case of benzodiazepines, induce unnecessary dependence. Simple reassurance as to the nature of the symptoms which are experienced is often all that is required to bring about their resolution.

As distinct from a phase of denial, it is possible that **no response** occurs following loss, either because the relationship had little emotional value or the bereaved's support system is entirely complementary. Those with strong religious beliefs may see the loss as merely transitory until they are reunited with their loved ones in an after life.

ABNORMAL GRIEF

It is important to know which factors are associated with an atypical response to loss, so that help may be offered to those at significant risk of its development. Abnormal grief usually refers to a condition in which there is **prolonged denial or repression** of the expression of feeling, or where grief continues well beyond a time when it would be expected to have resolved (**chronic grief**). A number of **risk factors** have been identified.

1. Ambivalent Relationships

These are distinguished by the frequent expression of conflicting emotions (such as love and hate) by one or both partners. Relationships of this kind are often typified by fierce quarrelling and passionate reconciliations. When covert, one partner may admit to fantasies or fears of the other being killed or injured (an expression of wish fulfilment). When the bond is eventually ruptured, the surviving partner might initially experience a sense of relief, and feel little need to grieve. In time, intense feelings of loss and guilt develop, often accompanied by a sense of despair concerning the prospects for happiness in future relationships. The bereaved's behaviour may become self-punishing in response to a sense of failure and the inability to find an end to grieving.

2. Dependent Relationships

These are characterised by feelings of total helplessness without the other partner, often coexisting with bitter resentment of such dependency needs. The ending of such a relationship can result in the development of chronic grief, which is fully expressed from the outset but tends to be abnormally protracted.

3. Unexpected Losses

Unexpected losses may lead to prolonged shock or denial, following which the bereaved occasionally experience vivid feelings of the presence of the deceased for some time afterwards. This is often accompanied by symptoms of anxiety and an overwhelming sense of obligation towards the departed, resulting in guilt and recrimination at any attempt to disengage. Reactions of this kind are particularly common if relatives have been unable to see the deceased, which may occur after accidents or disasters where the victim is badly mutilated or the body is not discovered.

A 49-year-old man died suddenly and unexpectedly, during an admission to hospital for a routine cholecystectomy scheduled for the following day. As it was a Sunday afternoon, the body was quickly transferred to the hospital mortuary, and although his wife was telephoned immediately, she arrived too late to see the deceased on the ward. The nursing staff noted with some apprehension how calm and composed she initially seemed on receiving the news, but nevertheless attempted to comfort and console her. Unfortunately, the mortuary could not be reopened immediately, and while awaiting the arrival of the porter, the woman became increasingly agitated and started demanding to be allowed to see her husband, as she very much doubted he was dead. When she eventually viewed the body several hours later, she took only a cursory glance, insisted that it was not her husband, and stormed angrily out of the hospital.

She was visited at home later that evening by her general practitioner, and although she was at first unwilling to talk about the events of the day, she eventually acknowledged that her husband was dead. Over the next few weeks, she was seen regularly by her doctor, and began to express her anger with the hospital and her feelings of guilt for not being with her husband when he died. She felt very tense and anxious, but said she had been unable to cry. She strongly felt her husband's presence in the house, and had taken to periodically searching the rooms with the expectation of finding him there. She realised the irrationality of this behaviour, but confided that she sometimes heard her husband's voice while in the kitchen, and on two occasions had fleetingly seen him standing in the doorway.

4. Children

Children of preschool age (and those entering adolescence) who lose a parent are particularly vulnerable to the development of abnormal grief. **Young spouses**, **young parents** who lose a child, and **unmarried adults** whose elderly parents die may be similarly affected.

5. The Constitutional Profile

The constitutional profile of the bereaved can significantly influence the response to loss. The development of pathological grief is more likely in those who are physically ill or have a previous history of psychiatric disorder. People with inadequate or vulnerable personalities, and those who adopt a 'stiff upper lip' attitude to emotional circumstances, are similarly at risk.

6. Environmental Factors

Environmental factors which predispose to the occurrence of abnormal grief include financial hardship, social isolation, unemployment and circumstances which block a review of the relationship or the expression of emotion.

> An 81-year-old woman was admitted to hospital, having taken an overdose of sleeping tablets. Her husband had died 12 months beforehand, after the couple had been married for 60 years. She had received considerable support from her family and friends, but despite this, her distress appeared to increase with the passage of time, culminating in her suicide attempt.
>
> When seen by the duty psychiatrist, she appeared guilt-ridden, and constantly apologised for her behaviour and for wasting the doctor's time. She made repeated references to not being able to 'put right the terrible thing I've done', although any attempt to obtain an explanation resulted in her bursting into tears. During the following week she was seen twice more by the psychiatrist, and on the last occasion felt able to share her secret.
>
> Her husband's final illness had lasted several months, and although she spent much of the time at his bedside, he eventually died in hospital in the early hours of the morning, at a time when she had not been with him. She went to see his body a few hours later, and was accompanied to the chapel of rest by a kindly and well-meaning nurse who stayed with her. She had desperately wanted to kiss her husband goodbye, but felt too embarrassed to do so in the presence of her companion. She eventually left, experiencing a terrible sense of guilt at her failure to overcome her inhibitions, and this feeling had intensified as the weeks went by, culminating in her suicide attempt.
>
> Over the next few months, she was seen regularly by a bereavement counsellor, and by talking about her loss and the events following her husband's death, was gradually able to come to terms with her feelings. At follow-up one year later she was markedly improved and was living quite contentedly with one of her daughters.

Other situations which can complicate the expression of grief include multiple losses, and circumstances which result in a rapid orientation away from the event (e.g. remarrying within weeks of the death of a spouse).

The Management of Abnormal Grief

Where the loss has been denied or the expression of feeling has been repressed, interventions which facilitate the mourning process may be useful. At a basic level, these might involve listening sympathetically and encouraging talk about the loss. A more structured approach is that of **guided mourning**, in which a spouse or close relative may be encouraged to visit the grave, alter the arrangement of the contents of rooms, and handle photographs and possessions of the deceased. This aims to provoke **grief work** and to 'confirm' the reality of the change in circumstances.

Chronic grief may be dealt with by a **psychotherapeutic approach** which should attempt to bolster self-esteem and explore the possibilities of a new and meaningful life without the partner. It is also sometimes necessary to give 'authorisation' for grieving to stop, thereby allowing the acceptance of recovery.

Drugs should only be used where there is clear evidence of psychiatric illness, or when symptoms of anxiety are so intense or distressing that to withhold them would be unreasonable. If anxiolytics are prescribed, it is important that they are administered in low dosage and for relatively short periods, in order to avoid dependence or attempts at self-harm. Admission to hospital is sometimes indicated when distress is overwhelming and support systems are poor.

The Prevention of Abnormal Grief and Care of the Dying Patient

Where death can be **anticipated**, efforts should be made to reconcile estranged family members so that guilt can be minimised or prevented. Seriously ill patients and their families often want to know the truth, and to be told what is happening in language that they can understand. Withholding information when it is requested, or couching it in terms which are likely to be misleading, frequently creates additional problems. Relatives need the emotional support of care givers after receiving bad news, and may require several opportunities to talk to staff in order to assimilate information accurately. By helping them to anticipate the loss, the shock of bereavement will be considerably diminished.

Psychological symptoms are commonly experienced during terminal illness, and their management is just as important as that of physical problems, such as pain or vomiting. **Anxiety** may be related to fears of suffering intractable pain or sudden death, or worries about a loss of control and dignity. Such anxieties might be allayed by explaining to the patient the nature of the symptoms he is likely to experience, and offering reassurance that they can and will be adequately controlled. Allowing dying patients to share in decisions about their management, such as the timing and amount of analgesia they receive, increases their sense of having some command over their destiny. The presence of relatives or friends is often a source of great comfort, and regular contact should be encouraged. Anxiolytic drugs may sometimes be necessary to help control intolerably high levels of distress.

Low self-esteem, exaggerated feelings of guilt and psychomotor retardation are reliable indices of **depression** in terminal illnesses, and they often respond well to treatment with antidepressants or ECT. When depressive symptoms are refractory, they might be due to suppressed anger, the facilitation of which may bring about some improvement in the mental state. Paranoid reactions are also encountered, in which the blame for the illness is projected onto relatives or professional care givers. Mental confusion can be distressing for both the patient and the family, and in some cases is remediable. In such instances, a check should be made for untreated infections, or drugs being given unnecessarily.

If the illness is prolonged, some patients will have had time to adjust to their situation before they die. Some adapt well to enforced role changes, while others need help in making the transition. As death approaches, many patients withdraw and may not wish to see anyone. Families sometimes feel rejected, but it should be explained to them that this is often a normal part of preparing for death. If patients express a wish to **die at home** they should be allowed to do so, on the assumption that symptoms can be adequately controlled and sufficient nursing and medical support is provided. This may lead to greater cohesion among the family and the facilitation of grief after the death, because of the familiarity of the environment. **Hospices** offer expertise in dealing with the physical and psychological care of the dying. They are of particular benefit to people whose families are in need of extra support, many of whom will then be able to cope with the patient at home for at least some of the terminal period.

Surgical procedures which result in visible loss or disfigurement (such as amputation or mastectomy), or those in which the loss is mainly symbolic (e.g. losing the ability to have further children after hysterectomy), often provoke the development of grief. Adequate preparation before the operation and allowing the expression of grief during the postoperative period, are both important factors in minimising the likelihood of an abnormal emotional response ensuing. Support and counselling may need to be continued throughout the period of rehabilitation.

Counselling can be of particular benefit to those at risk of developing pathological grief, and may be provided by doctors, trained counsellors or voluntary organisations such as CRUSE. Its aim is to promote the grieving process, and to provide support and reassurance about the normality of the various symptoms and emotions experienced. In addition, it offers an opportunity to monitor the risk of suicide and intervene where necessary. At a later stage, counselling should concentrate on promoting re-engagement with the outside world, by helping the bereaved to rebuild their lives and cultivate new interests and relationships. It is important that support does not lead to dependence, so that the bereaved should be encouraged to help themselves as much as possible and to believe in their own abilities.

SUMMARY

1. **Bereavement** is the condition which usually follows loss. Because response to loss is highly variable in terms of its mode of expression, duration and outcome, 'normal grief' is difficult to define. Commonly, shock and denial are rapidly followed by acute 'pangs of grief', in which symptoms of anxiety and a sense of yearning are often accompanied by motor restlessness. Pseudohallucinations and illusions are sometimes experienced. Irrational feelings of anger towards the self, the deceased or his care givers may subsequently result in the development of guilt.

Between episodes of acute grief, a chronic background disturbance is recognised, marked by a persistent sense of helplessness and despair, and functional changes. For a time disengagement from the outside world occurs. The manner in which grief is expressed varies widely from culture to culture. In some communities the expression of grief is highly ritualised, while in others it is a personal and private matter. Where people are deprived of social support they may adopt the sick role in order to derive comfort from the medical profession. Recovery is followed by re-engagement with the outside world, in which former interests and acquaintances are resumed, and new relationships are made.

2. Other responses which may occur following loss include an alteration in the physical health of the bereaved, the development of psychiatric disorder and behavioural changes. **Abnormal grief** refers to a state in which there is prolonged denial or repression of the expression of feeling, or grief continues well beyond a time when it would be expected to have resolved. Its development is associated with the ending of ambivalent or dependent relationships, unexpected losses, children and young spouses who are bereaved, young parents who lose a child or unmarried adults whose elderly parents die. Abnormal grief is also more likely in those who are physically ill, have a past psychiatric history or a vulnerable personality. Environmental precipitants include financial hardship, social isolation, unemployment, and circumstances which block a review of the relationship.

3. Therapeutic intervention should aim to facilitate the mourning process where the loss has been denied or the expression of feeling suppressed. The management of chronic grief involves improving self-esteem and exploring possibilities for a new and meaningful life without the deceased. Drugs should only be used when there is clear evidence of psychiatric illness, or symptoms of anxiety are intolerable.

4. Where death can be anticipated, the development of morbid grief may be prevented by encouraging the reconciliation of estranged family members to minimise subsequent guilt. The relatives of seriously ill patients should be helped to anticipate the loss, in order to minimise the shock of bereavement when the death eventually occurs. Psychological symptoms, notably anxiety and depression, are common in terminally ill patients, and should be treated as vigorously as physical problems, such as pain or vomiting. Some patients adjust well to the prospect of death, while others need considerable help and support in coming to terms with their situation. Patients who wish to die at home should be allowed to do so. Hospices are often able to help families look after their relative at home for at least some of the terminal period.

REFERENCES AND FURTHER READING

Parkes, C. M. (1965). Bereavement and mental illness. *British Journal of Medical Psychology*; **38**: 1–12 and 13–26.
Parkes, C. M. (1972). *Bereavement: Studies of Grief in Adult Life*. London: Tavistock.
Parkes, C. M. (1985). Bereavement. *British Journal of Psychiatry*; **146**: 11–17.

8 SCHIZOPHRENIA AND PARANOID STATES

To most lay people, **schizophrenia** means a split personality, a 'Jekyll and Hyde' character who sometimes behaves quite normally and at other times is evil or mad. Unfortunately, this is a misinterpretation of a term which literally means 'split mind', and refers to a shattering or disintegration of the various mental functions which allow us to lead fulfilling and purposeful lives, rather than a division of the personality into two opposing types.

Because schizophrenia is a very complex disorder, many students find it difficult to understand how such a wide variety of patients with differing symptoms and problems can all be diagnosed as suffering from the same condition. This is because in its acute form, schizophrenia can produce severe mental disturbance that may later progress to chronic functional disability and an entirely different clinical picture.

In order to provide a framework for understanding this condition, it is necessary not only to look at its characteristics, but also to consider how knowledge of its causation and treatment continues to develop. Schizophrenia is classified as one of the major functional psychoses along with the affective disorders (mania and depression) which are dealt with in Chapter 5.

The term **psychosis** is frequently used in a number of different ways, so that its meaning has become imprecise and vague. Its use here is applied to those conditions in which there is an impairment of mental function of such a degree that it interferes with the ability to meet the demands of everyday life and maintain adequate contact with reality. Distortion of the environment can occur through individuals harbouring abnormal beliefs which are demonstrably false (**delusions**), and experiencing deceptions and misinterpretations of their senses known respectively as **hallucinations** and **illusions**. Consequently insight* is diminished or lost.

*Insight is another term which is poorly defined and has a number of meanings. It can refer to:

1. the degree of correct understanding that the patient has as to the nature of his condition (does he understand that he is mentally ill?)
2. the degree of correct understanding of the underlying cause of the disorder and its implications regarding treatment and outcome.

DEVELOPMENT OF THE CONCEPT OF SCHIZOPHRENIA

In order to gain a clearer understanding of the condition, it is helpful to consider how the concept of schizophrenia has developed over the last 100 years. In the early nineteenth century, when doctors first began to take a serious interest in the mentally disturbed, one theory held that all patients who exhibited gross abnormalities of behaviour or speech were suffering from a single form of mental illness, the 'unitary psychosis'. Others attempted to differentiate 'insanity' into discrete disorders, and as a result, a confusing array of conditions were described, including katatonia and hebephrenia.

Later in the century, the German psychiatrist **Kraepelin** attempted to bring some order to the system of classification by regarding katatonia and hebephrenia as variants of a single disorder, dementia praecox (*see below*). He also proposed a division of psychosis into organic and functional types. **Organic psychoses** were those in which it was possible to demonstrate a physiological disturbance (such as infection) or alteration in the structure of the brain or other body organ (e.g. a tumour), which as a consequence produced mental illness (*see* Chapter 9). **Functional psychoses**, by contrast, were those in which no such change was evident. Kraepelin further divided functional psychoses on the basis that some patients with mental illness showed a progressive deterioration of psychological functioning, while in others illness occurred in bouts, in between which they felt well and functioned normally. Illnesses in which disorders of thinking, emotional blunting, delusions and hallucinations seemed to progress to a dementia-like state were termed **dementia praecox** by Kraepelin. Since the main symptoms of the non-progressive, episodic illnesses were mania and depression, he called these **manic-depressive psychoses** (Fig. 8.1).

Kraepelin's classification was therefore concerned with **prognosis.** It is now evident that his differentiation was an over-simplification, as many patients with psychoses do not fit neatly into one or other category.

Bleuler a Swiss physician, became interested in the mechanism of **symptom formation** in dementia praecox. He considered that this disorder was due to a splitting of the mind (in much the same way that a large rock shatters or disintegrates when it is struck by a great force), and in 1911 he coined the term **schizophrenia** to describe graphically the separation of the various components of mental functioning which occurs (Fig. 8.2). This term has now completely replaced 'dementia praecox'.

Bleuler believed that a number of **fundamental symptoms** existed in schizophrenia, from which all others were derived. The diagnosis came to be based upon the presence of one or more of the symptoms known as the **four 'A's**. These were:

1. loosening of **associations** — more commonly known as 'thought disorder', in which thinking processes become disconnected so that

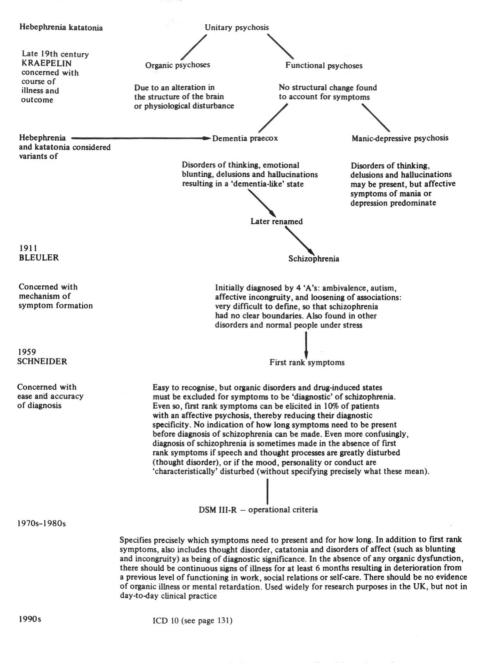

Fig. 8.1 Development of the concept of schizophrenia

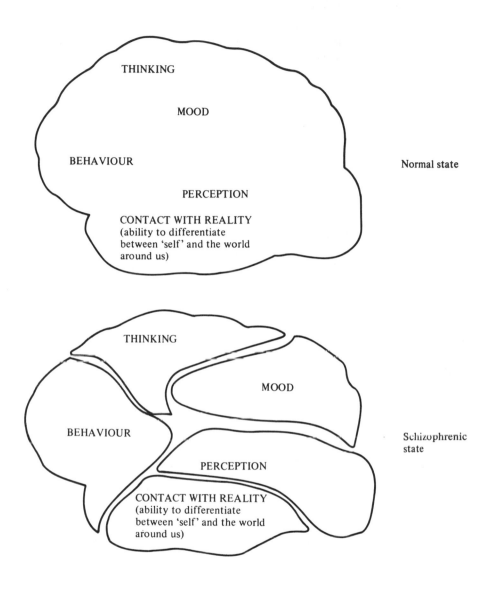

Fig. 8.2 Diagrammatic representation of the splitting of mental
functions in schizophrenia

speech loses its sense and meaning
2. **affective** incongruity or blunting of emotion — giggling at bad news or not responding to an emotionally charged situation
3. **autism** — withdrawal from reality into an inner world of fantasy
4. **ambivalence** — the co-existence of strongly conflicting attitudes, ideas feelings or drives, resulting in ambivalence of intellect, emotion or the will.

The diagnosis did not depend upon the presence of delusions or hallucinations, because Bleuler felt that these were secondary to the fundamental symptoms outlined above. However, it was apparent that when based on the four 'A's, schizophrenia had no clear boundaries. This was because of the indefinite characteristics of the symptoms which resulted in poor consistency in their detection. Furthermore, they were frequently considered to be present in other forms of mental disorder, and could be provoked by stress in some normal people. This led to a widening of the concept of schizophrenia, so that by the 1950s, the term was rapidly becoming devoid of useful meaning.

In order to make the diagnosis more reliable, attempts were made to identify a group of symptoms characteristic of schizophrenia, but rarely found in other disorders. In 1959, **Schneider**, a German psychiatrist, defined a number of symptoms which he considered to be of first rank importance in making the diagnosis of schizophrenia, provided organic disease or drug intoxication were absent. Their importance lies in their easy recognition, so that **first rank symptoms** are widely used diagnostically by psychiatrists in the UK and Europe. They are summarised in Table 8.1.

The presence of first rank symptoms makes the diagnosis of schizophrenia likely, but not definite. For example, it is now well recognised that they can be elicited in about 10% of patients suffering from affective psychoses. Furthermore, under certain circumstances, the diagnosis of schizophrenia is sometimes made in their absence (*see later*). No allowance was made by Schneider for the length of time they are present; whether first rank symptoms are noted on just one occasion or persist for several months, the diagnosis would be schizophrenia in both cases. This is a controversial issue, because many psychiatrists believe that the duration of illness is important in deciding whether or not a person has schizophrenia.

To overcome this last problem, several workers in the USA have devised **operational criteria** for diagnosing schizophrenia, which include longitudinal factors (i.e. a specified length of time for which symptoms must be present), symptom content and evidence of deterioration from a previous level of functioning. These are included in the Diagnostic and Statistical Manual for the diagnosis and classification of diseases (DSM III-R). In addition to first rank symptoms, other phenomena such as thought disorder, changes of affect and catatonia (discussed later) are also

Table 8.1 First rank symptoms of schizophrenia

Schizophrenia is the most likely diagnosis if any of the following are present in the absence of organic disease or substance abuse:

1. thought insertion
2. thought withdrawal
3. thought broadcasting
4. 'made' feelings
5. 'made' actions
6. 'made' impulses
7. delusions of somatic passivity
8. audible thoughts
9. auditory hallucinations in the third person talking or arguing about the subject
10. auditory hallucinations in the third person commenting on the subject's actions
11. delusional perception

These symptoms are discussed in detail later in the text, but for the present it should be noted that they concern abnormal psychological features such as delusions and hallucinations.

considered to be of diagnostic significance by DSM III-R. Symptoms should not be attributable to organic dysfunction, and there should be continuous signs of illness for at least 6 months, resulting in deterioration from a previous level of functioning in such areas as work, social relations and self-care.

Although DSM III-R is widely used in the UK to select patients for research purposes, everyday practice still relies upon the **clinical judgement** of the examining doctor in deciding whether or not the patient has schizophrenia. The diagnosis of schizophrenia must always be considered if first rank symptoms are elicited, but it should be remembered that they can occur in other illnesses, such as mania, depression, drug-induced states and organic disorders. When these symptoms persist, schizophrenia can be diagnosed with more confidence, and if they are accompanied or followed by deterioration of the personality and level of functioning, then few would dispute the nature of the condition (Fig. 8.3).

ICD 10 is likely to introduce operational criteria for the diagnosis of schizophrenia based upon the presence of Schneiderian first rank symptoms or bizarre

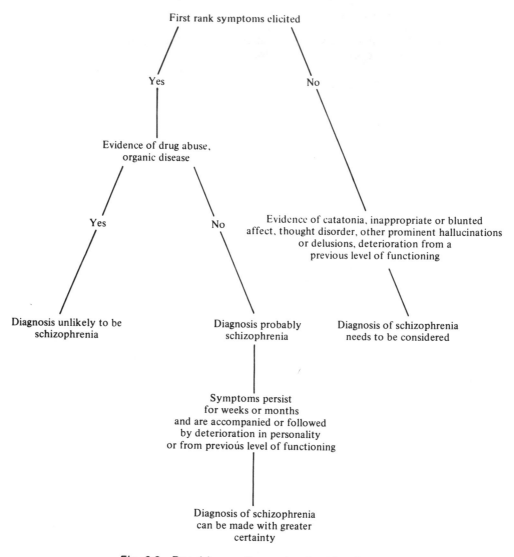

Fig. 8.3 Reaching a diagnosis of schizophrenia

delusions of other kinds which have been clearly present for at least one month or more. Any hallucinatory voices which continue for weeks or months on end are also expected to be considered diagnostically significant. In the absence of these symptoms, the diagnosis can still be made if symptoms from two of the following three categories are present:

1. delusional ideas of any content accompanied by hallucinations in any modality
2. the negative symptoms of schizophrenia (blunting of affect, apathy and poverty of speech)
3. breaks or interpolations in the train of thought.

Conditions meeting such symptomatic requirements, but of a duration less than one month, will probably be diagnosed as a schizophreniform episode, and reclassified as schizophrenia if the symptoms persist for longer periods of time.

In summary, many different concepts of the illness have been proposed in the past century, some of which persist to this day, so that schizophrenia remains a difficult condition to define and at times, to diagnose accurately.

EPIDEMIOLOGY

The **prevalence** of schizophrenia is approximately **1%** and is fairly constant among different populations, with only a few minor regional variations worldwide. The **incidence** is of the order of 15-20 new cases per 100 000 of the population per year. Men and women are affected equally, with the average age of onset in the early twenties.

Initially, there is no social class variation, although as the illness progresses, many sufferers inevitably drift down the social scale. Interestingly, more schizophrenics are born during the winter months in both the northern and southern hemispheres, although the reasons for this remain unknown.

CLINICAL FEATURES OF ACUTE AND CHRONIC SCHIZOPHRENIA

Schizophrenia describes two seemingly unrelated states, often referred to as the acute and chronic forms of the illness. The terms not only apply to the rate of onset and duration of the condition, but also to symptom content.

In **acute schizophrenia**, patients typically experience gross psychological disturbance in the form of abnormal beliefs (delusions) and/or hallucinations. They may be preoccupied with hearing voices which talk about them when nobody else is present, or believe that external forces, such as laser beams, control their actions. In contrast, **chronic schizophrenia** characteristically produces problems of social interaction and motivation, so that sufferers are often apathetic, withdrawn and isolated. In addition, they are sometimes troubled by the kind of phenomena which occur in the acute state. The relationship between acute and chronic schizophrenia is shown in Fig. 8.4.

ACUTE SCHIZOPHRENIA

The characteristic features seen in this condition are often referred to as the **positive symptoms** of schizophrenia (Fig. 8.4).

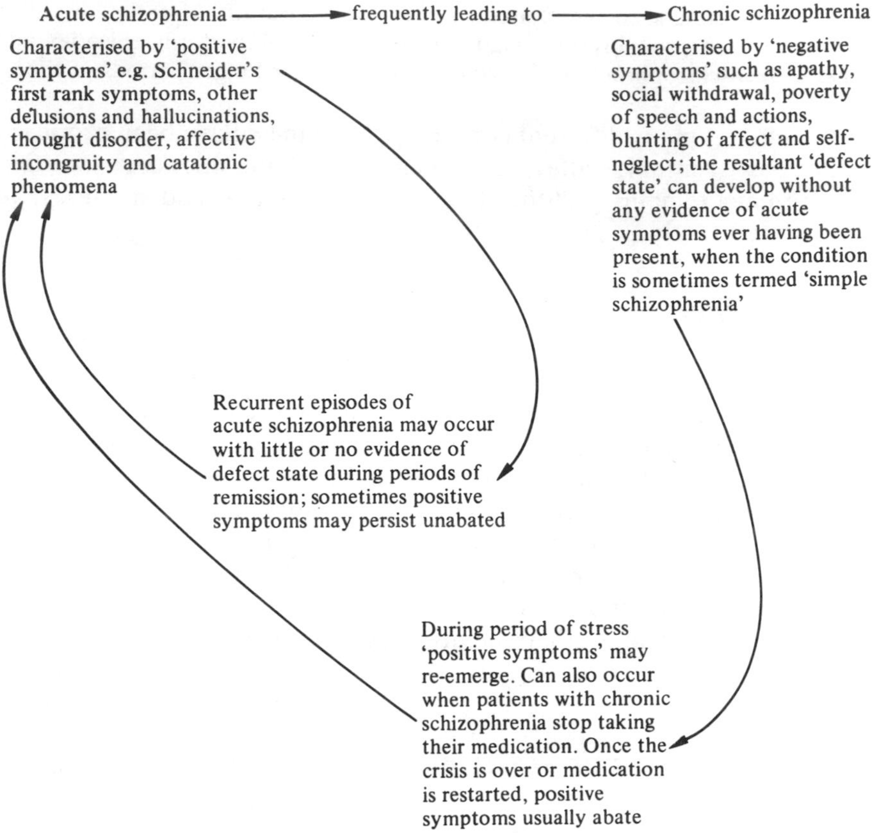

Acute schizophrenia ————————►frequently leading to ————————►Chronic schizophrenia

Characterised by 'positive
symptoms' e.g. Schneider's
first rank symptoms, other
delusions and hallucinations,
thought disorder, affective
incongruity and catatonic
phenomena

Characterised by 'negative
symptoms' such as apathy,
social withdrawal, poverty
of speech and actions,
blunting of affect and self-
neglect; the resultant 'defect
state' can develop without
any evidence of acute
symptoms ever having been
present, when the condition
is sometimes termed 'simple
schizophrenia'

Recurrent episodes of
acute schizophrenia may occur
with little or no evidence of
defect state during periods of
remission; sometimes positive
symptoms may persist unabated

During period of stress
'positive symptoms' may
re-emerge. Can also occur
when patients with chronic
schizophrenia stop taking
their medication. Once the
crisis is over or medication
is restarted, positive
symptoms usually abate

Fig. 8.4 The relationship between acute and chronic schizophrenia.
The terms 'acute' and 'chronic' signify symptom content as well as the
course of the illness

Appearance and Behaviour

Some patients dress bizarrely or show obvious signs of self-neglect. They
may laugh inappropriately or talk to themselves. Others remain immobile
or show sudden unexpected behavioural changes. They might be socially
awkward, preoccupied and withdrawn, or outwardly appear and behave
quite normally.

A 22-year-old man with no previous psychiatric history had worked as a
painter and decorator until 6 months before his admission to hospital. At that
time, his attendance at work became sporadic and he took to his bed for long
periods of the day. His parents reported that he became increasingly
withdrawn and uncommunicative, and noted at times that their son would
smile inappropriately or appear to be listening to something which only he was
aware of.

Speech

This may reflect an underlying **thought disorder**, which presents as an indistinct abnormality of the construction and use of language, resulting from a basic disturbance of thinking. In its earliest stages, thought disorder may be apparent when the patient converses but the listener realises that he has understood little of what is being said. Unclear or irrelevant answers to questions where the individual constantly wanders off the point is known as **knight's move thinking** or **derailment**. In very severe forms of thought disorder, the patient can be completely incomprehensible, talking jumbled nonsense referred to as a **word salad**.

> In response to the question, 'Are you being troubled by any strange thoughts or ideas?', a patient gave the following reply:
> 'Being troubled is a relative consequence of what is or isn't new meaning. How I interpret my feelings isn't interpreted by us or God in this or any other form. Assess us if you must, but take no trouble to liken me to coal.'

Other forms of thought disorder which have been described include **concrete thinking** (an inability to deal with abstract ideas) and **over-inclusiveness** (a failure to maintain boundaries around topics, so that irrelevant information continually enters into conversation). Schizophrenic patients may use ordinary words in unusual ways (**paraphasias**) or invent entirely new words (**neologisms**).

> A schizophrenic patient, when asked how he felt, replied 'I'm a bit swavy' while gesticulating with his hands that this meant 'up and down'. He would also point to his stomach and refer to it as his 'tavern'.

Mood

The patient's mood may be normal or entirely **incongruous**, such as greeting bad news with inappropriate laughter. **Perplexity** or **fear** are sometimes evident, especially if the individual is tormented by delusions or hallucinations (*see below*).

Thought Content

Abnormalities of thought content may take the form of **paranoid delusions**, which are frequently persecutory in nature. **Delusions of reference** can also occur, which are false beliefs entertained by the subject that other people, events or objects have a particular and unusual meaning specifically for him. He may say that people in the street take special notice of him, or that he sees reference to himself on the television, in newspapers or on advertising hoardings. When the individual realises that the feelings originate within himself, they are known as ideas (as opposed to delusions) of reference (*see* Chapter 2).

A 34-year-old man believed he was wanted by the police for molesting children. Despite visiting a number of police stations and being reassured that no such charges were held against him, he persisted with this notion. He was certain that officers were following him in their vehicles, and every time he heard a car horn sound, he believed this was a signal to indicate their presence (a delusion of reference). Eventually, he was sure there was a conspiracy against him, and in confirmation, reported hearing the voices of two policemen discussing his case in the flat next door.

In **thought alienation**, the subject has the experience that his thoughts are under the influence of some outside force, or that others are participating in his thinking.

Passivity experiences are also first rank symptoms in which the subject has a delusional belief that impulses, actions, emotions or sensations which he experiences are not his own, but are being imposed on him by some outside force or influence against his will. These phenomena are forms of **ego boundary disturbance**, in that the subject is no longer able to determine where his own internal world of thoughts, drives and emotions ends and the external world begins.

Thought alienation and passivity experiences include:

1. **Thought withdrawal**: the subject experiences his thoughts being taken out of his mind against his will by some external force or agency. Sometimes, he may be observed to stop in mid-sentence, and on resuming his conversation might report that his mind was completely emptied of all thoughts — a very frightening experience. This objective manifestation of the experience is known as **thought block** and is not to be confused with interruption in the train of thought, a common occurrence in which one is momentarily lost for words and cannot think of what to say next.

   A 30-year-old man reported that while filling his car at a service station, his thoughts were suddenly sucked out of his mind by the petrol pump, thereby leaving it totally empty.

2. **Thought insertion**: the subject experiences thoughts which he does not recognise as a product of his own mind, and which he believes have been put there by some outside force or agency. Once again, the experience occurs against his will, so that he is a passive recipient.

   A 26-year-old woman reported that the thoughts of a man, whom she had met briefly some time ago, were repeatedly put into her mind by him.

They consisted of his views and sexual fantasies about other women, which she knew were not her own thoughts. When asked how this occurred, she replied 'He treats my mind like a screen and flashes his thoughts onto it.'

3. **Thought broadcast**: the subject experiences his unspoken thoughts as being known to, or shared by, those around him, so that he believes that they are not contained within his own mind.

   A 23-year-old audio-typist claimed that her thoughts were being shared by all of her colleagues in the typing pool at her office. She believed that her thoughts travelled through the earphones of her dictating machine, and were then transmitted via the electric wiring into the headsets of other secretaries.

4. **Made feelings**: the subject experiences feelings or emotions which he does not recognise as his own. They are attributed to some external force and are believed to be imposed upon him.

   A 28-year-old woman said 'Although I look happy and I laugh, inside I feel a cold anger because it is Charlie Chaplin who is laughing and not me. He puts his happiness into my brain for no reason, and you have no idea how awful it is to feel this way when it is not you.'

5. **Made impulses**: the subject is overcome by a sudden impulse which he does not believe to be his own, but on which he subsequently acts.

   A 34-year-old patient broke every window in the psychiatric unit where he was resident. When questioned by the irate hospital administrator he said 'A sudden impulse came over me to get more oxygen. It was not my wish, it came to me from God who wanted it done as soon as possible.'

6. **Made acts**: the subject experiences his actions as being completely under the control of an external influence that initiates and directs the movements throughout. He feels like a robot, the passive observer of his own actions.

   A 21-year-old man said 'I see my arms and legs move but it is not me moving them. I am just a puppet, a plaything for them to use.'

7. **Somatic passivity**: the subject believes he is a passive and reluctant recipient of bodily sensations imposed upon him by some external influence.

   A 22-year-old man reported that he sometimes became very angry, because he could feel a man and a woman having sexual intercourse on his back. He knew this was happening, since he experienced his spine rocking back and forth with their copulatory movements. He found this very distressing and it would occasionally wake him at night. Although he said he had never seen the couple, he knew he would recognise them when they met, and he planned to kill the man because of the constant harassment.

Delusional perception is the final abnormality of thought content described by Schneider as a first rank symptom. A normal perception is followed by an abnormal and false interpretation of that perception, which is immediate, overwhelming and usually self-referential.

A 27-year-old accountant, with no previous psychiatric history, looked out of the window of his flat and felt a sense of unease that something frightening was about to happen. He saw some birds pecking at cherries on a tree and immediately realised that this meant he was the subject of a 'death plot' by FBI agents, who were conspiring to eliminate him.

In this case, the normal perception is that of the birds pecking at the cherries, which is followed by the abnormal interpretation, namely the false belief that he is the subject of a conspiracy. Because the abnormal belief appears suddenly and fully formed in the mind like a 'brain wave', so that its development is not understandable in terms of previous thoughts or other experiences, it is described as a **primary (autochthonous) delusion**.

The delusional perception is sometimes preceded by a **delusional mood**, in which the subject has a conviction that there is something going on around him which concerns him, but he does not know what it is. The delusional mood often dissipates following the occurrence of the delusional perception.

Perceptual Abnormalities

Schneider described three first rank symptoms which are special forms of **auditory hallucinations**. These are audible thoughts, voices arguing about the subject in the third person, or voices commenting on his actions.

1. **Audible thoughts** are the repetition, in the form of auditory hallucinations, of thoughts which have occurred a short time before, so that the patient experiences voices speaking his thoughts aloud.

   A 19-year-old woman reported hearing the voice of her favourite pop star coming from a cupboard in her room. The voice would repeat all her thoughts, which she found very distressing. For example, she would think 'I must wash my hair tonight' and almost immediately afterwards, she would hear the voice repeating 'I must wash my hair tonight'.

2. **Voices arguing about the subject** involve two or more hallucinatory voices discussing or arguing about him in the third person.

> A 23-year-old law student described hearing two voices arguing about his prospects in the forthcoming examinations. He believed the voices came from his home, several miles away. One would say 'He'll never get through, he's useless', while the other would retort, 'He's OK, he knows his stuff.'

3. **Voices commenting on the subject's actions** are a description of the patient's activities as they occur, by one or more voices referring to him in the third person.

> A 32-year-old housewife heard a voice coming from her garden, which continually described her actions. From the moment she awoke, she was subjected to a running commentary such as 'She's getting up now. . . she's going to the bathroom. . . she's brushing her teeth.'

Hallucinations may also take the form of noises, music and singing. **Visual hallucinations** are experienced in schizophrenia, but are uncommon and should always raise the suspicion of an organic disorder. Hallucinations of **taste**, **smell** and **touch** are also occasionally encountered.

Perception is sometimes disturbed in other ways, so that colours or sounds appear unduly vivid or altered in quality. Irrelevant features of ordinary things may seem more important than the whole object or situation.

Catatonic Phenomena

A number of abnormalities of movement, posture and speech are sometimes observed together in schizophrenia (in varying combinations) which are features of **catatonia** (Table 8.2). Catatonic phenomena can occur in other psychiatric disorders (such as affective illnesses and hysterical states), as well as in some organic conditions (e.g. lesions of the basal ganglia or temporal lobe). Their causation is unclear, but they probably represent a disorder of voluntary muscle control.

Insight

Insight is nearly always lost in the acute syndrome, so that the patient is unable to attribute any of his experiences to being mentally ill. Orientation and memory are usually normal, although concentration and attention may well be impaired.

Table 8.2 Features of catatonia

Complex disorders
Stupor

Disorders of movement and posture
Obstruction
Mannerisms
Stereotypies
Opposition
Negativism
Ambitendency
Automatic obedience
Perseveration
Grimacing
Cooperation (mitmachen, mitgehen)
Echopraxia
Catalepsy

Disorders of speech
Echolalia
Manneristic speech
Stereotypies of speech
Verbigeration
Perseveration of speech

(*see* Glossary for definition of terms)

CHRONIC SCHIZOPHRENIA

In the period before effective drugs were available to treat the positive symptoms of schizophrenia, prolonged 'acute' phases of the condition were more frequently observed. Although hallucinations and delusions often persisted for months or years, in time they tended to become less florid or eventually disappeared completely. In cases where an illness was brief, sudden in onset and clearly precipitated by an adverse event, complete recovery sometimes occurred following resolution of the positive symptoms. However, when the onset was insidious, and the illness long-lasting or recurrent, this invariably led to lasting personality damage, and the development of a **defect state**. Although drugs which are effective in treating the acute stage of the illness have been available since the 1950s, their use appears to have had little bearing on preventing the evolution of the defect state. Consequently, patients exhibiting features of chronic schizophrenia are still commonly seen in clinical practice, and their management remains a major therapeutic problem.

In minor cases, the defect state may result in a slight impairment of liveliness and general interest in life, which is only discernible to those who knew the individual before his illness. However, in general, the effects are more severe and conspicuous, presenting as the **negative symptoms** of schizophrenia (Table 8.3).

Table 8.3 The negative symptoms of schizophrenia

1. Lack of initiative and drive
2. Slowness of action
3. Poverty of speech
4. Social withdrawal — loss of interest in other people and impaired capacity to form enduring relationships
5. Blunting of emotional expression
6. Deterioration of social behaviour and self-neglect

All or some of the above can result in a **permanent change in personality**. The patient is handicapped in every aspect of life, including work, leisure and relationships.

Acute psychotic episodes can recur, particularly during times of stress, with a return of delusional beliefs and hallucinations. **Thought disorder** may persist, and abnormalities of movement (such as **mannerisms** and **stereotypies**) sometimes develop.

Depression is a common feature of chronic schizophrenia, but emotional blunting can make its detection difficult. It may be due to partially regained insight after taking medication or to a side-effect of the drugs themselves. It is also possible that depression is an integral part of the chronic syndrome. Compared with the general population, there is an increased rate of suicide amongst people suffering from schizophrenia.

DIFFERENTIAL DIAGNOSIS

Schizophrenic-like symptoms can occur in association with drug abuse (especially amphetamines and cannabis), chronic alcoholism, temporal lobe epilepsy, head injury, cerebral tumour and encephalitis (*see* Chapter 9). Affective psychoses and certain paranoid states may also resemble schizophrenic illnesses.

VARIETIES OF SCHIZOPHRENIA

A number of these were defined by the early psychiatrists, and some of the terms are occasionally used in current clinical practice if the symptoms clearly approximate to the subtypes that Kraepelin and Bleuler described. **Hebephrenic schizophrenia** has an early onset, often in late adolescence. Thought disorder and affective symptoms form a prominent part of the clinical picture. In **catatonic schizophrenia**, characteristic disturbances of movement, speech and posture occur (*see* Table 8.2). **Paranoid schizophrenia** describes those illnesses where hallucinations and/or delusions of *any* type are prominent in the absence of any gross deterioration of personality (it is *not* specific to delusions of persecution). In **simple schizophrenia**, there is progressive deterioration akin to a defect state in the absence of acute psychotic symptoms.

Schizoaffective illness is a disorder in which features of schizophrenia are intermingled with those of mania or depression, the latter being more common. Illnesses in this category do not usually result in permanent damage to the personality. Episodes tend to be recurrent, with periods of complete remission in between. The diagnosis should only be made when both schizophrenic and affective symptoms are pronounced. Family studies of these patients show a lower incidence of schizophrenia than of affective illness, suggesting that they have more in common with the latter.

Schizoaffective illnesses differ from those cases in which depression occurs in association with chronic schizophrenia, in that with the latter:

1. symptoms of schizophrenia have frequently been present for some time before the onset of depression (ICD 10 is likely to classify this condition as post-schizophrenic depression)
2. negative symptoms of schizophrenia often predominate
3. personality deterioration is commonplace.

Cycloid psychosis is a term originating from Scandinavia, and is used to describe a disorder which shares features with both affective and schizophrenic illnesses. Characteristically, the condition has a sudden onset, fluctuations of mood being associated with paranoid delusions and episodes of ecstasy. Other features, such as perplexity, anxiety or changes in the level of activity, may also be evident. The prognosis is generally good, and personality deterioration does not usually occur.

AETIOLOGY

1. Genetic Factors

A genetic influence in the development of schizophrenia is supported by the findings of **family**, **twin** and **adoption** studies (*see* p. 7). Table 8.4 shows that the closer the relationship to the schizophrenic patient, the higher the risk a relative has of developing the illness.

However, not only genetic factors are involved, since the co-twin is not always affected when one member of an identical pair develops schizophrenia. This possibly suggests that a **vulnerability** to develop the disorder is inherited, rather than the condition itself, and that certain environmental factors need to be present before the illness becomes manifest.

Table 8.4 Family risk of schizophrenia

Relationship to schizophrenic patient	Lifetime expectancy of developing schizophrenia (expressed as a % risk)
No relationship	1
Second-degree relative (aunt, uncle, grandparent)	3
Parent	4
Sibling (brother or sister)	9
Non-identical twin	9–12
Child of schizophrenic	12
Child with both parents schizophrenic	36
Identical twin	40–45

2. Environmental Factors

Environmental factors which may interact with a genetic predisposition to schizophrenia include the influence of family relationships, life events, birth trauma and infection.

The influence of **family relationships** on the rate of relapse in schizophrenia has been carefully studied. It was noted that some patients who were discharged from hospital to home appeared to relapse more rapidly and frequently than those who went to live in hostels — a somewhat surprising finding. Further investigation revealed that patients with an increased rate of relapse seemed to come from families with **high expressed emotion (HEE)**. In these HEE families, which are a minority, relatives tend to be over-involved with the life of the schizophrenic member, and also express an excessive amount of critical comment. In contrast, **low expressed emotion (LEE)** families do not exhibit these traits, and consequently, the patient has a reduced rate of relapse.

This finding has important implications for the management of schizophrenia by social intervention. By educating family members about the illness, encouraging them to be less critical and to spend fewer hours with the patient, it is possible to lower the amount of expressed emotion and subsequently reduce relapse rates.

Other abnormal family processes have been identified in the past as being instrumental in the causation of schizophrenia (schizophrenogenic mothers, double-bind theory, marital skew and schism — *see* glossary). However, their aetiological significance is not proven by experimental findings, nor do they appear to be specific to families with a schizophrenic member. Consequently, it is likely that they merely reflect the difficulties created in the family by the patient.

Many schizophrenic patients who suffer a relapse of their illness have been shown to experience an excess of both favourable and unfavourable **life events** in the 3-week period prior to their admission to hospital (c.f. life events in the aetiology of depression; p. 88). It therefore seems that both acute (life events) and chronic (expressed emotion) stresses are associated with relapse in schizophrenia.

A number of neurological abnormalities have been identified in some patients with schizophrenia, most notably an increase in the size of the ventricles within the brain. In addition, it is known that patients who suffer with temporal lobe epilepsy may have symptoms similar to those found in schizophrenia. It has been suggested that these organic and electrical abnormalities might result from **injury** to the brain at birth or **viral infections** in the neonatal period, which subsequently give rise to schizophrenia in adulthood. However, at present there is no direct evidence to support either of these proposals.

3. Psychodynamic Theories

Although dynamic psychotherapy is very rarely used in treating schizophrenia, a number of psychodynamic theories of causation have been proposed. All of them attempt to make sense of the abnormal patterns of thinking and behaviour which are frequently encountered in this condition. **Freud** saw schizophrenia as an indrawing of life energy or 'libido' into the self, so that the outside world became meaningless and was replaced by a meaningful inner world of fantasy and false beliefs. **Melanie Klein** saw the disorder as being due to incomplete psychological development. Her view was that it results from perpetuation of a failure by the child in early life to recognise that his mother, who at times is 'good' by satisfying his needs and at other times 'bad' by denying them, is one and the same person (paranoid-schizoid position).

4. Biochemical Theories

Numerous biochemical theories have been postulated as to the cause of schizophrenia, but only the **dopamine hypothesis** is widely accepted. This theory proposes that the disorder is due to an excess and overactivity of the neurotransmitter dopamine in the **mesolimbic pathway** of the brain, and originated from post-mortem findings in schizophrenic patients. Supporting evidence is derived from the knowledge that **amphetamines**, which increase dopamine release, can cause a psychotic illness that is clinically indistinguishable from acute schizophrenia, and can also exacerbate the existing disorder.

Antipsychotic drugs (neuroleptics), which are used in the treatment of schizophrenia, are found to block dopamine receptors. The degree of their antipsychotic potency is directly proportional to their dopamine receptor binding capacity.

MANAGEMENT

As with all psychiatric disorders, physical, social and psychological aspects of management need to be considered.

1. Physical Treatments

Neuroleptic drugs are the mainstay of treatment in the acute phase of the illness and are discussed more fully in Chapter 12. These compounds have been shown to be consistently more effective than placebo in treating the positive symptoms of schizophrenia, such as delusions and hallucinations. It is probably worthwhile keeping most patients on a maintenance dose of medication for at least one year after recovery, because relapse is most likely to occur during this period. The effectiveness of drugs on the negative symptoms of chronic schizophrenia is less well established, but in some patients they are clearly beneficial in preventing further relapse and the reappearance of the acute phase of the illness.

A wide variety of neuroleptic drugs is available and choice will depend upon the needs of the patient, a consideration of the side-effects of each preparation, as well as personal preference. For example, **chlorpromazine** has useful sedative properties for controlling excitable or violent patients, but it also tends to lower the blood pressure, often making it unsuitable for use in the elderly or those with cardiac problems. By contrast, **haloperidol** is not as sedating, nor does it cause significant hypotension. However, it may produce severe extrapyramidal side-effects, particularly in the young and elderly. The properties of a number of commonly used neuroleptic drugs are shown in Table 8.5.

Because there is a wide variation in absorption when taken orally, the dose of neuroleptic required to control psychotic symptoms differs from one patient to another. In addition, following uptake from the gastro-intestinal tract, the drug must pass through the liver, where a significant proportion is inactivated by the so-called **first pass metabolism** before reaching the general circulation. This is avoided when drugs are given intramuscularly, so that a neuroleptic administered in this way has a greater potency than an equivalent oral dose.

Ensuring that schizophrenic patients take their medication can be a major problem, because many lack insight into their condition and they can see no reason to take drugs. Even if insight is retained, some will not accept that there is a risk of suffering a relapse, which further compounds the problem of compliance. For these reasons, **depot preparations** have been developed, in which the neuroleptic is suspended in an oily base and injected deep into muscle. The drug is gradually released into the blood stream over the course of a few weeks, and so maintains serum levels to ensure a therapeutic effect. Providing the patient agrees to attend for his injection, the problem of daily compliance is overcome.

Table 8.5 Characteristics of some commonly used neuroleptic drugs

Drug (generic/trade name)	Route of administration	Characteristics
Chlorpromazine (Largactil)	Orally or intramuscularly, rarely intravenous	Sedating, can produce postural hypotension and extrapyramidal effects
Haloperidol (Haldol)	Orally or intramuscularly, rarely intravenous	Less sedating than chlorpromazine, but tends to produce more marked extrapyramidal effects
Thioridazine (Melleril)	Usually orally	Sedating, with few extrapyramidal effects, popular for use with disturbed behaviour in the elderly
Trifluoperazine (Stelazine)	Usually orally	Similar effects to chlorpromazine, but produces less sedation and postural hypotension
Flupenthixol decanoate (Depixol)	Depot medication given by deep intramuscular injection	Long-acting preparation used in maintenance therapy of chronic schizophrenia
Fluphenazine decanoate (Modecate)	Depot medication given by deep intramuscular injection	Long-acting preparation used in maintenance therapy. Suggested that it may cause depression

Because of their dopamine-blocking actions, neuroleptic drugs also produce extrapyramidal side-effects, including pseudoparkinsonism, acute dystonic reactions, akathisia and tardive dyskinesia. These are discussed more fully in Chapter 12, along with other adverse reactions.

Anticholinergic (antiparkinsonian) drugs, such as **benztropine** and **procyclidine**, are used to treat some of these extrapyramidal side-effects, but should not be routinely prescribed with neuroleptics. This is because they can produce unpleasant reactions of their own, such as dry mouth and blurred vision, as well as cause excitement and confusion when excessive amounts are taken. There is also some indication that they increase the risk of developing tardive dyskinesia.

Electroconvulsive therapy is sometimes used in the treatment of schizophrenia, especially when catatonic symptoms are present. Its use in alleviating other acute symptoms remains controversial, although it may be beneficial in combination with neuroleptics where these alone are ineffective. Depression which develops in association with chronic schizophrenia often responds to ECT.

The management of **schizoaffective illness** usually relies on a combination of physical treatments. Patients with schizodepressive disorders often show a more favourable response to ECT and/or neuroleptics than to antidepressant drugs. Both sets of symptoms tend to improve simultaneously regardless of the treatment used. Neuroleptics and lithium are equally effective in treating schizomanic illnesses.

2. Social Management

Environmental stimulation needs to be carefully controlled during the acute phase of the illness, since too much can result in a worsening of symptoms, with an exacerbation of delusions and hallucinations. Therefore, if the patient is hospitalised, caution needs to be exercised over his attendance at group meetings, occupational therapy and ward activities, at which times stress and confrontation should be kept to a minimum. Once his condition is stable, a well planned **occupational therapy programme** is essential. An initial assessment should be made of his level of functioning before the illness, in terms of his work capability and social aptitude. A graded approach to **rehabilitation** is then undertaken using facilities within the hospital, and where needed, progressing to the day hospital, sheltered workshops, hostels, day centres and half-way houses (*see* Chapter 14).

Manipulating the family environment, by lowering expressed emotion to prevent relapse in schizophrenia, has already been considered. However, inactive and impoverished surroundings are just as harmful as overstimulation to these patients, and can produce a number of social handicaps. This was ably demonstrated in a well known study which compared patients from three hospitals. The first provided an environment in which patients led as normal an existence as possible, and were actively rehabilitated. In contrast, patients at the second hospital had little contact with the outside world, few personal possessions and spent much of the day unoccupied and unstimulated. They were looked after by staff with rigid and authoritarian attitudes, who held little expectation for their recovery. The third hospital offered an environment somewhere between the other two.

In comparing patients whose initial illness had been similar in type and severity, the results showed that the extent of social withdrawal, poverty of conversation and socially deviant behaviour correlated closely with the degree of impoverishment of their environment and lifestyle. The above characteristics, known collectively as the **institutionalisation syndrome**, suggest that some of the disabilities seen in chronic schizophrenia are preventable by the provision of an appropriate therapeutic milieu.

3. Psychological Management

Psychotherapy has a place in the management of schizophrenia in a general supportive role, rather than using a dynamic approach. Behavioural techniques, such as **token economies**, are used in some hospitals to encourage motivation and activity (*see* p. 279).

PROGNOSIS

Both patients and their relatives need to have some idea of the likely prognosis of the disorder. When the illness begins at an early age and runs a slow progressive course, there is a greater risk of a poor outcome. Rapid onset after a clear precipitating stress, and evidence of mood disturbance, suggest a better prognosis. Patients who are unmarried or lack a supportive relationship are more prone to relapse, as are those living in families with high levels of expressed emotion. The results of a 5-year follow-up study of treated schizophrenic patients are shown in Table 8.6.

Despite the apparently poor outlook demonstrated by these figures, one longer-term study conducted over 22 years suggests that schizophrenics do not deteriorate significantly beyond the initial 5-year period, and that a higher proportion of cases have a benign outcome than was once generally considered.

Table 8.6 Results of a 5-year follow-up study of treated schizophrenics

Recovered fully and remained well on medication	40%
Improved to some degree, but suffered at least one relapse during the follow-up period	20%
Persisted with symptoms despite treatment, but condition stable enough to live in the community	30%
Remained severely ill, showing little or no response to medication and requiring long-term hospitalisation	10%

Community Care in Schizophrenia

The decision to close large mental hospitals is at least partly due to a desire to prevent the institutionalisation of chronic schizophrenics. Unfortunately, such problems can develop in almost any setting, including hostels. Current policy aims to provide high-quality, community-based residential and recreational centres as an alternative to hospitalisation. Whether this will be achieved remains to be seen, but there are already misgivings that these vulnerable individuals will end up in prison or become vagrants if discharged from the hospitals, unless adequately financed community care facilities are available.

The Future

Despite a great deal of research, the cause of schizophrenia remains unknown. Although drugs are helpful in controlling some of the acute symptoms of the illness, they do little to prevent the development of the chronic phase. Consequently, many patients become severely handicapped, both socially and emotionally, so that they are unable to function without considerable support either in hospital or in the community.

The search for new and better drugs needs to continue, particularly as existing medication used in the treatment of schizophrenia can produce side-effects, which in some cases are as incapacitating as the illness itself. Some of the debilitating aspects of the disease have been shown to be caused or accentuated by caring for patients in an impoverished environment. Sufficient funding should therefore be available to ensure the continued development of social aspects of treatment, and the provision of an adequate number of rehabilitation units, both in hospitals and in the community.

PARANOID STATES

The term **paranoid** is widely used in psychiatry to describe a group of symptoms or beliefs, a personality type (*see* p. 47), a variety of schizophrenia and a group of disorders known as paranoid states. Although the expression is commonly employed as a synonym for 'persecutory', its application in psychiatry is broader than this.

Paranoid beliefs include ideas and delusions of reference, grandeur, jealousy and love, as well as of persecution. The common feature of all of these symptoms is the distorted manner in which the subject views himself in relation to other people. These beliefs occur in a number of psychiatric disorders, notably schizophrenia, affective illnesses and organic states. However, paranoid delusions are sometimes elicited in individuals in whom there is no evidence of any of these conditions.

Under these circumstances, the psychosis is referred to as a **paranoid state**, of which paranoia and paraphrenia are the most commonly encountered forms.

In the case of **paranoia**, the delusions gradually develop to form a whole system of false beliefs which are 'logically' constructed. Even so, they normally remain encapsulated, so that other aspects of thinking, behaviour and reality testing remain unaffected and personality deterioration does not occur. Consequently, the individual is usually able to work normally and maintain a social life, although this may be limited to some extent by his belief system. Hallucinations are absent in paranoia, but when they form a prominent additional part of the clinical picture, the disorder is referred to as **paraphrenia**. The relationship between paranoia, paraphrenia and paranoid schizophrenia is summarised in Table 8.7.

Where persecutory beliefs are the prominent feature of a paranoid state, the subject may say that he is being picked on, talked about, referred to or noticed by others, offering evidence which is highly unlikely or totally improbable. He might be convinced that there is a plot to kill or harm him, and this may be associated with beliefs of being spied on, drugged or hypnotised. Not surprisingly, many patients become fearful and profoundly depressed over their perceived harassment. Others become angry and excitable, and feel compelled to take action against their persecutors, especially if their allegations have been investigated and dismissed by the police or other authorities.

Hallucinations in paraphrenic illnesses are frequently auditory and may take the form of voices or noises. For example, one patient in hospital complained of hearing two nurses plotting against her, while another

Table 8.7 Paranoid states and paranoid schizophrenia

	Paranoia	Paraphrenia	Paranoid schizophrenia
Age of onset	30–40	50+	Late teens or early 20s
Personality	Well preserved	Well Preserved	Frequently deteriorated
First rank symptoms of schizophrenia	Absent	Absent	Usually present
Paranoid delusions	Present	Present	Usually present
Hallucinations	Absent	Present	Usually present

described the sound of a drill which she thought a neighbour was using to destroy her house. Visual hallucinations, such as seeing intruders or burglars, are sometimes described, while tactile hallucinations may be cited as evidence of physical molestation, often of a sexual nature. Olfactory and gustatory sense deceptions take the form of bad smells and unpleasant tastes. Auditory and visual misperceptions also occur, and all perceptual abnormalities tend to worsen at night.

A 38-year-old unmarried marketing manager sought help from his general practitioner because he felt generally unwell. Routine questioning by the doctor revealed that the patient thought his discomfort was due to his food being adulterated with powder by people unknown to him. He believed this had continued for at least 8 years, dating from an occasion when he had seen someone 'slip something into my drink' in a pub. From that time, he became convinced that somebody readily gained access to his home and added 'something' to the food and drink in his cupboards, although he was unable to explain how or why this occurred. He had made no attempt to report the matter, because until recently he had been certain that it had a beneficial effect on his energy and mood, and was probably 'some sort of drug'. Apart from this false belief, no other abnormality of thought content was elicited nor did he describe any hallucinations. He was successful at work and the only obvious effect that his delusional beliefs had on his life was that he rarely drank in pubs and only ate meals with people he knew well. Investigations revealed no organic abnormality and a drug screen was negative.

A 74-year-old widow, who lived alone, had made repeated appeals to the police for help, because she believed that her neighbour in the flat above was planning to kill her. She claimed to hear the woman plotting with her husband in bed at night, and was convinced that the loose plaster on her ceiling was due to holes being drilled into the floor of the upstairs flat, through which poisonous gas would be passed. She came to the attention of the psychiatric services when she was found sleeping in a shop doorway, having left her home for fear of what might happen to her. Enquiries revealed that the day before she had pushed some lighted newspaper through her neighbours' letterbox, with the intention of killing them. When she realised that she had failed, she fled in terror.

Delusions of grandeur, in the absence of a sustained mood disturbance, may be expressed in the form of special abilities or talents, frequently attributed to some divine force such as God or Jesus. Sometimes, the patient feels inspired to put them to spectacular use, such as ridding the world of disease or meeting with political leaders to discourage them from war. Grandiose identities are encountered in which the subject believes that he is rich, famous, related to royalty or in some way special.

Delusions of jealousy usually centre around a false belief that a partner is being unfaithful. The condition of pathological jealousy and other rare paranoid states are discussed further in Chapter 23.

Aetiology

Paranoid states are more likely to occur in individuals who have an underlying **paranoid personality**. Freud viewed the development of paranoid symptoms as a defence against feelings of inadequacy, inferiority and lack of self-trust. By attributing devious motives to the words and actions of others, unacceptable feelings about oneself can be denied.

Some authorities regard paranoia and paraphrenia as variants of paranoid schizophrenia, because of the similarity of clinical features. This viewpoint is further supported by the observation that relatives of patients with paraphrenia have an increased risk of developing schizophrenia when compared with the general population. Individuals who develop paraphrenia frequently live in **social isolation** and are often unmarried or childless. Forty per cent suffer from **impairment of sight or hearing**, which increases the likelihood of the misinterpretation of sensory stimuli.

Management

Patients who harbour paranoid delusions are often suspicious of the intentions of those who are trying to help them, and consequently, will not reveal the nature of their beliefs. The content of their thoughts may have to be deduced from their general behaviour and attitude towards questioning. Some people reveal beliefs which are sufficiently bizarre to be obviously false; one woman alleged that her neighbour pushed a screwdriver into her ear every night while she slept. Other claims which might be credible will require verification, such as when neighbours or local children are accused of harassing the patient.

The degree of fixity of the delusion should be determined by asking the individual if there is any possibility that his expressed problem could be a figment of his imagination. It is equally important to ascertain whether there is a likelihood of him acting on his beliefs. Acts of violence against the person or property of alleged persecutors sometimes occur, particularly if the patient is convinced that the police and others do not believe him. Other paranoid subjects can become profoundly depressed or frightened, and might contemplate or attempt suicide. **Compulsory detention** may then be necessary, particularly if the patient refuses to accept treatment. If paranoid beliefs arise as part of another disorder, such as schizophrenia, affective illness or an organic state, treatment is then of the underlying condition.

Because many patients who develop paranoid states live in social isolation, **increasing support and contact with the community** may improve their condition to some extent. This can be achieved by regular visits from community workers or by offering a place at a day centre or day hospital. Even so, medication in the form of **neuroleptics** is nearly always required. In many cases, this does not result in a total disappearance of the delusions, but patients often report that they are no longer bothered by them, nor feel compelled to act on them. Hallucinations usually respond well to drug treatment, but further misinterpretation of sensory stimuli can be minimised by ensuring that, where possible, **defects of sight or hearing are corrected** (such as through the provision of a hearing aid or removal of cataracts). Many patients fail to take their medication once they are out of hospital, and it may be necessary to give them regular depot injections to ensure compliance. In many cases, the illness runs a chronic, non-fluctuating course.

SUMMARY

1. **Schizophrenia** is one of the major psychoses, involving a disintegration of the various mental functions which affect thinking, behaviour, perception and mood; insight is diminished or lost.

2. **Historical development**: Kraepelin (1896) first classified psychoses into organic and functional types, the latter being further subdivided according to prognosis into dementia praecox and manic-depressive illness. Bleuler (1911) coined the term schizophrenia (which rapidly replaced dementia praecox), and based the diagnosis upon the four 'A's — autism, affective incongruity, ambivalence and loosening of associations. Schneider (1959) defined first rank symptoms of schizophrenia in an attempt to make the diagnosis more reliable. These involve thought alienation, passivity experiences regarding impulses, feelings, sensations and actions, auditory hallucinations and delusional perception. Further developments in the diagnosis of schizophrenia have included the use of operational criteria which specify symptom content, longitudinal factors and deterioration from a previous level of functioning.

3. **Epidemiology**: schizophrenia has a prevalence of approximately 1% worldwide, and an incidence of 15–20 new cases per 100 000 population per year. Men and women are affected equally, with the average age of onset in the early twenties.

4. **Clinical features**: schizophrenia describes two seemingly unrelated states, referred to as the acute and chronic forms of the illness. These terms signify symptom content, as well as the rate of onset and duration of the condition. Acute schizophrenia is characterised by 'positive symptoms', including Schneider's first rank symptoms, other delusions and hallucinations, thought disorder and affective incongruity. Chronic schizophrenia is characterised by 'negative symptoms' which culminate in the development of a 'defect state', resulting in lack of drive, social withdrawal, poverty of speech and action, blunting of affect and self-neglect; depression may also be common.

5. **Schizoaffective illnesses**: involve symptoms of mania or depression intermingled with those of schizophrenia, and do not normally result in permanent damage to the personality.

6. **Aetiology**: evidence from family, twin and adoption studies suggests that a vulnerability to develop schizophrenia is probably inherited, and that the influence of environmental factors is required before the illness becomes manifest. Factors that have been implicated include abnormal family processes, high expressed emotion, life events, birth trauma and infection. The biochemical substrate of the genetic predisposition is thought to involve an excess of the neurotransmitter, dopamine, in the mesolimbic pathway of the brain.

7. **Management**: neuroleptic drugs are the mainstay of treatment in schizophrenia. They are effective orally, but can be administered by depot injection to aid compliance. Troublesome side-effects are common and include pseudo-parkinsonism, acute dystonia, akathisia and tardive dyskinesia. Rehabilitation is important to prevent institutionalisation, but needs to be gradual, since excessive environmental stimulation may cause a relapse of the illness.

8. **Prognosis** in schizophrenia is variable. Maintenance drug therapy is beneficial to some, but not all patients. Effective community care requires adequate provision of facilities for work, accommodation and recreation.

9. **Paranoid states**: paranoid beliefs include ideas and delusions of persecution, reference, grandeur, love and jealousy. A common feature of these symptoms is the distorted manner in which the subject views himself in relation to other people. They may be features of schizophrenia, affective illnesses or organic states. However, psychoses in which paranoid delusions occur in isolation are known as paranoid states, and these include paranoia and paraphrenia.

10. In **paranoia**, a delusional system gradually develops, which is often encapsulated, so that the individual is usually able to function relatively well. A paranoid state in which hallucinations form a prominent part of the clinical picture is known as **paraphrenia**. In both disorders, personality is preserved. Hallucinations in paraphrenia occur in all modalities, but are most frequently auditory.

11. **Aetiology and management**: an underlying paranoid personality, social isolation and defects of sight or hearing are all predisposing factors in the development of paranoid states. Social support and the correction of sensory defects may improve the condition, but most patients will require neuroleptic medication. Compulsory detention might be necessary if the patient refuses treatment and is likely to harm himself or others. The illness often runs a chronic and non-fluctuating course.

REFERENCES AND FURTHER READING

Bleuler, E. (1911) Dementia praecox or the group of schizophrenias. English translation by J. Zinkin 1950. New York: International University Press.

Bleuler, M. (1974). The long-term course of the schizophrenic psychoses. *Psychological Medicine*; **4**: 244–54.

Crow, T. J., Deakin, J. F. W., Johnstone, E. C., Longden, A. (1976). Dopamine and schizophrenia. *Lancet*; **i**: 563–66.

Gottesman, I. I., Shields, J. (1976). Critical review of recent adoption, twin and family studies. *Schizophrenia Bulletin*; **2**: 360–400.

Guirguis, W. H. (1981). Schizophrenia: the problem of definition. *British Journal of Hospital Medicine*; **25**: 236–40.

Hirsch, S. R. (1983). Psychosocial factors in the cause and prevention of relapse in schizophrenia. *British Medical Journal*; **286**: 1600–1.

Kraepelin, E. (1896) *Psychiatrie, ein Lehrbuch für studierende und Ärzte*, 5th edn. Leipzig: Barth.

Mellor, C. S. (1970). First rank symptoms of schizophrenia. *British Journal of Psychiatry*; **117**: 15–23.

Procci, W. R. (1976). Schizoaffective psychosis: fact or fiction? *Archives of General Psychiatry*; **33**: 1167–78.

Schneider, K. (1959) *Clinical Psychopathology*. New York: Grune and Stratton.

Spitzer, R., Endicott, J., Robins, E. (1975). Clinical criteria for psychiatric diagnosis and DSM III. *American Journal of Psychiatry*; **132**: 1187–92.

Vaughn, C. E., Leff, P. J. (1976). Influence of family and social factors on the course of psychiatric illness. *British Journal of Psychiatry*; **129**: 125–37.

Wing, J. K. (1966). Five year outcome in early schizophrenia. *Proceedings of the Royal Society of Medicine*; **59**: 17–18.

Wing, J. K., Brown, G. W. (1961). Social treatment of chronic schizophrenia: a comparative survey of three mental hospitals. *Journal of Mental Science*; **107**: 847–61.

9   ORGANIC PSYCHIATRY

Organic psychiatry is concerned with those conditions in which mental disorder arises as a result of demonstrable structural disease of the brain or physiological disturbance affecting cerebral function. In some instances, mental functioning is extensively impaired, and contact with reality is diminished. Under these circumstances, the disorder may be referred to as an **organic psychosis** (*see* Chapter 1).

CLASSIFICATION

Classification can be considered in terms of:

1. **acute** and **chronic** organic reactions, which differ according to the rate of onset, course and duration of symptoms, and whether or not there is impairment in the level of consciousness
2. **focal** and **diffuse** lesions, depending upon the site and extent of pathological changes in the brain
3. **specific** or **global** impairment of brain function; whether isolated aspects of cerebral functioning are affected, or the impairment is generalised.

Acute and Chronic Organic Reactions

In an **acute organic reaction**:

1. impairment in the level of consciousness occurs (Fig. 9.1)
2. the onset of the condition is usually rapid and tends to run a fluctuating course, lasting at most a few weeks
3. impaired consciousness can also be distorted by perceptual abnormalities and changes in mood (when the disorder is known as a **delirium**)
4. evidence of underlying structural brain damage is uncommon. In most cases, the disorder resolves spontaneously or is potentially

Impairment of consciousness is obvious when there is evidence of drowsiness or sleepiness during examination. Minor degrees may be more difficult to elicit. Consciousness exists on a continuum extending from full consciousness at one extreme to coma at the other.

CONSCIOUSNESS
|
A state of awareness of the self and the environment. The individual is
bright and alert and appears to function well.

|

CLOUDING OF CONSCIOUSNESS
|
Slight impairment of clarity of thinking, attention, awareness or memory, which may not be
apparent unless specifically tested for (*see* Chapter 2).

|

DELIRIUM
|
Consciousness is not only impaired, but is also distorted by illusions, hallucinations, delusions
and changes in mood. The level of arousal is high, and psychomotor activity is frequently increased.

|

DROWSINESS
|
Further impairment of consciousness with lack of attentiveness and awareness, which is usually
obvious on direct observation.

|

SEMICOMA
|
Subject appears unconscious, but can be roused by painful stimuli.
There may be evidence of uncoordinated movement.

|

COMA
|
'Unconsciousness'. No response to external stimuli, absent reflexes, no spontaneous movement
(other than those of respiration). No sign of mental activity.

NB   The term 'stupor' is sometimes used by neurologists to refer to a state of akinetic mutism resulting from lesions in the upper brain stem in which consciousness is probably impaired. In psychiatry, stupor refers to a state in which speech and spontaneous movement are absent, but consciousness is preserved.

Fig. 9.1 Impairment of consciousness

reversible, although some can progress to a chronic irreversible stage.

The term 'confusion' is sometimes used to describe the impairment of consciousness which occurs in acute organic reactions — otherwise referred to as 'acute confusional states'. Because of the ambiguity which surrounds its application, the term is best avoided in descriptions of the mental state, and as an alternative 'perplexity' should be used (*see also* Glossary for 'confusion').

Irrespective of their cause, the clinical features of acute organic reactions are remarkably constant (*see later*).

Chronic organic reactions:

1. involve an acquired global impairment of cerebral functions, which occur in a setting of clear consciousness. Impairment of **intellect** is the essential feature (evident as problems with memory, attention, thinking or comprehension), although other mental functions (mood, personality and social behaviour) are usually affected simultaneously and may sometimes be the prominent or presenting aspect. Chronic organic reactions are also known as **dementia**.
2. characteristically have a gradual onset and tend to run a progressive, irreversible course.
3. structural brain damage is frequently present.

The division between acute and chronic reactions is somewhat artificial, and features of both may sometimes coexist clinically (Table 9.1).

Focal and Diffuse Cerebral Lesions

Some organic reactions result from **diffuse** cerebral pathology, such as the widespread atrophy and degeneration of brain tissue associated with senile dementia. Other conditions, such as tumours or strokes, produce **focal** or localised lesions within the brain at one or more sites.

Both cerebral hemispheres are differentiated into several lobes, each of which subserves a number of specific functions (Fig. 9.2). It follows that a focal lesion in one lobe or hemisphere may produce specific psychological or neurological signs and symptoms, which will help to localise the site and extent of the underlying pathology.

The **frontal lobe** contains the motor cortex, as well as the speech area in the dominant hemisphere. It also influences aspects of the personality associated with social skills and motivation. Consequently, personality changes can occur with frontal lobe lesions, resulting in disinhibition, euphoria, apathy, poor concentration and lability of mood. There may also be evidence of physical dysfunction in the form of contralateral spastic paresis, gait disturbance and motor dysphasia. On examination, a grasp reflex is sometimes present. Anosmia and optic atrophy can result from inferior lesions that encroach on the orbit, and incontinence due to loss of sphincter control may be troublesome.

The **parietal lobe** contains the sensory cortex, and is also concerned with linguistic and arithmetical ability, body image and visuospatial function. Certain parietal dysfunctions are specific to the dominant or non-dominant hemisphere, while others are common to lesions in either hemisphere. The latter include:

Table 9.1 Summary of the typical features of acute and chronic organic reactions

	Acute organic reaction	Chronic organic reaction
Onset	Rapid	Insidious
Course	Fluctuating, usually reversible or spontaneous recovery	Progressive over a long time scale; tends to be irreversible in most cases
Structural brain damage	Usually none	Frequently present
Consciousness	Impaired — the subject may be overtly drowsy or sleepy (*see Fig. 9.1*)	Clear
Orientation	Disorientation in time and place — clouding of consciousness disrupts processing of information from external senses. Differentiation between thoughts, memories and real events becomes disturbed	Disorientation in time, place and eventually person — due to memory failure, and declining intellectual ability to integrate information meaningfully (not due to clouding of consciousness)
Memory	Variable — immediate, recent and long-term may all be impaired	Variable — initially immediate and recent impaired, long-term affected as memory loss progresses
Deterioration of intellect and personality	Absent	Present, collateral information from other informants often necessary to confirm early changes
Thought content	Disorganised, thought content abundant, may develop delusions as a result of perceptual abnormalities	Disorganised, thought content often impoverished, leading to a failure of communication. Memory loss sometimes leads to development of paranoid delusions
Perceptual abnormalities	Commonly present, illusions and hallucinations (particularly visual)	Not uncommon — can occur in the early stages and may be less prominent as illness progresses

Overlap is common and 'acute-on-chronic' reactions can develop. It is essential to obtain information about the history and clinical features from another informant.

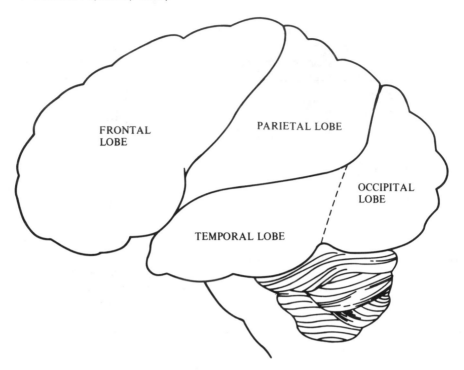

Fig. 9.2 The lobes of the external surface of the cerebral hemispheres

1. constructional apraxia (inability to copy or construct three-dimensional figures)
2. topographical disorientation (difficulty in finding one's way about, even in familiar surroundings)
3. atopognosia (inability to locate a sensation correctly)
4. agraphognosia (inability to recognise numbers or letters written on the skin).

Lesions of the **dominant** lobe can result in:

1. motor or sensory dysphasia
2. motor apraxia (the inability to perform voluntary movements in the absence of motor or sensory deficit)
3. visual agnosia (a failure to recognise an object by sight, which is not due to visual or intellectual deficit)
4. Gerstmann's syndrome: a rare phenomenon involving dyscalculia (impairment of numerical skills), dysgraphia (impairment of the ability to write), finger agnosia (inability to recognise or name individual fingers, so that the patient cannot discriminate which digit is being touched when the eyes are closed) and right–left disorientation.

Non-dominant parietal lobe lesions may cause:

1. disorders of body image, such as contralateral neglect
2. dressing apraxia (inability to dress oneself)
3. prosopagnosia (inability to recognise familiar faces)
4. anosognosia (inability to recognise disability caused by disease).

Parietal lobe damage can also produce cortical sensory loss, resulting in difficulty with the correct location of stimuli, recognising objects by touch (astereognosis) and discerning two-point discrimination.

The **temporal lobe** is mainly associated with the functions of memory and the comprehension of language, as well as influencing certain aspects of emotion. Lesions in this region may result in personality changes (such as increased aggressiveness and emotional lability), receptive dysphasia (impairment of the ability to comprehend speech and writing) and memory disturbance. Verbal memory is affected by dominant lobe dysfunction, while non-verbal memory (for music, faces and pictures) is impaired with non-dominant lobe lesions.

The **occipital lobe** contains the visual cortex, and lesions in this area can lead to complex disturbances of visual function.

Brain stem lesions can result in a dysmnesic syndrome (*see below*), hypersomnia and emotional lability.

Specific or Global Impairment of Cerebral Function

A global impairment of cerebral function occurs in dementia, eventually resulting in gross behavioural, intellectual and personality deterioration. However, in certain organic conditions only specific aspects of psychological functioning are affected. For example, in the dysmnesic syndrome (Korsakoff's psychosis) a profound defect of memory occurs, but with relative preservation of other intellectual abilities (*see* Chapter 11).

ACUTE ORGANIC REACTIONS

Acute organic reactions are more likely to occur in those who are particularly susceptible to cerebral disturbance — the very young, the elderly, postoperative cases and those with pre-existing physical illness.

Aetiology

There are many causes of acute organic reactions (Table 9.2), the commonest of which are peripheral infections, drugs, alcohol withdrawal, cerebral hypoxia and head injury. Some of these are discussed in greater detail later in this chapter.

Table 9.2 Some causes of acute organic reactions

Vascular	Transient ischaemic attacks, cerebral infarcts (often secondary to hypertension), subarachnoid haemorrhage, transient global amnesia, systemic lupus eyrythematosus
Trauma	Head injury
Epilepsy	Psychomotor seizures and postictal states
Vitamin deficiencies	Particularly B_1, B_{12}, nicotinic acid
Metabolic abnormalities	Hepatic or renal failure, water and electrolyte disturbances, acute intermittent porphyria
Endocrine abnormalities	Thyroid, parathyroid and adrenal disorders, hypo- and hyperglycaemia, hypopituitarism, phaeochromocytoma
Cerebral hypoxia	May be secondary to cardiorespiratory failure or severe anaemia, leading to reduced arterial oxygen concentration; also post-anaesthesia
Toxins	Alcohol (excessive consumption or acute withdrawal — *see* Chapter 11), carbon monoxide poisoning, industrial metals such as lead, mercury or manganese; drugs — illicit substances or prescribed medication (*see* Table 9.7)
Space-occupying cerebral lesions	Brain tumour, subdural haematoma, cerebral abscess
Infections	Cerebral (meningitis, encephalitis) or peripheral (respiratory, urinary tract)

Clinical Features

The onset is typically acute, impairment of consciousness being associated with disorientation, poor concentration and distractability. The subject tends to be restless, emotionally labile, anxious and perplexed, especially when he fails to comprehend either his surroundings or what is happening to him. Acute organic reactions characteristically have a fluctuating course, with periods of clouded consciousness interspersed with lucid intervals. Symptoms are often worse at night, when darkness or poor lighting exacerbate misinterpretation of sensory stimuli. Delirium is associated with gross disturbance of perception, namely illusions and hallucinations, as a result of which delusional ideas may develop. Following recovery, the individual frequently has little or no recollection of events during his illness.

A general practitioner was called to the home of one of his elderly patients by the police, after they had received a call from her requesting help. On arrival, he found the woman hiding in her garden shed, insisting that she had seen Vietnamese Boat People climbing out of the lavatory bowl and overrunning her house. A history obtained from a neighbour confirmed that the woman had appeared perfectly well when she was seen 2 days beforehand. The patient was too distraught to examine further, as she kept screaming that she could see 'the invaders' standing behind the doctor. In view of the absence of any previous psychiatric history, and the apparently rapid onset of symptoms, the doctor suspected that the most likely cause of her hallucinations and persecutory beliefs was a delirium. He arranged for the woman to be admitted to the local psychogeriatric unit, which she readily agreed to, in order to escape from the horde she believed was occupying her home. On admission, she was found to be febrile and a urine sample which she provided was noted to be blood-stained and foul-smelling. Culture later confirmed the presence of an *Escherichia coli* infection. Antibiotic treatment resulted in the resolution of her urinary and psychiatric symptoms within 7 days.

Management

The basic principle of management involves the identification and treatment of the underlying cause. Nursing care should include reassuring the patient during periods of confusion, and maintaining a well-lit and uncluttered environment to avoid increasing his disorientation. Simple measures, such as regularly reminding him of the time, his whereabouts and who is caring for him can considerably reduce distress. Similarly, unnecessary noise should be kept to a minimum, and the patient is best cared for in a single room, ideally being attended by the same nurse on each shift.

Disturbances of fluid and electrolyte balance will need to be corrected, while the administration of psychotropic drugs is preferably kept to a minimum, as they may increase the level of confusion. However, if the patient is very restless and disturbed by day, sedation may be needed, in which case small doses of haloperidol can be given. Benzodiazepines or chlormethiazole are often used as sedatives in delirium tremens and as a general measure to help induce sleep. The prognosis will to an extent depend on the underlying cause, and although in most cases recovery is complete, some acute organic reactions progress to a chronic phase or have a fatal outcome.

CHRONIC ORGANIC REACTIONS (DEMENTIA)

Chronic organic reactions are otherwise referred to as dementia. (In addition to describing a clinical syndrome which can have many causes, the term **dementia** is also used to label a group of specific degenerative conditions, the presenile and senile dementias, which are discussed later.)

Dementia is defined as an acquired global impairment of memory, intellect and personality, without impairment of consciousness. In dementing illnesses, deterioration can sometimes extend over several years, often with profound consequences for both patients and their families. The organisation of psychiatric services for people with dementia (who form the bulk of the 'elderly severely mentally ill' population) is discussed in Chapter 10.

Aetiology

There are various causes of chronic organic reactions (Table 9.3), but it is estimated that the underlying pathology is treatable in only 5–10% of cases. In such instances, early intervention may arrest the dementing process.

Prevalence

Current estimates suggest that 5% of the over-65s and 20% of the over-80s in the UK suffer from dementia. However, the total number is probably greater than this, since many mild forms of the illness go undetected, while others with more advanced symptoms may be supported by relatives at home and remain unknown to psychiatric services. Inevitably, numbers will increase as the elderly population grows larger, so that the demands on the Health Service are likely to escalate accordingly. Senile and multi-infarct dementia are by far the commonest forms of chronic organic reactions encountered in the elderly, and in some cases the two disorders may coexist (*see later*).

Clinical Features

Dementia usually has an insidious onset, and in the initial stages there might be little evidence of disability other than the occasional lapse of recent memory, which is often interpreted as normal forgetfulness. Premorbid personality traits are sometimes exaggerated; e.g. the person who has always been 'set in his ways' may become increasingly rigid and inflexible in his manner. Insight is often retained during this early phase, so that the sufferer can become anxious and depressed at the realisation of his failing mental faculties. As further deterioration develops, diminishing intellectual capacity and memory loss are more apparent. This can sometimes lead to the development of persecutory delusions, particularly if misplaced articles are assumed to have been stolen.

Wandering (especially at night) and neglect of personal hygiene, diet and clothing are often major causes of concern for relatives and other care givers. Other changes which occur in speech and behaviour include perseveration (the inappropriate repetition of words or actions), confabu-

Table 9.3 Some causes of chronic organic reactions

Degenerative conditions	Senile dementia (SDAT), Alzheimer's disease, Pick's disease, Huntington's chorea, Creutzfeldt-Jakob disease, Parkinson's disease
Vascular	Multi-infarct dementia, cerebrovascular accident, systemic lupus erythematosus, subarachnoid haemorrhage
Trauma	Severe head injury, 'punch-drunk' syndrome
Epilepsy	Dementia more likely when epilepsy is chronic and severe (? repeated hypoxia) or where there is underlying brain damage
Vitamin deficiencies	B_1, B_{12} and folate, nicotinic acid
Metabolic abnormalities	Wilson's disease, chronic uraemia
Endocrine abnormalities	Hypothyroidism, parathyroid disorders, hypopituitarism, hypoglycaemia, diabetes
Cerebral hypoxia	Post-cardiac arrest, respiratory failure, severe anaemia
Toxins	Prolonged alcohol consumption, carbon monoxide poisoning, exposure to heavy metals such as lead, mercury, silver or aluminium
Space-occupying cerebral lesions	Brain tumour, cerebral abscess, subdural haematoma
Infections	Encephalitis, neurosyphilis, meningitis, human immunodeficiency virus (AIDS)
Miscellaneous causes	Multiple sclerosis, normal pressure hydrocephalus, non-metastatic cancer

lation (a falsification of memory), nominal aphasia (the inability to name objects) and catastrophic reactions (explosive displays of emotion in response to demands beyond the subject's capabilities). Thinking becomes slow and restricted, and is associated with a diminution of the range of activities in which the subject engages.

In the later stages of the illness, there is a progressive deterioration of the personality, associated with a lack of emotional response, apathy and loss of insight. Hallucinations can occur in all sensory modalities. Socially unacceptable behaviour, such as aggressiveness, sexual disinhibition and incontinence often increases, and is eventually accompanied by a general deterioration in physical health. Ultimately, the subject becomes bed-ridden, with death frequently resulting from intercurrent physical illness.

It is important when contemplating a diagnosis of dementia to distinguish the condition from a depressive illness. This can sometimes be difficult, especially if depressed mood is denied or the patient is uncommunicative. Furthermore, the psychomotor retardation and poor concentration occasionally found in affective disorders may be interpreted as being due to memory impairment, personality deterioration and intellectual deficit (depressive pseudodementia). It is estimated that 10% of individuals in whom a diagnosis of dementia is initially made, have later been shown to suffer from a depressive illness. A correct diagnosis is more likely where a history is obtained from a relative or friend, behaviour is observed over a period of time on the ward or in the home, and information is recorded concerning sleep pattern, weight change and eating habits. Psychometric testing may be useful in confirming or refuting the provisional diagnosis, but where doubt persists, a trial of anti-depressant medication or ECT might help resolve the dilemma. It must also be remembered that depression and dementing illnesses are not mutually exclusive and may coexist. Indeed, there is evidence that depression is a not infrequent component of early dementia.

Management

Because it is essential to identify treatable causes of dementia, initial management should include the following investigations:

1. haematological profile — full blood count, ESR, serum folate and B_{12}
2. biochemical profile — urea and electrolytes, serum creatinine, calcium and phosphorus, liver function tests, blood glucose
3. thyroid function tests
4. treponemal antibodies (VDRL/TPHA)
5. urine microscopy and culture
6. skull and chest x-rays
7. electrocardiogram.

More sophisticated investigations are sometimes necessary and may include an electroencephalogram (EEG) and computerised axial tomography (CAT scan) of the brain.

The primary aim of management in a case of irreversible dementia is to maintain the quality of the subject's life and standard of functioning at an optimal level for as long as possible. The patient should preferably be kept at home, so as to minimise the confusion and disorientation which is likely to occur if he is placed in an unfamiliar environment. The maintenance of good physical health is important to prevent accelerated deterioration, although drugs should be used sparingly to reduce the likelihood of precipitating an 'acute-on-chronic' organic reaction.

People with dementia rarely ask for help themselves, and it is usually left to distraught relatives and other care givers to enlist professional support. Consequently, it is often useful to consider the demented patient together with those who support him in the community as a unit, and deal with their collective needs accordingly. The assessment and care of the elderly mentally ill within the community and in hospital is discussed in Chapter 10.

A 76-year-old woman was found by the police walking along the road in the early hours of the morning, wearing only a nightdress and slippers. She told the patrolman that she was going shopping and seemed oblivious to the fact that it was the middle of the night. She was able to give her name and address, and was taken home. Her husband had been unaware that she had got up and left the house, but he told the policeman that he had become increasingly concerned about his wife's behaviour and forgetfulness during the past few months, and was finding it hard to cope. She had always been a neat and fastidious person, and although she still attempted to do the housework, their home had become progressively untidy despite his efforts to maintain some sense of order. Although she was generally pleasant and cheerful, he had noticed that whenever she found herself unable to perform simple tasks around the house, she would become very emotional, and once or twice when he had tried to help her, she had reacted explosively, screaming and sobbing uncontrollably for some time afterwards. On numerous occasions she had left things burning on the stove, and only the day before had left the gas unlit, until the smell had alerted him to the danger. He had suggested to his wife that she should go and see the doctor, but she said she felt quite well, and he assumed her forgetfulness was just part of growing old.

Later that morning she was visited by her general practitioner, who had not seen her for many months since she was an infrequent attender at surgery. Although he noted that the woman was apparently bright and alert, she failed to recognise him, and was unable to remember any of the events that had taken place in the early hours, insisting that she had slept well throughout the night. She did not know the day of the week, and thought the month was February even though it was mid-summer and very warm. Cognitive testing showed that her short-term memory was clearly impaired, although her husband confirmed that events she recalled from the past were accurate.

Because of the difficult domestic situation, and the need to carry out further assessment, it was decided to admit the woman to the local psychogeriatric unit, which she agreed to with some persuasion. She became extremely agitated shortly after admission, and that night broke the fire alarm on the ward in an effort to get help, insisting that she was being held in prison. With considerable effort, the nurses managed to calm her down and persuaded her to stay. During the next week, it was apparent to the nursing staff that she was incapable of finding her way around the ward, although she was able to dress and feed herself with some assistance. Results of investigations excluded any treatable cause for her condition, and in view of the overall findings, she was diagnosed as suffering from senile dementia.

The remainder of this chapter is devoted to specific causes of both acute and chronic organic reactions.

DEGENERATIVE DISORDERS

These conditions arise from primary degenerative processes within the brain. Four of them (Alzheimer's disease, Pick's disease, Creutzfeldt-Jakob disease and Huntington's chorea) generally have an onset before the age of 65 years and are known collectively as **presenile dementias**. The pathology of one of the presenile conditions, Alzheimer's disease, is indistinguishable from that of senile dementia, and many authorities consider them to be the same disorder occurring in different age groups. Consequently, the latter is often referred to as senile dementia–Alzheimer's type (SDAT).

Senile Dementia-Alzheimer's Type (SDAT)

This is the commonest form of dementing illness with an onset usually between 70 and 75, and a female to male ratio of 2:1. There is some evidence of a genetic predisposition to its development, but the mode of inheritance is unknown. The clinical features have been outlined earlier, and the course is invariably progressive, with death commonly resulting from a physical complication, such as bronchopneumonia. The period over which deterioration occurs can vary widely. In some cases, there is a rapid decline, culminating in death 2–5 years from the time of diagnosis. However, a protracted course of up to 10 years or more is sometimes seen.

Pathological changes include cortical atrophy, dilated ventricles and widened sulci. Microscopy reveals 'senile plaques' in the cerebral tissue, which are silver-staining and contain amyloid. They are associated with neurofibrillary tangles, and the numbers of both are increased in relation to the clinical severity of the condition. Other features include loss of neurones (particulary cholinergic) and glial proliferation.

Acetylcholine precursors (such as choline or lecithin) and cerebral vasodilators have been used in an attempt to halt or reverse the progressive deterioration of senile dementia, but results so far have proved inconclusive.

Alzheimer's Disease

Alzheimer's disease is the most frequently encountered form of presenile dementia, with an age of onset between 40 and 60 years and a female to male ratio of 2:1. Excessive concentrations of aluminium have been discovered in the brains of some patients suffering from Alzheimer's disease, although as yet no definite aetiological significance has been attributed to this finding. The pathological changes, clinical features and prognosis are otherwise identical to those of SDAT, except that focal changes (especially involving the parietal lobe) and epileptic seizures are more common, and the decline is often rapid.

Pick's Disease

This is an uncommon disorder, affecting twice as many women as men, with a peak age of onset between 50 and 60 years. It is probably transmitted by a single autosomal dominant gene. Characteristic pathological changes result in a proliferation of 'Pick's cells', which are balloon-like in appearance and contain silver-staining inclusion bodies. Circumscribed frontal and temporal lobe atrophy occurs, as a result of which the gyri take on a typical 'knife-blade' appearance.

The clinical features tend to be less severe than with Alzheimer's disease, particularly as the parietal lobes are usually unaffected. Early changes involve personality deterioration of the frontal lobe type (*see* p. 158), with memory loss a relatively late feature. The illness tends to run a progressive course, with death occurring after 2–10 years.

Creutzfeldt-Jakob Disease (subacute spongiform encephalopathy)

The most interesting aspect of this very rare condition is that it is thought to be caused by a **transmissible viral agent**, similar in nature to that responsible for Kuru, a brain disease affecting certain tribes of Papua New Guinea, that are known to have practised cannibalism.

Pathological features include neuronal loss, ventricular dilatation, gliosis and cystic changes resulting in a characteristic sponge-like appearance of the grey matter. The onset of the illness is relatively sudden, followed by rapid deterioration in association with various neurological abnormalities. The final stage is one of severe dementia, and death occurs within two years of diagnosis.

Huntington's Chorea

First described in the nineteenth century, this disorder is characterised by a dementia associated with abnormal choreiform movements. It is caused by a single autosomal dominant gene, although cases without a family history also occur, presumably due to spontaneous mutation.

Huntington's chorea affects approximately one in 20 000 of the population with an equal sex incidence. The onset is most commonly between 35 and 45 years of age, although the condition has been diagnosed in both childhood and old age. Pathological features include generalised cortical atrophy, with the most extensive changes occurring in the frontal lobes and basal ganglia. The movement disorders (*see below*) probably result from a deficiency of the inhibitory neurotransmitter gamma-amino-butyric acid (GABA), leading to a relative excess of dopamine in the basal ganglia.

The onset tends to be insidious and psychiatric symptoms are often prominent in the early stages, sometimes leading to a delay in the correct diagnosis. Clinical features include lability of mood, antisocial and aggressive behaviour, and occasionally a paranoid psychosis. Choreiform movements usually develop at a later stage, although they can sometimes be the presenting feature of the illness. Initially, the face, head and upper limbs are involved, but eventually the whole body can be affected. Tremor, rigidity and ataxia may also be present. The development of dementia is slow and progressive, with death usually occurring 12–16 years after the onset of the illness.

Dopamine-depleting drugs, such as tetrabenazine, or the phenothiazines, may help to alleviate the choreiform movements, but the only effective form of treatment at present lies in **prevention** through offering genetic counselling to families at risk.

Parkinson's Disease

This common condition of the elderly results from cellular degeneration of dopamine-producing cells in the basal ganglia, and is recognised clinically by the triad of bradykinesia, rigidity and tremor. Psychiatric problems are encountered in nearly half of all patients suffering from Parkinson's disease, the most common being depression. Although the latter may be explained as an emotional response to suffering a chronic physical illness, it has also been suggested that the depressive symptoms have an organic basis, since they sometimes occur before physical disabilities are present.

Patients receiving L-dopa treatment for the illness occasionally develop depression or a paranoid psychosis, while the use of anticholinergic drugs sometimes results in agitation and excitement. A mild or moderate dementia develops in about one-third of those with Parkinson's disease, particularly in the very elderly, although it is not always progressive and appears unrelated to the severity of any physical disability.

VASCULAR DISEASE

Multi-Infarct Dementia (MID)

Formerly known as **arteriosclerotic dementia**, this condition is mainly caused by thromboemboli (originating in extracranial vessels damaged by atherosclerosis), which produce numerous cerebral infarcts in association with cystic necrosis and gliosis. It is the second most commonly encountered form of dementia after SDAT, with a peak onset between 60 and 70 years, and is slightly more prevalent in males.

Unlike senile dementia, in which impairment of cerebral function is both insidious and progressive, deterioration in MID tends to occur in a stepwise fashion, correlating with repeated episodes of cerebral infarction over a length of time. As a result, periods of relative stability may be observed, during which no significant decline of mental function occurs. The mood is often labile and nocturnal confusion is a common feature, although characteristically, personality and insight are preserved until the later stages of the illness. There may be evidence of arteriosclerotic

Table 9.4 A summary of the clinical and pathological differences between multi-infarct dementia (MID) and senile dementia–Alzheimer's type (SDAT)

	MID	SDAT
Pathology	Cerebral infarction arising from thromboemboli in extracranial vessels	Cortical atrophy, senile plaques and neurofibrillary tangles seen microscopically in cerebral tissue
Sex ratio	More common in males	More common in females
Average age of onset	60–70 years	70–75 years
Course	Stepwise progression, death in 4–5 years	Steady decline; in some cases, there is a 'rapid' deterioration with death occurring 2–5 years from the time of diagnosis. However, a more protracted course of up to 10 years or more is sometimes seen
Impairment of intellect and personality	Occur late	Occur early
Retention of insight	Often retained until late stages	Insight lost early on in course of illness
Focal neurological signs	Frequently present	Few
Hypertension	Frequently present	Inconstant
Physical symptoms	Headache, dizziness, tinnitus often present	Inconstant

changes elsewhere in the body and hypertension is a common finding. Focal neurological signs are frequently present, and there may be a history of headaches, dizziness, epileptic seizures, cerebral ischaemic attacks or strokes.

In addition to general aspects of management, treatment should be directed towards the control of hypertension, although this needs to be cautiously handled in the elderly to avoid causing further cerebral ischaemia if the blood pressure falls too low. The prognosis is generally poor, death occurring within 5 years of diagnosis, usually from other complications such as ischaemic heart disease or cerebrovascular accident. A summary of the clinical and pathological differences between MID and SDAT is shown in Table 9.4.

Cerebrovascular Accidents

Acute **subarachnoid haemorrhage** is frequently fatal, while those who survive often show signs of cognitive impairment, personality change and depressed mood. Similar changes may be observed following other types of cerebrovascular accident. Depression is particularly common in **stroke** victims, whose capacity for independent living is diminished due to paralysis or communication difficulties.

Transient Global Amnesia

This is a disorder of middle and old age, and is seen more often in men. A sudden loss of recent memory occurs, accompanied by an inability to store new information, although recall of distant events and other cognitive functions are unaffected. There is no impairment in the level of consciousness, and the subject is usually able to continue talking and functioning normally, although he may be perplexed by his memory loss. Attacks typically last for several hours, after which memory function recovers completely, although there is an amnesic gap for the episode. The cause of the condition is uncertain, but is probably due to cerebral ischaemia.

Systemic Lupus Erythematosus (SLE)

SLE is a connective tissue disorder producing widespread inflammatory changes of blood vessels, with the extensive development of vasculitis and multiple microinfarcts. Cerebral vessels are affected in more than 50% of cases, so that epileptic seizures and psychiatric disorders are common. Both acute and chronic organic reactions can occur, as well as personality changes, neurotic symptoms and psychotic illnesses. Treatment with steroid drugs may cause further psychiatric complications.

HEAD INJURY

Each year over 100 000 people in the UK are admitted to hospital with head injuries, mostly as a result of road traffic accidents. The vast majority undergo no more than temporary concussion and are discharged home, having suffered no lasting damage. However, in the minority of cases where more severe head injuries are sustained, long-term organic, psychiatric or social sequelae can develop, sometimes resulting in permanent disability. The degree of impairment will depend on many factors: the circumstances of the accident, the site and extent of any brain damage, the age and personality of the individual, and the social dysfunction which results from the injury.

1. Organic Complications

Even in the absence of overt complications, such as a depressed skull fracture or intracranial bleeding, **prolonged impairment of consciousness** following trauma decreases the likelihood of full recovery. The most useful prognostic indicator after a head injury is the duration of **post-traumatic (anterograde) amnesia (PTA)**, this being the interval of time between the head injury and the return of normal, continuous memory (Fig. 9.3). However, there may be 'islands' of memory which are retained prior to full recovery. Unlike retrograde amnesia (*see below*), the duration of PTA does not usually diminish with time. Furthermore, it can extend beyond the return of clear consciousness, and is likely to be prolonged in the elderly. As a general rule, PTA of less than 12 hours indicates the likelihood of a full recovery. When it exceeds 24 hours in duration, there is an increased risk of residual disability such as brain damage, epilepsy, psychiatric disorder or intellectual deficit. PTA is an unreliable prognostic indicator in the case of penetrating head injuries, where serious complications can occur even though loss of memory is minimal or non-existent.

The length of **retrograde amnesia** represents the time between the moment of injury and the last clear memory before the incident (Fig. 9.3). Although it frequently occurs, it is a poor indicator of prognosis. Irrespective of its initial length, retrograde amnesia invariably shrinks over a period of time, so that its final duration is usually less than a minute.

Repeated head injuries, such as those sustained by boxers, can result in a chronic progressive encephalopathy known as **'punch-drunk' syndrome**. Pathological changes involve cerebral atrophy in association with brain-stem and cerebellar damage. The clinical features include ataxia, tremor, spasticity, a shuffling gait, personality changes and a progressive dementia.

HEAD INJURY

TIME

| Continuous memory prior to head injury | Retrograde amnesia: variable in length but tends to diminish with time. Final duration is often less than a minute. A poor indicator of prognosis | Post-traumatic amnesia (PTA): time interval between head injury and the return of normal, continuous memory. Duration is fixed, and is a good indicator of prognosis. PTA of less than 12 hours indicates the likelihood of full recovery. | Continuous memory |

Fig. 9.3 Memory impairment after head injury

2. Psychiatric Complications

The development of mental disorder following a head injury is more likely when trauma is severe, especially if it is associated with brain damage or epilepsy. Other risk factors include an abnormal premorbid personality, or a personal/family history of psychiatric disorder. **Personality changes** and **neuroses** occur in about one-fifth of severe head injuries, while 10% of cases develop schizophrenic-like, paranoid or affective **psychoses**. **Cognitive impairment** is seen in a small proportion of subjects, especially if the PTA is of more than 24 hours duration.

Post-traumatic stress disorder is a term applied to a constellation of symptoms which occasionally follow relatively trivial head injuries, and are not attributable to any demonstrable organic pathology. The symptoms include headaches, dizziness, fatigue, poor concentration, irritability and intolerance to noise, and are sometimes disproportionately severe to the injury sustained. In some instances, such as following an industrial injury or road traffic accident, victims may resort to litigation to obtain compensation for their disabilities, and it was for this reason that the disorder was initially termed **compensation (or accident) neurosis**. The issue of whether symptom production occurs consciously (malingering) or unconsciously (hysteria) remains undetermined, but there is little evidence to support the concept that the majority of cases resolve once compensation is paid. Indeed, in many instances, symptoms persist despite treatment and a successful outcome to litigation, and can lead to long-standing functional disability.

3. Social Complications

Both organic and psychiatric impairment may result in time off work following a head injury, and this can extend to long-term sick leave or redundancy. Relationship difficulties may also develop, and sometimes lead to marital breakdown and social isolation.

EPILEPSY AND PSYCHIATRIC DISTURBANCE

Epileptic seizures affect approximately one in every 200 people and can be generalised or focal (particularly of the temporal lobe). There is a much greater prevalence of epilepsy among psychiatric inpatients and those with mental retardation when compared with the general population. Mental disorder is especially common in those with **temporal lobe epilepsy**, where convulsions are rare, the seizures being characterised by complex psychomotor manifestations such as automatisms, fugues, mood changes and other phenomena.

The reasons for the increased rate of psychiatric disturbance among epileptics remain unclear, although possible causes include undetected 'brain damage', abnormal mental functioning during the interictal period (between seizures), the side-effects of anticonvulsant drugs, and the stigma associated with the condition. The concept of a specific 'epileptic personality' is no longer accepted.

Preictal Phenomena (before the seizure)

Certain individuals have a tendency to develop **prodromal** moodiness and irritability for several hours or days prior to a seizure. An **aura** is often experienced immediately before the epileptic attack, and may involve hallucinations or illusions, mood changes and feelings of unreality, including the phenomenon of **déjà vu**. This is a sudden feeling of familiarity with a place or situation which the individual knows he has not previously encountered.

Ictal and Postictal Phenomena (during and after the seizure)

These are most commonly associated with temporal lobe seizures, usually in the absence of a convulsion. **Automatisms** involve the performance of simple or complex actions in a state of clouded consciousness, so that the subject is unaware of his behaviour. Episodes rarely last for more than a few minutes, and often commence with the individual seeming dazed and staring vacantly ahead. This may be followed by complex facial movements, such as repetitive blinking, chewing or lip-smacking. Sometimes, the subject wanders about in an apparently purposeful manner, and might pick up objects or move items of furniture around. Once the automatism is completed, he may appear confused and suspicious, since he has no memory of the incident. Very rarely, criminal acts are judged in court to have taken place during an automatism, as a result of which the defendant is not considered fully responsible for his behaviour (*see* Chapter 24).

Fugues involve wandering behaviour during a seizure, and are associated with amnesia for the episode. There is clouding of consciousness and those affected have been known to travel great distances from their point of origin. Fugues can also occur in the setting of a depressive illness or hysterical disorder.

Twilight states involve a subjective alteration of awareness, so that emotionally significant experiences and perceptions have a dream-like quality. The episode usually lasts for several hours, during which time psychomotor retardation and perseveration of movements or speech occur.

Transient hallucinatory experiences are quite common in temporal lobe epilepsy, and may involve any of the sensory modalities.

Interictal Phenomena (between seizures)

Psychiatric disturbance is common during the interictal period (especially between temporal lobe seizures), with **neuroses**, such as anxiety, minor depressive and phobic states being the most frequently encountered forms of mental disorder. By comparison, **psychoses** are relatively rare; illnesses which are clinically indistinguishable from schizophrenia have been reported as occurring in the interictal phase in those with temporal lobe epilepsy of the dominant lobe, and are said by some authorities to be more common when the frequency of seizures is diminished. This may explain why psychotic symptoms develop, or are sometimes exacerbated, when fits are well controlled with anticonvulsant drugs. Interictal affective psychoses, which are most commonly depressive, are thought to be associated with non-dominant temporal lobe seizures.

Epileptics do not differ from the general population with regard to intelligence, but in a small proportion of cases, a **dementia** develops involving diffuse cerebral atrophy and personality deterioration. This seems to be more likely where there is underlying brain damage, or where the epilepsy is chronic and severe. It has also been proposed that the dementia is related to long-term administration of anticonvulsant drugs, but so far this theory remains unproven.

There is no definite link between epilepsy and **criminal behaviour**, although the prevalence of the disorder among prisoners is slightly greater than in the general population. The reasons for this are undetermined.

VITAMIN DEFICIENCIES

Thiamine (vitamin B₁) deficiency is most commonly associated with alcohol abuse, and may result in the development of Wernicke's encephalopathy or Korsakoff's psychosis. Both conditions are discussed in detail in Chapter 11.

Nicotinic acid deficiency can result in the condition known as pellagra, characterised by dermatitis, diarrhoea and dementia. During the acute stages, the individual may be emotionally labile and delirious.

Folate deficiency is sometimes seen in patients receiving anticonvulsant medication. It can cause a macrocytic anaemia and, in severe untreated cases, dementia.

Vitamin B$_{12}$ deficiency is associated with the development of pernicious anaemia and subacute combined degeneration of the spinal cord. However, these physical manifestations may be preceded by apathy, depression and occasionally, a paranoid psychosis. In common with other vitamin deficiencies, acute or chronic organic reactions can occur.

METABOLIC AND ENDOCRINE DISORDERS

Several metabolic and endocrine conditions may cause psychiatric organic reactions (Tables 9.5 and 9.6).

CEREBRAL HYPOXIA

An impaired oxygen supply to the brain may result from a number of cardiorespiratory and vascular disorders. These include acute myocardial infarction, cardiac failure, severe anaemia, blood loss, bronchopneumonia and chronic obstructive airways disease. Acute hypoxia, particularly in the elderly, can lead to confusion or delirium, whereas chronic hypoxic states may cause irreversible brain damage and dementia.

TOXIC REACTIONS

Various prescribed and illicit drugs (Table 9.7) can produce an acute organic reaction in susceptible individuals. A toxic reaction can also occur following the inhalation of **carbon monoxide**, which may lead to cerebral hypoxia resulting in confusion, delirium and, if prolonged, dementia. Excessive **lead** ingestion can produce a toxic state, which might eventually progress to dementia. The characteristic clinical picture in **mercury poisoning** is one of irritability, anxiety and a coarse tremor, occasionally accompanied by features of an acute organic reaction.

SPACE-OCCUPYING LESIONS

The characteristics of any psychiatric or neurological symptoms which develop in association with space-occupying lesions of the brain will

Table 9.5 Metabolic disorders

Disorder	Psychological symptoms and other features
Hepatic failure	Acute encephalopathy arises from failure to prevent toxins entering the general circulation and reaching the brain. Psychological symptoms include drowsiness and delirium, sometimes progressing to coma. The condition runs a fluctuating course, and during periods of remission, personality and mood changes may be evident (such as emotional lability, apathy and disinhibition)
Renal failure	Presenting features include drowsiness, fatigue, low mood and poor concentration. Where uraemia is severe, there may be additional memory impairment and psychomotor retardation. Subsequently, epileptic seizures or (rarely) a paranoid psychosis can develop
Acute intermittent porphyria	An inherited defect of haemoglobin metabolism, transmitted by an autosomal dominant gene, resulting in the formation of the metabolite, porphobilinogen. Attacks may occur spontaneously or be precipitated by infection, pregnancy or drugs (barbiturates, alcohol, anticonvulsants, oral contraceptives, anti-inflammatory agents and hypoglycaemics). Mild cases often go unrecognised, and the condition is commonly seen in young adults. As well as gastrointestinal and neurological symptoms, psychiatric complications include lability of mood, confusion, delirium and schizophrenic-like psychoses
Wilson's disease (hepatolenticular degeneration)	An inherited defect of copper metabolism, transmitted by an autosomal recessive gene, which results in a deficiency of the enzyme, caeruloplasmin. Excessive copper is deposited in the liver, kidney, basal ganglia and eye. Psychiatric manifestations include personality changes, affective and schizophrenic-like psychoses, as well as intellectual decline which may progress to dementia
Fluid and electrolyte disturbances	Sodium or potassium depletion are the most frequent disorders encountered, resulting in fatigue, apathy, depression, anxiety or an acute organic reaction

Table 9.6 Endocrine disorders

Disorder	Psychological symptoms and other features
Hypothyroidism	Psychiatric complications are common and the condition may be mistaken for a primary mental disorder. Features include depressed mood, fatigue, apathy, poor concentration and psychomotor retardation. Severe hypothyroidism may result in the development of 'myxoedema madness', in which delirium is sometimes associated with a paranoid psychosis. Epilepsy, ataxia and coma can also occur, while dementia may develop in chronic cases
Thyrotoxicosis	Frequently misdiagnosed as a primary psychiatric disorder. The mood is usually anxious and agitated, although depression or (rarely) mania may also occur. Extreme overactivity of the thyroid can result in the development of delirium as part of a 'thyrotoxic crisis'. Schizophrenic-like psychoses are sometimes seen
Cushing's syndrome	May result from overactivity of the adrenal cortex or the prolonged use of steroid drugs. Depression is common, but sometimes the mood is elevated. Delirium or a paranoid psychosis can also occur
Addison's disease	Adrenal failure may result from primary atrophy, infection, surgery or sudden cessation of steroid drugs after prolonged use. Psychiatric symptoms are common and include anxiety, depression, apathy and mild memory impairment. In an 'Addisonian crisis', adrenal hormone levels fall rapidly and can result in the development of delirium
Parathyroid disease	Psychiatric symptoms develop in over half of those with excess or deficiency of parathyroid hormone. The commonest features include anxiety, depression, fatigue or apathy. With very high or low serum calcium levels, impairment of consciousness and seizures may occur
Hypopituitarism	May follow pituitary failure resulting from postpartum haemorrhage, tumour or head injury. Psychiatric symptoms are common and can include irritability, depression, lack of drive and memory impairment. In cases of acute pituitary damage, delirium or coma may ensue
Hypoglycaemia	Most commonly occurs in diabetics who use excessive insulin or omit meals, although rarely may be due to an

continued overleaf

Table 9.6 *Continued*

Disorder	Psychological symptoms and other features
	insulinoma. Symptoms of anxiety are often prominent and may be associated with bizarre or aggressive behaviour. Failure to correct blood glucose levels results in progressive impairment of consciousness and eventual coma. Prolonged periods of hypoglycaemia can lead to irreversible brain damage
Hyperglycaemia	Very high blood glucose levels in diabetics can produce delirium and eventual coma. The development of cerebral arteriosclerosis may result in a slowly progressive dementia
Phaeochromocytoma	Adrenaline and noradrenaline secreted by chromaffin cell tumours of the adrenal medulla or sympathetic ganglia. Episodes of severe anxiety occur in association with hypertension, tachycardia and other signs of autonomic overactivity. It is a rare cause of an acute organic reaction.

depend upon the site and extent of the abnormality, and the nature of the pathological changes which occur (*see* p. 158).

Cerebral Tumour

Psychiatric symptoms are frequently present, and sometimes precede the onset of neurological signs. Raised intracranial pressure is more likely to occur with rapidly growing tumours, often resulting in the development of an acute organic reaction. By contrast, neoplasms which grow slowly are more commonly associated with the development of insidious cognitive impairment. In addition to symptoms of organic reactions, patients with cerebral tumours may present with seizures, features resembling functional illnesses (affective, neurotic or schizophrenic), as well as changes in personality. However, in some cases, relatively large tumours (such as frontal meningiomas) can develop 'silently' and remain undetected for many years.

Cerebral Abscess

A cerebral abscess may develop following a penetrating head injury or secondary to an infection in the middle ear, sinuses, lungs or a more distant site. Rapid formation is associated with an acute onset of delirium, headache, vomiting, pyrexia and evidence of focal neurological signs. By

Table 9.7 Drugs which may cause a toxic organic reaction

Alcohol	Lithium
Amphetamines	LSD
Anticholinergic compounds	MAOI antidepressants
Barbiturates	MARI antidepressants
Benzodiazepines	Neuroleptics
Beta-blockers	Opioids
Cannabis	Oral hypoglycaemics
Cocaine	Phenacetin
Digoxin	Phencyclidine
Isoniazid	Salicylates
L-dopa	Steroids

contrast, a cerebral abscess which develops gradually may be less obvious, and is more likely to go undetected. In such instances, the patient may present with non-specific features of ill health, changes in temperament and mild impairment of consciousness. Neurological signs are often minimal or absent.

Subdural Haematoma

A chronic subdural haematoma can develop following relatively minor head injuries (especially in the elderly), sometimes trivial enough not to be remembered. Because of its slow rate of formation, clinical features may not be apparent for several months after the initial trauma. The condition is characterised by a fluctuating level of consciousness, vague headaches, general slowness and difficulty with concentration or memory. Neurological signs are infrequent.

INFECTIONS

Peripheral infections involving the chest or urinary tract are a common cause of confusion in the elderly. Intracranial infections, notably neurosyphilis, encephalitis, cerebral abscess and meningitis, are much less frequent.

Neurosyphilis

Neurosyphilis is now a rare complication of spirochaetal infection. Three types are recognised: **meningovascular syphilis** produces inflammation of the meninges and cerebral arteries, resulting in irritability, headaches, lethargy and labile mood. **Tabes dorsalis** involves atrophy of the dorsal roots and posterior columns of the spinal cord, and is characterised by ataxia, pain and paraesthesia of the lower limbs. The most important type from the psychiatric viewpoint is **general paresis**, which may develop up to 25 years after the initial infection. Pathological changes comprise thickening of the dura mater, cerebral atrophy (particularly of the frontal lobe), as well as inflammatory and degenerative changes of the cerebral cortex. Psychiatric manifestations include depression, mania, personality changes of a frontal lobe type (apathy and disinhibition), paranoid psychosis and a slowly progressive dementia. Serological testing of the blood or cerebrospinal fluid should be considered in all individuals who show evidence of organic brain disease or any unexplained psychiatric disorder.

Encephalitis

Encephalitis can follow viral infections, such as herpes simplex, influenza and measles (including vaccination), or occur secondary to bacterial meningitis, cerebral abscess and blood-borne infections. Clinical features include a rapid onset of headache, pyrexia and vomiting, often associated with photophobia, neck stiffness, and sometimes papilloedema. An acute organic reaction can develop and may be accompanied by seizures. Those who survive the initial infection may be left with residual neurological deficits, personality changes and cognitive impairment. Epidemics of encephalitis have occasionally been reported, such as the outbreak of **encephalitis lethargica** shortly after the First World War. Following resolution of the acute phase, which was marked by daytime drowsiness and visual disturbance, many sufferers were left with residual features of parkinsonism, as well as undergoing personality changes or developing schizophrenic-like illnesses.

MISCELLANEOUS DISORDERS

Multiple Sclerosis

Psychiatric symptoms frequently develop in association with this remitting condition, in which there is disseminated demyelination throughout the central nervous system, primarily affecting the white matter of the brain and spinal cord. Approximately one-quarter of sufferers become depressed, particularly in the early stages of the illness, often soon after learning the diagnosis. In the later stages, some patients become inappropriately cheerful or frankly euphoric, possibly resulting from a combination of organic brain damage and denial of the disease's implications. Personality changes sometimes occur, and in over 50% of cases some degree of intellectual impairment is evident.

Normal Pressure Hydrocephalus

Early recognition and treatment of this condition are important in order to prevent the development of a dementia. The primary cerebral lesion involves an obstruction in the subarachnoid space (rather than in the ventricles), which prevents the normal circulation of cerebrospinal fluid. Consequently, ventricular dilatation develops, but CSF pressure remains normal. The disorder is more common in the elderly and often of unknown aetiology, although some cases can result from subarachnoid haemorrhage, meningitis or head injury. Characteristic features include the insidious onset of psychomotor retardation, urinary incontinence, an unsteady broad-based gait and progressive dementia. A brain scan reveals enlarged ventricles, although there is no air present in the subarachnoid space. Treatment consists of the insertion of a ventriculo-caval shunt, with some patients showing a good recovery of their intellectual function.

Neuropsychiatric Complications of Non-Metastatic Cancer

Neoplastic lesions are sometimes associated with neuropsychiatric disorders occurring in the absence of cerebral metastases, or developing some time before there is clinical evidence of the disease. Manifestations include encephalopathy, motor or sensory neuropathies and muscular disorders. Some authorities have suggested a metabolic or hormonal basis to account for these complications, while others have implicated some form of immunological disturbance or an associated viral infection. However, at present their cause remains unknown.

SUMMARY

1. **Organic psychiatry** is concerned with those conditions in which mental disorder arises as a result of structural disease of the brain or physiological disturbance affecting cerebral function. Organic reactions may be acute or chronic, while the underlying cerebral lesion can be focal or diffuse, resulting in specific or global impairment of brain function.
2. In **acute organic reactions** there is impairment in the level of consciousness which can also be distorted by perceptual abnormalities (delirium). Onset is rapid and the condition tends to run a fluctuating course. The commonest precipitants are alcohol withdrawal, illicit or prescribed drugs, peripheral infection and cerebral hypoxia. In addition to identification and treatment of the underlying cause, management should aim to minimise confusion and disorientation, and correct disturbances of fluid or electrolyte balance.
3. **Chronic organic reactions** are characterised by a global impairment of

all cerebral functions in a setting of clear consciousness. Onset is gradual, and the condition tends to run a progressive, irreversible course. There is frequently evidence of structural brain damage. Senile (SDAT) and multi-infarct dementia (MID) are the commonest forms of the disorder. In SDAT, a progressive decline in intellect, memory and personality may be accompanied by wandering, self-neglect and socially unacceptable behaviour. Associated physical deterioration usually results in death from an intercurrent illness. In MID, deterioration tends to be stepwise, with intermittent periods of relative stability. The presenile dementias include Alzheimer's disease, Creutzfeldt-Jakob disease, Pick's disease and Huntington's chorea. Parkinson's disease results from degeneration of dopamine-producing cells in the basal ganglia, and is commonly associated with depressive symptoms and occasionally dementia.

Those who show signs of dementia should be fully assessed to exclude treatable causes. In irreversible cases, management is directed towards preserving the quality of life, and maintaining the subject at an optimal level of functioning for as long as possible, preferably at home.

4. **Head injuries** can result in the development of long-term physical, psychological or social problems. Neurotic symptoms and personality changes are the most common psychiatric sequelae. Prolonged impairment of consciousness following a head injury decreases the likelihood of full recovery. Post-traumatic amnesia is the best indicator of prognosis, a duration in excess of 24 hours being associated with residual disabilities such as brain damage, epilepsy or intellectual impairment. Mental disorder is more common in those with **epilepsy**, especially temporal lobe seizures. In the latter, convulsions are rare and seizures are characterised by automatisms, perceptual abnormalities, fugues, and other phenomena. Psychiatric disturbance is sometimes evident between seizures.

5. Vascular disorders, vitamin deficiencies, metabolic and endocrine dysfunction, cerebral hypoxia and toxins can all give rise to either acute or chronic organic reactions. Space-occupying lesions of the brain (tumour, abscess or haematoma) may produce both psychiatric and neurological symptoms. Depending on the nature, site and extent of the lesion, organic reactions, personality changes and disorders resembling functional illnesses can all occur. Similar manifestations may be seen with neurosyphilis, encephalitis, multiple sclerosis, and non-metastatic cancer. The early detection and treatment of normal pressure hydrocephalus can sometimes lead to a good recovery of intellectual function.

REFERENCES AND FURTHER READING

Byrne, J., Arie, T. (1985). Rational drug treatment of dementia? *British Medical Journal*; **290**: 1845–46.

Cohen, R. I., Pfeffer, J. M. (1987). Accident neurosis revisited. *Medicine, Science and the Law*; **27**: 177–80.

Davison, K. (1985). Drug treatment of organic brain syndromes. *British Journal of Hospital Medicine*; **34**: 112–15.

Flor-Henry, P. (1976). Epilepsy and psychopathology. In *Recent Advances in Clinical Psychiatry-2* (Granville-Grossman, K. L., ed.), Edinburgh: Churchill Livingstone.

Lishman, W. A. (1987). *Organic Psychiatry: The Psychological Consequences of Cerebral Disorder*, 2nd edn. Oxford: Blackwell.

Mulley, G. P. (1986). Differential diagnosis of dementia. *British Medical Journal*; **292**: 1416–18.

Scott, D. F. (1978). Psychiatric aspects of epilepsy. *British Journal of Psychiatry*; **132**: 417–30.

10 PSYCHIATRY IN THE ELDERLY

The psychiatry of old age has become increasingly important in recent years due to the relative growth in the number of elderly people within the total population, and the resultant increase in those over the age of 65 who suffer from psychiatric disorder.

THE SIZE OF THE PROBLEM

Fifteen per cent of the population in the UK (currently about 7.5 million people) are aged over 65, but this figure will probably rise to 20% by the year 2000. This is a consequence of an almost static birth rate, combined with improved health care measures, leading to an increasingly aged society.

The psychogeriatrician is concerned with the management of mental illness occurring for the first time in old age, and in some regions, with the continuing care of those suffering from long-standing psychiatric disorders who have reached the age of 65. Studies have indicated that more than a quarter of the over-65s have some type of psychiatric disorder (Table 10.1), the majority living outside hospital, either in their own homes or in some form of residential accommodation. The remainder, however, still occupy a significant number of acute or long-stay psychiatric hospital beds. Consequently, although the planning and organisation of psycho-

Table 10.1 Prevalence of psychiatric disorder in the over-65s

Disorder	Prevalence
Dementia and other organic brain disorders	5% severe 5% mild
Functional psychoses	5% approx.
Neuroses and personality disorders	12%

geriatric services is largely **community orientated**, it also entails the provision of facilities for those in need of hospital care (*see later*).

AETIOLOGY

Although psychological problems in the elderly are frequently multi-factorial in origin, the influence of **physical illness** and **social stressors** is often greater than in younger age groups. Because the likelihood of cerebral and systemic disease increases with advancing age, the elderly are more prone to develop organic brain disorders (dealt with in Chapter 9, which should be read in conjunction with this section). In addition, when illness results in physical dysfunction or immobility, the capacity for independent living is frequently diminished, and dependence on others may cause a loss of self-esteem and a predisposition towards the development of psychiatric disorder.

Old age is a time when other **losses** must inevitably be faced. The death of a spouse can lead to loneliness and isolation, while retirement may result in financial hardship, loss of status and a diminished sense of purpose in life. Living off a pension or fixed income forces many elderly people to make economies which can be detrimental to their mental and physical health. Consequently, homes are frequently heated inadequately or allowed to fall into disrepair, and shopping bills are reduced by buying less food or only poor-quality items. Any of these factors may act to precipitate or accentuate psychological problems.

The elderly are less able to adjust to social and other changes which often have to be dealt with, and this **lack of adaptability** tends to increase the amount of stress to which they are subjected. Even seemingly positive steps can have adverse consequences. For example, moving from unsuitable accommodation to a warm and pleasant residential home sometimes results in unhappiness or depression due to a perceived loss of independence or a feeling of isolation, especially if this involves a move away from family or friends. A **vulnerable premorbid personality** or a **past history of psychiatric disorder** are additional factors which can predispose to the development of mental illness.

ASSESSMENT OF PSYCHOLOGICAL PROBLEMS IN OLD AGE

Normal ageing produces a gradual, but slight, deterioration of memory, as well as a decrease in the speed at which both physical and psychological tasks are performed. Less interest tends to be shown in contemporary events and the outside world, and conversation often focuses on the past rather than the present. The ability to make or accept changes in lifestyle also diminishes, and unfavourable personality traits (such as meanness or egocentricity) may become accentuated to intolerable proportions. Consequently, it is sometimes difficult to distinguish between the physical and psychological changes of normal ageing, and those which indicate the onset of illness.

Although thorough history-taking and examination of the mental and physical state are important aspects of assessment, some additional information is usually required when evaluating problems in this age group. Management decisions concerning the elderly are largely determined by an individual's ability to cope in his current environment, the extent and effectiveness of his support system, and the presence of any factors which constitute a risk to personal safety or that of others. For these reasons, it is preferable to conduct the initial assessment in the subject's home or current dwelling. The **domiciliary visit** not only presents an opportunity to observe living conditions, but also allows a determination of how the person functions in familiar surroundings. Relatives or neighbours are often available to provide collateral information, which is particularly important if memory problems or failing intellectual abilities prevent the subject from giving a coherent and reliable account of his difficulties.

In deciding whether or not the patient can be managed at home, it is necessary to determine if his basic needs (warmth, food, personal hygiene and finances) are adequately catered for, and if any behavioural problems (such as leaving on the gas, wandering, antisocial conduct) present an unacceptable risk to his safety. It is also important to consider how much support the individual is receiving from relatives, neighbours or professional agencies, and whether any further input is required.

Special attention should be paid in the **history** to determine the onset of the presenting problem, and to identify any likely precipitants, such as adverse life events. Sometimes, this information can only be obtained from relatives or the general practitioner, who may also give details of past psychiatric and physical disorders, as well as any medication the patient is taking. Finally, it is helpful to know how the person spends a typical day, in order to gain an overall impression of his level of functioning and the impact any current problems have on his life.

The **mental state examination** should always include a detailed assessment of cognitive function. It is often helpful to supplement clinical examination with some form of **psychometric testing**. Although many tests are essentially the realm of the clinical psychologist, others can be readily administered by ward staff with only minimal training. The Clifton Assessment Procedure for the Elderly (CAPE) is a brief method for evaluating mental and behavioural competence in the elderly. Using scores obtained from tests of basic skills (such as orientation, counting, reading and drawing) and observations of behaviour, subjects can be graded to indicate their level of disability and the degree of care they are likely to need. Information of this kind is not only useful for diagnostic purposes, but also for assessing progress following treatment. Other similar tests which are used include the Mini-Mental Score, the Kendrick Battery and the Roth-Hopkins test for dementia (*see* glossary).

A **physical examination** should be performed to identify any major systemic disorder, as well as to establish whether there are any defects of sight or hearing. A rectal examination is particularly important, since the discomfort caused by faecal impaction is often a cause of agitation or apparent confusion. **Investigations** for suspected organic disorders are discussed on p. 166.

GENERAL ASPECTS OF TREATMENT

Where possible, elderly people with psychiatric disorders should be treated at **home** rather than in hospital, since the majority value their independence and function better in their own environment. **Hospital admission** is sometimes necessary for further assessment of the case or may be required if the individual's social supports are inadequate. Additional indications are when treatment in the community has failed or is not feasible, or when the patient's mental disorder is of a nature or degree which constitutes a significant risk to his well-being or the safety of others. Because psychological and physical problems commonly coexist, many units caring for the elderly are jointly run by geriatricians and psychiatrists.

When prescribing **psychotropic drugs** for the elderly, certain precautions should always be borne in mind:

1. A careful assessment of possible physical contraindications to drug therapy should be made prior to commencing treatment. If treatment with antidepressants is contemplated, it is usually advisable to perform an ECG to exclude arrhythmias, conduction defects or evidence of myocardial infarction. Similarly, renal and hepatic function should be adequate before drug therapy is commenced.
2. Drugs should be prescribed in lower doses than for younger adults because of the risk of toxic reactions and an increased tendency to develop side-effects.
3. Dosages should be increased slowly because of the small difference between therapeutic and toxic effects.
4. In order to improve compliance, it is preferable to make drug regimens as simple as possible (once or twice daily), to involve community care workers or relatives in the supervision of medication if the patient is confused or forgetful, to give written and verbal instructions regarding the correct dosages and to see the patient at regular intervals.

5. It is advisable to avoid polypharmacy, in order to minimise the likelihood of dangerous or unpredictable drug interactions. The prescriber should limit his therapeutic repertoire to a small number of compounds with which he is familiar.

Psychological treatments in the elderly emphasise the role of supportive psychotherapy and practical advice, rather than analytical interpretations. Aims should be clearly defined and attention given towards improving self-esteem. Seeing the patient together with other family members may help to identify areas of conflict and frustration, as well as define individual needs and reduce levels of stress. Behavioural modification can sometimes be of help in reducing undesirable behaviour (such as aggressiveness or constant shouting) or improving control over basic physical functions (e.g. incontinence in demented patients may be reduced by regular toileting). Reality orientation is often used with confused patients, and involves the regular provision of basic information (such as the time of day or their whereabouts) in an attempt to minimise disorientation and distress.

Social measures aim to reduce isolation and increase opportunities for independent functioning. It is essential to liaise with social services at an early stage in planning home care, since support is available through a number of facilities. These include the provision of a home help, meals-on-wheels, laundry incontinence services, 'twilight nurses' and financial aid for carers in the form of an attendance allowance. It may sometimes help to arrange for the patient to attend either a day centre or day hospital where multidisciplinary assessment and care can be organised. Regular visits from voluntary workers or members of the primary care team are also an important feature of community support (*see later*). Occupational therapy can help to improve physical mobility, as well as teach self-care, social and domestic skills.

Elderly people who are no longer able to live in their own home (but are still capable of some degree of independent living) may be offered **sheltered accommodation** in a warden-controlled flat, residential home or unit for the elderly mentally ill. For those with mild impairment in mental and behavioural functioning, warden-supervised accommodation is often appropriate. In this setting, elderly people live in a complex of self-contained flats, sometimes centred around a large communal area, such as a lounge or television room. This serves to preserve independence and privacy, but also overcomes the problems of loneliness and isolation by allowing residents to socialise with one another when they wish to do so. Each home is usually equipped with an alarm linked directly to the warden's on-site flat, so that help is readily at hand when needed. Residential homes for the elderly are suitable for those people who have retained certain basic social skills, but are no longer capable of independent living. Residents are expected to be ambulant and continent, and require only minimal assistance with dressing, washing and feeding themselves. Homes of this type are sometimes referred to as **Part III accommodation**, named after that part of the 1948 National Assistance Act which requires local authorities to provide such establishments for the care of the elderly.

AFFECTIVE DISORDERS IN THE ELDERLY

Depression is a common disorder of late life, and although the initial response to treatment is often favourable, the long-term prognosis is generally poor with a high rate of relapse. Despite an overall predominance of females, elderly men are much more likely to become depressed than those in younger age groups, and they frequently present a significant suicidal risk.

The aetiology of depression is discussed in detail in Chapter 5. Its development in the elderly is more likely to be associated with cerebral disease or systemic illness, and is sometimes caused or exacerbated by the drugs used to treat these conditions. Life events, such as bereavement or retirement, are other common precipitants, while social isolation and loneliness may serve to perpetuate depressive symptoms.

Elderly people who become depressed do not always readily complain of low mood, but instead may describe feelings of emptiness or lack of emotion. Worries or preoccupations about physical health, financial status or social circumstances are other presenting features of a depressive illness. Anorexia and weight loss can be severe, while constipation and disrupted sleep are frequent complaints. Agitation is common, although sometimes the picture is one of apathy and psychomotor retardation. When the latter is severe, self-neglect and refusal to eat or drink can lead to a life-threatening situation. Delusions and hallucinations may be associated with depressed mood, centring around ideas and feelings of persecution, ill-health, guilt, nihilism and worthlessness. Suicidal thoughts and feelings of hopelessness are often expressed (*see* Chapter 7 for details of asssessment and management).

A 74-year-old woman was referred to her local psychogeriatric unit with a 3-month history of difficulty in swallowing and weight loss. Extensive physical investigations had revealed no abnormality, and although she denied any psychological symptoms, a psychiatric opinion was sought. At interview, she appeared tense and unhappy, insisting that she was not mad and that there was definitely a lump in her gullet which she could feel on swallowing. Detailed assessment of her mental state was not possible since she refused to answer questions, and she angrily terminated the interview by walking out after only a few minutes.

The psychiatrist liaised with the woman's general practitioner, who agreed to review her regularly. Three weeks later, he reported a marked deterioration in her condition. She had attended surgery in a state of great distress, complaining that her throat and bowels were now completely blocked, and that she was unable to eat or drink anything. She apologised repeatedly for the 'foul stench' which she believed she gave off, attributing it to the trapped and rotting contents of her stomach. When reassured by the doctor that he could smell nothing unpleasant, she became tearful and began talking about the pointlessness of her life. She expressed a wish to die since no one would help or believe her.

She was subsequently reassessed by the psychogeriatrician who was unable to persuade her to come into hospital. He considered that she was suffering from a depressive illness marked by hypochondriacal delusions and associated olfactory hallucinations. In view of her refusal to eat or drink and the presence of suicidal ideation, she was compulsorily admitted to hospital. Following admission, she declined all forms of treatment, expressing a wish either to have her throat cut open or be left to die. In view of the clinical features with which she presented, and the risk of serious deterioration in her mental and physical condition, ECT was considered to be the most appropriate form of treatment. Since the patient was unwilling to give consent, a second opinion was sought, and following a consideration of the case by an independent doctor from the Mental Health Act Commission, authorisation was given for ECT to be administered. After two treatments, she began to eat and drink with only minimal persuasion, although she still insisted that her throat was obstructed. She continued to improve steadily as the course of ECT progressed, and after ten treatments her symptoms had completely resolved.

Distinguishing symptoms of a depressive illness from feelings of unhappiness, which are commonly experienced by elderly people who are lonely and isolated, can sometimes be difficult. In the case of the latter, the capacity to enjoy life is often retained, even if the opportunity to do so has been lost. The presence of biological features of depression may also be helpful in establishing the diagnosis. However, care must be taken when interpreting the significance of symptoms such as anorexia and weight loss, since they may be a manifestation of physical illness. The importance of differentiating between affective disorder and dementia is discussed on p. 165. In most cases, the correct diagnosis can be reached by a careful appraisal of the history and mental state, as well as the results of any physical and psychometric investigations.

The diagnosis of **mania** and **hypomania** in the elderly can present a difficult problem because the core features of elation, hyperactivity and flight of ideas are frequently absent. Instead, the clinical picture is often one of irritability and overtalkativeness, associated with paranoid ideas, aggressiveness and disinhibited behaviour. Mixed affective states are more common in this age group, where manic behaviour may be seen in association with a depressed mood.

The **management** of affective disorders is fully discussed in Chapter 5.

Summarised below are those aspects of treatment which are especially important in the elderly.

1. Co-existing physical illness should be vigorously treated.
2. Antidepressant medication needs to be prescribed cautiously (and often in lower dosages) because of the increased risk of toxicity and unwanted side-effects.
3. Lithium can be useful in the management of bipolar affective disorder, although particular care should be taken in supervising its administration, and in ensuring that renal and thyroid function are adequate.
4. ECT may be considered the treatment of choice in cases of severe depression, especially if the patient is deluded, retarded, suicidal or not eating and drinking adequately. It might also be appropriate in those instances where antidepressant medication has failed or is contraindicated.
5. It is important to identify and deal with any adverse social factors which may have contributed to the present illness, or are likely to increase the risk of relapse following recovery, such as poor housing or social isolation.

OTHER FUNCTIONAL DISORDERS

Neuroses rarely occur for the first time in old age, and are more likely to be a resurgence of disorders present earlier in life, or associated with the development of physical illness.

The diagnosis and management of **schizophrenia** and **paranoid states** are discussed in Chapter 8.

PSYCHIATRIC SERVICES FOR THE ELDERLY

Psychogeriatric services should aim to provide care for patients with all types of mental disorder, and not concentrate solely on the needs of the demented. A **multidisciplinary approach** to patient care (*see* Chapter 1) is particularly appropriate in the psychogeriatric setting. The team usually consists of the psychogeriatrician and junior medical staff, clinical psychologist, social worker, hospital-based and community psychiatric nurses, and occupational therapist. From time to time, other professionals or key workers are included in the assessment and management of patients, such as the geriatrician, general practitioner and field social worker.

In addition to the provision of community services and residential accommodation discussed earlier, **hospital-based facilities** are also required. Long-stay beds are necessary to meet the needs of those with dementia and other chronic conditions who cannot survive in the community. Some beds are assigned for holiday admissions, in order to give relatives and other care givers respite from their responsibilities for a few weeks during the year. Acute beds may be used for the purposes of assessment or for the treatment and rehabilitation of those with remediable psychiatric disorders. Day hospital facilities provide a similar range of functions, but are more appropriate for those whose condition does not warrant inpatient care. Follow-up of patients is often conducted by community nurses and general practitioners, as well as at hospital out-patient clinics.

SUMMARY

1. Approximately 15% of the UK population is currently aged over 65, and of this group, about one-quarter have some form of psychiatric disorder. The **causation** of psychological problems in the elderly is frequently multifactorial, although physical illness and social stressors have a greater influence than in younger age groups. The majority of the elderly mentally ill live outside of hospital, so that the planning of psychogeriatric services is largely community orientated.

2. The domiciliary visit is an important aspect of **assessment** which permits an appraisal of living conditions, the patient's level of functioning and coping resources, and the existence of any risk factors, as well as an opportunity to obtain further information from relatives or friends. Examination of the mental state should always include a detailed assessment of cognitive function, which may need to be supplemented by psychometric testing. Physical examination is particularly important, and should look for evidence of a neurological or other systemic disorder, as well as identifying defects of sight or hearing.

3. A multidisciplinary approach to patient care is particularly appropriate in the psychogeriatric setting. Elderly patients are best managed at **home**, providing their basic needs are catered for and their support system is adequate. **Hospital admission** is sometimes necessary for further assessment, or when treatment in the community has failed or is not feasible. Long-stay admission wards provide a high degree of nursing supervision for those whose disabilities are severe. Other hospital-based facilities include holiday and acute admission beds and day hospital care. **Psychotropic drugs** should be prescribed with care because of the risk of toxic reactions and side-effects. To improve compliance, dosage regimens need to be simple, drugs should be supervised by relatives or friends if the patient is confused or forgetful and medication reviewed at regular intervals.

4. **Psychological treatments** should emphasise the use of simple supportive

techniques as a way of improving self-esteem. Family meetings are often useful to identify areas of conflict and reduce stress. Behavioural modification can help to reduce undesirable behaviour, or improve control over basic physical functions. Reality orientation may help to minimise disorientation and distress. **Social measures** aim to reduce isolation, and increase independent functioning through the use of day centres, community services, visits by voluntary and primary health care workers and occupational therapy. For those people no longer capable of independent living, **sheltered accommodation** may be offered.

5. **Depression** is a common disorder of late life, the overall prognosis being poor with a high rate of relapse. Depressed mood is not always the presenting feature, and worries about health, finances or social circumstances may be the overriding complaint. Agitation is common, although apathy and retardation may be marked, and can result in a life-threatening situation. Biological features are sometimes severe. Delusions and hallucinations may occur, and the risk of suicide (especially in elderly single men) should always be considered. **Mania** and **hypomania** can cause diagnostic problems in the elderly, because hyperactivity and elation are frequently absent. Hospital admission is often necessary for the treatment of affective disorders in the elderly, and antidepressants, lithium and ECT all have a place in management. It is important to identify and deal with any adverse social factors which may have precipitated the illness or increase the risk of subsequent relapse following recovery.

REFERENCES AND FURTHER READING

Health Advisory Service (1982). *The Rising Tide: Developing Services for Mental Illness in Old Age.* Sutherland House, Sutton, Surrey SM2 5AN.

Kay, D. W., Beamish, P., Roth, M. (1964). Old age mental disorders in Newcastle-on-Tyne. Part 1, a study of prevalence. *British Journal of Psychiatry*; **110**: 146–58.

Murphy, E. (1983). The prognosis of depression in old age. *British Journal of Psychiatry*; **142**: 111–19.

Pattie, A. H., Gilleard, C. J. (1979). *Manual for the Clifton Assessment Procedures for the Elderly (CAPE).* Sevenoaks: Hodder and Stoughton Educational.

Williamson, J., Stokoe, I. H., Gray, et al. (1964). Old people at home: their unreported needs. *Lancet*; **i**: 1117–20.

11

THE ABUSE OF ALCOHOL
AND OTHER DRUGS

The abuse of alcohol and other drugs is increasing worldwide, so that virtually every government is now concerned with the control of drug trafficking and the spread of addiction. Alcohol is still the most widely abused drug in Europe, but because it forms an integral part of the social activities, business life and religious practice of many cultures, it is generally thought of as being far less harmful than other addictive substances which are obtained and used illicitly. Despite this, alcohol dependence is the biggest public health problem in the UK, resulting in immeasurable human suffering and costing industry over one billion pounds a year in lost revenue. The abuse of other drugs and the specific problems associated with them follow in the second part of this chapter.

It is helpful at this stage to consider some of the terms which are frequently used in association with the problems of substance abuse and dependence. A **drug** is any substance that is taken into a living organism and modifies one or more of its functions. **Drug abuse** is persistent or occasional excessive use of a drug which is out of keeping with accepted medical practice.

After a while tolerance and dependence may develop. **Tolerance** refers to the way the body adapts to the repeated presence of a drug, so that the user has to increase the dose to achieve the original effect. **Dependence** describes a compulsion to take the drug following its repeated administration.

Dependence is of two types, physical and psychological. **Physical dependence** is said to exist when a specific group of symptoms occur after the individual stops taking the drug. These **withdrawal symptoms** have a well-defined course and are unpleasant, but they can be stopped or prevented by further drug-taking.

Psychological dependence is present when a craving for the drug exists in order to experience its psychic effects, and sometimes to avoid the discomfort of its absence. This may result in 'drug-seeking behaviour', such as pressurising doctors for drugs or embarking on a life-style exclusively aimed at obtaining supplies, and at times resorting to criminal behaviour to do so.

ALCOHOL ABUSE

Used in moderation, alcohol confers a number of apparent advantages, such as increased confidence, a sense of well-being and temporary respite from stress. The vast majority of drinkers experience no long-term ill effects, but in a minority, problems develop through misuse.

The term **alcoholic** has serious limitations because the problems associated with alcohol abuse are so diverse and can occur with widely varying levels of consumption. This is evident in the World Health Organisation's definition of alcoholics:

> Those excessive drinkers whose dependence on alcohol has attained such a degree that it shows noticeable disturbance or an interference with their bodily and mental health, their personal relationships and smooth economic functioning, or who show prodromal signs of such a development. They therefore require treatment.

A more useful and practical descriptive system uses the term **alcohol-related disabilities**, which can manifest as physical, psychological and social difficulties. The proportion of people who develop these problems within a given population has been shown to rise in relation to total alcohol consumption.

Epidemiology

The number of drinkers and the amount they consume is obviously difficult to determine accurately. In the UK approximately 2 million people are **excessive drinkers**, of whom one half are thought to be **problem drinkers**, a subgroup of these being **dependent** on alcohol (estimated between 250 000 and 500 000).

Excessive drinkers are men who regularly consume more than 21 units, or women who consume more than 14 units of alcohol/week (*see below*). Even though their drinking may not affect their personal relationships or functioning at work, they are at increased risk of developing many of the physical complications associated with prolonged heavy drinking (*see* Table 11.1), as well as becoming dependent on alcohol.

The **standard unit of alcohol** is an important concept to understand, as it allows reasonably accurate quantification of alcohol consumption, irrespective of the type of beverage.

1 standard unit of alcohol = 10 g of absolute alcohol = half a pint of beer = one single spirit = one glass of wine = one small glass of sherry. A

bottle of spirits contains 28 units, and a bottle of wine 7 units of alcohol*.

The above measures are obviously approximations. By definition, a man who drinks on average more than 10 pints of beer or 10 double measures of whisky per week is an excessive drinker. There is considerable debate as to the levels of consumption which constitute an upper limit for 'safe drinking', but many authorities consider this to be an average of 3 units/day for a man, and 2 units/day for a woman.

Problem drinkers are those in whom alcohol consumption is either continuously or intermittently out of control, thereby causing physical, psychological or social damage to themselves or other people.

Dependent drinkers are those in whom signs or symptoms of alcohol withdrawal develop when they stop drinking. The term **alcoholic** is commonly applied to this group, but currently, the expression **alcohol dependence syndrome** is used in a wider context to describe not only a state of mental or physical disturbance when alcohol is withdrawn, but also recognisable patterns of drinking behaviour. These include:

1. narrowing of the drinking repertoire: drinking takes on a set pattern to avoid withdrawal symptoms, as opposed to the day-to-day variation which occurs in those not dependent on alcohol
2. increased tolerance to alcohol: large amounts of alcohol can be consumed with only minimal signs of intoxication
3. prominence of drink-seeking behaviour: drinking becomes the principal activity at the expense of other pursuits
4. repeated withdrawal symptoms (*see later*)
5. relief or avoidance of withdrawal symptoms by further drinking
6. subjective awareness of loss of control over drinking: further alcohol is consumed despite any desire to stop
7. reinstatement after abstinence: drinking after a period of abstention is likely to result in a rapid recurrence of the alcohol dependence syndrome.

The **prevalence** of alcohol abuse may be determined in a number of ways, including the estimation of mortality rates from cirrhosis of the liver, the number of hospital admissions for alcohol-related disabilities, and by measurement of per capita (average) consumption of alcohol in a population. In all age groups, men outnumber women by approximately 2:1, although consumption among females is increasing more rapidly.

Certain **occupations** are associated with a higher risk of alcohol abuse.

---

*In the UK spirit strength is given as 'proof' — that mixture of alcohol and water which when added to gunpowder would just permit it to ignite — 70° proof = approximately 40% alcohol. Wine contains about 15% alcohol, sherry and fortified wine about 18–20% alcohol.

These include people who work with alcohol (barmen or waiters), those who entertain with alcohol (executives or salesmen), those who work unsocial hours (doctors or journalists), heavy industrial workers (e.g. miners and steelworkers) and members of the merchant navy or armed forces.

Aetiology

A diversity of opinion exists as to whether alcohol abuse is an 'illness', or arises as a result of moral weakness or a lack of self-discipline. The issue has important therapeutic and legal implications, both in determining the attitude and approach of care givers, and the degree of responsibility the habitual drinker must accept for the consequences of his behaviour. At present, the controversy remains unresolved, but it is nevertheless useful to look at the evidence supporting the relative contributions of inherited, organic, psychological and environmental factors in the development of alcohol abuse.

1. GENETIC FACTORS

It is known that alcohol abuse has a tendency to run in families, and a genetic influence is supported by the findings of twin and adoption studies (*see* p. 7). The mode of inheritance is uncertain, but several genes are possibly involved (polygenic model).

2. BIOCHEMICAL THEORIES

Changes involving neurotransmitters within the brain have been postulated in those who become dependent on alcohol. The theory has evolved from the observation that these individuals develop higher blood acetaldehyde levels than non-dependent subjects when they drink. This metabolite then interacts with catecholamines to produce complexes (tetrahydro-isoquinolines) which are similar in structure to morphine alkaloids, and their binding to specific receptor sites in the brain is postulated as stimulating the urge to drink further.

Animal studies indicate that tolerance and dependence may result from an adaptive change in nerve cell membranes.

3. PERSONALITY

There is no firm evidence to support the concept of a unique alcoholic 'character', although certain personality disorders (e.g. psychopathy) are associated with alcohol abuse.

4. LEARNING THEORY

This considers drinking alcohol and its subsequent abuse as a type of learned behaviour derived from:

a. **modelling**: in which drinking habits are based upon those of parents and peer groups
b. **operant conditioning**: whereby the enjoyable effects of alcohol positively reinforce further drinking
c. **classical conditioning**: the sights and sounds associated with drinking become coupled with pleasant alcohol-induced feelings.

5. SOCIOCULTURAL DETERMINANTS

Alcohol abuse is more prevalent in those countries, such as France and Italy, where wine is inexpensive, widely available and forms an integral part of social life. In the UK, the highest rate of alcohol-related problems occurs in Scotland. Worldwide, certain ethnic groups have a low rate of consumption. In the case of the Japanese, for example, this is possibly attributable to the finding that a large percentage of the population have an atypical form of the enzyme alcohol dehydrogenase. This leads to the formation of relatively high levels of acetaldehyde, with resultant unpleasant facial flushing, when only small amounts of alcohol are consumed.

From an early age, peer group pressure is often an important factor in initiating the onset of alcohol abuse; e.g. by encouraging excessive drinking in the form of 'round buying' in public houses. Less adequate individuals may turn to drink to boost their confidence and reduce anxiety about failure and rejection.

ALCOHOL DEPENDENCE

Once dependence is established, a wide spectrum of symptoms can occur when alcohol is withdrawn. These eventually disappear with continued abstinence or if further drinking occurs. They may be conveniently divided into simple withdrawal phenomena, withdrawal fits and delirium tremens.

1. Simple Withdrawal Phenomena

These usually commence a few hours after the last drink and reach a peak within the next 24 hours. Symptoms include tremulousness and agitation, sweating, nausea or vomiting, choking or retching (the 'dry heaves'), hyperacusis and tinnitus, itching, muscle cramps and early morning wakening. Feelings of panic or guilt may also occur.

2. Withdrawal Fits

These occur in about 10% of those dependent on alcohol, and are most likely 24–48 hours after the last drink. They are indistinguishable from epileptic seizures and can be prevented by the prophylactic administration of anticonvulsant drugs.

3. Delirium Tremens

Delirium tremens characteristically begins 2–4 days after cessation of drinking in approximately 5% of those with alcohol dependence. This syndrome has a rapid onset, with impairment and fluctuation in the level of consciousness, resulting in profound confusion and disorientation. The patient also experiences perceptual abnormalities in the form of **illusions** and **hallucinations** which are commonly visual. Typically, these consist of rapidly moving small animals, such as rodents or snakes. **Delusional beliefs** may also develop, particularly with a persecutory content.

Other features of this syndrome include marked insomnia, agitation and restlessness. **Autonomic disturbance** can occur in the form of sweating, tachycardia, dilated pupils and hypertension. **Tremor** is frequently prominent and ataxia might be evident if the patient attempts to walk. **Gastrointestinal disturbances** include nausea, vomiting, diarrhoea and anorexia, which may result in dehydration and electrolyte imbalance. **Infection** and **pyrexia** can be present from the onset in up to half of all cases, so that prophylactic antibiotic cover is frequently necessary.

Delirium tremens often begins at night and persists for several days, with symptoms worse during the hours of darkness. The episode usually ends with a period of deep prolonged sleep, and on awakening, all symptoms have disappeared, with the subject remembering little of the preceding events.

This syndrome is a disorder of the reticular activating system of the brain, which is responsible for arousal and wakefulness. Because alcohol suppresses rapid eye movement (REM) or dream sleep, when drinking ceases there is a rebound of REM manifested by the perceptual abnormalities seen in this condition.

The **management** of delirium tremens must begin with hospitalisation, followed by the prompt administration of some form of sedation, such as **chlordiazepoxide** (Librium) or **chlormethiazole** (Heminevrin). Large doses may initially be required to prevent withdrawal fits and to control overarousal, but should then be gradually tailed off over the course of the next 5–7 days to avoid the development of dependence on the drug. Major tranquillisers are best avoided because they lower the seizure threshold. Frequent or continual observation is very important, and regular communication essential to keep the patient in touch with reality. Dehydration is a common finding and intravenous replacement of fluid and electrolytes is necessary if adequate oral intake is not possible. When infection is present or suspected, it should be treated vigorously with appropriate antibiotic therapy.

It is common practice to give large doses of **vitamin B complex** intramuscularly or intravenously to prevent the development of Wernicke's encephalopathy (*see* p. 203). Blood glucose levels should also be checked at regular intervals to look for hypoglycaemia. The patient is best nursed in a well-lit environment to avoid shadows and areas of darkness. This reduces the likelihood of perceptual abnormalities and confusion. It is important to remember that despite active intervention, delirium tremens carries a mortality rate of approximately 10%.

PSYCHOLOGICAL IMPAIRMENT DUE TO ALCOHOL ABUSE

1. Alcohol Intoxication

The features of alcohol intoxication are well known and the development of inebriation with its variable effects on behaviour, mood and conversation does not need further discussion. An **idiosyncratic response,** resulting in highly irrational or aggressive behaviour, has been described in certain individuals who have consumed only small amounts of alcohol (otherwise referred to as pathological intoxication). This may occur in chronic heavy drinkers who have underlying physical damage to the central nervous system. **Alcoholic blackouts** consist of a total loss of memory for specific events during heavy bouts of drinking, even though at the time the subject appeared fully conscious, and was behaving and conversing normally. Amnesia also occurs with very high levels of blood alcohol, when consciousness is grossly impaired. Because alcohol lowers the seizure threshold, **fits** can occur during drinking in those with an epileptic tendency or the established condition.

2. Alcoholic Dementia

Prolonged alcohol intake can lead to a generalised deterioration of mental functioning (evident on psychological testing), which may later progress to a clinically identifiable dementia. The latter bears the hallmark of all dementing illnesses, in that it is an acquired global deterioration of cerebral function involving intellect, memory and personality, in a setting of clear consciousness (*see* Chapter 9). The condition tends to have a gradual onset and there is usually a history of heavy drinking for many years. Cognitive impairment may be reversible in the early stages. Computerised axial tomography (CAT scanning) reveals cerebral atrophy and enlargement of the ventricles in about 60% of those subjects dependent on alcohol. However, cognitive impairment does not always parallel the degree of cerebral atrophy seen on a CAT scan, since it may arise from subcortical damage (as in the case of Korsakoff's psychosis).

3. Wernicke–Korsakoff Syndrome

Wernicke's encephalopathy and Korsakoff's psychosis represent different stages of the same disorder. **Wernicke's encephalopathy** is the acute reaction to severe **vitamin B₁** (thiamine) **deficiency**, which is most commonly (but not exclusively) encountered in those who abuse alcohol and therefore have a poor nutritional intake. (Other causes of thiamine deficiency are carcinoma of the stomach, malabsorption syndromes, pregnancy, intractable vomiting and malnutrition.) Pathological changes are evident in the walls of the third ventricle, floor of the fourth ventricle, thalamus, mamillary bodies, brain stem and cerebellum. The changes consist of cell loss, petechial haemorrhages and proliferation of blood vessels.

The principal **clinical features** of Wernicke's encephalopathy are: (1) nystagmus, (2) ophthalmoplegia (particularly of the lateral rectus muscle), (3) ataxia, (4) clouding of consciousness and cognitive impairment, (5) peripheral neuropathy. The onset is frequently sudden and may be missed because it shares several of the features of acute alcohol intoxication. Hypotension, tachycardia and abnormal liver function are sometimes evident. Over 80% of untreated cases progress to the chronic phase of **Korsakoff's psychosis**.

The onset of this disorder can be sudden or insidious. Unlike dementing conditions in which there is global impairment of cerebral function, Korsakoff's psychosis involves a specific defect of memory, with preservation of other aspects of intellect and personality. However, it is quite uncommon in its pure form, the clinical picture sometimes being complicated by features of a coexistent global alcoholic dementia.

Although immediate memory, as tested by digit span, is normal, short-term memory (e.g. tested by asking a subject to repeat a name and address after five minutes) is defective. The ability to learn new information is therefore severely impaired, and an **anterograde amnesia** develops. There is also a period of **retrograde amnesia** which extends for weeks, months and occasionally longer before the onset of the illness (Fig. 11.1), although beyond this, long-term memory is unimpaired.

Confabulation, which is a falsification of memory, is often present. It is best explained in terms of a mind devoid of a store of recent memories, drawing on more distant recollections, and therefore is not a deliberate attempt by the patient to deceive the examiner. For example, a patient

← Intact continuous long-term memory	← Retrograde amnesia extending back for weeks or months →	ONSET OF KORSAKOFF'S PSYCHOSIS	Anterograde amnesia becoming longer with time as no new memories are retrievable →

Fig. 11.1 Diagram representing memory defect in Korsakoff's psychosis

who gives an incorrect account of what he had for breakfast that morning may in fact be describing a meal he had some time ago. Some features of Wernicke's encephalopathy, such as nystagmus or peripheral neuropathy, may persist following the development of Korsakoff's psychosis. The memory disturbance is so incapacitating that the development of this condition is frequently devastating to both the patient and his family.

A 46-year-old clerical officer was sent home from work when he developed nausea and vomiting. He complained of some disturbance of vision and pains in his legs, and his wife became concerned when, during the course of the next 24 hours, her husband became increasingly confused and apathetic. He was unsteady on his feet and could only stagger to the toilet with assistance. He was visited by his doctor who decided to admit him to hospital where, on examination, he was noted to have a large tender liver, conjugate gaze paralysis, a grossly ataxic gait and angular stomatitis. In view of the physical findings and the gross level of disorientation he was diagnosed as suffering from Wernicke's encephalopathy. Although his physical condition improved slowly with treatment (see below), he was noted to have gross impairment of memory.

His wife became particularly distressed when she discovered that he had no recollection of her mother dying 3 months beforehand or of having moved house the year before. He described himself as having recently left the merchant navy, which in fact he had done 12 years beforehand. Whereas previously he had been an energetic individual with several hobbies and interests, he now appeared to be content to spend his day sitting quietly in a chair, totally unaware of his plight. Although he could be readily engaged in conversation, its content was limited, and he tended to ask incessantly about the weather and the state of the dahlias in the garden.

His wife described him as 'a man who had always liked a drink', but she was not aware that he had a problem with alcohol. She had noted recently that he ate very little at mealtimes, but she attributed this to the fact that he told her he had a large cooked meal in the pub at lunchtimes. Subsequent information from work colleagues revealed that his lunches were entirely of the liquid variety.

Prevention is the most effective form of treatment and is achieved by giving large doses of intramuscular or intravenous **thiamine** to all patients suspected of abusing alcohol, particularly if they have paid scant attention to their diet. It is often necessary to continue with vitamin supplementation for many months or longer to effect complete resolution of symptoms.

Infection, dehydration and electrolyte disturbance may all require attention in the treatment of Wernicke's encephalopathy.

The **prognosis** is variable, with an approximate mortality rate of 20% in the acute stage. Of those who go on to develop Korsakoff's psychosis, 25% will recover completely with treatment, 50% show partial improvement and the remainder no improvement at all.

Other causes of Korsakoff's psychosis include subarachnoid haemorrhage, hypothalamic tumours, carbon monoxide poisoning, tuberculous meningitis and bilateral occlusion of the posterior cerebral artery.

ASSOCIATED PSYCHIATRIC DISORDERS

1. **Alcoholic hallucinosis** is an uncommon condition in which auditory hallucinations occur in a setting of clear consciousness (in contrast to those of delirium tremens). They often commence with simple sounds such as buzzing, gradually evolving into voices which may be in the second or third person. The content is usually deprecatory or threatening and **paranoid delusions** can develop. Although the experiences are often transient, lasting at most a few days or weeks, 5–10% of cases may last for up to 6 months, in which case treatment with neuroleptic drugs is often helpful. At this stage, a diagnosis of schizophrenia should also be considered. (DSM III-R includes auditory *or* visual hallucinations as diagnostic criteria for alcoholic hallucinosis.)

2. **Affective disorders** have a circular relationship with alcohol abuse. Approximately 10% of those with depressive illnesses drink heavily to relieve their symptoms. On the other hand, many heavy drinkers become depressed, either out of remorse for their behaviour or because of difficulties arising from their abuse of alcohol. In depression which is secondary to drinking, the mood usually lifts within a week or two of stopping alcohol. The risk of suicide is 50 times greater among those who abuse alcohol when compared with the general population, and many acts of deliberate self-harm are carried out under its influence (*see* Chapter 6). Consequently, it is dangerous to give antidepressants to someone who is dependent on alcohol.

3. **Anxiety states** and **phobic disorders** can lead to increased alcohol intake, since anxiety levels are frequently lowered and self-confidence boosted after drinking.

4. **Personality deterioration** tends to occur following prolonged alcohol abuse, and is often characterised by egocentric, dishonest and irresponsible behaviour. **Morbid jealousy** is also associated with excessive drinking (*see* p. 398).

5. **Sexual dysfunction**, such as loss of potency, may result from chronic alcohol abuse. However, this can also be due to the toxic effects of alcohol causing a peripheral neuropathy.

PHYSICAL COMPLICATIONS OF ALCOHOL ABUSE

The abuse of alcohol is associated with numerous physical disorders which are summarised in Table 11.1. Some complications occur before dependency is established and should be actively sought to aid early recognition of the problem drinker.

The Fetal Alcohol Syndrome

Women who drink heavily during pregnancy, particularly in the first 3 months, are at risk of giving birth to babies suffering from this condition. Affected infants tend to be of **low birthweight** and **short in stature.** The skull is small (**microcephaly**) and is frequently associated with mild to moderate **mental retardation**. The **facial appearance** is characteristic, with small eyes, prominent forehead, maxillary hypoplasia and a short upturned nose. Poor muscle tone and incoordination can also occur. The full features of the syndrome are not always present, and some cases of mental retardation without associated physical abnormalities may be attributable to heavy maternal drinking in pregnancy.

The question as to what constitutes 'safe' drinking in pregnancy remains unresolved. In view of the relative lack of knowledge on this subject, the Royal College of Psychiatrists recommends that women abstain completely from alcohol once pregnancy is confirmed. However, this in itself may not prove to be an effective means of prevention because of the higher risk of teratogenicity through drinking alcohol during the first few weeks after conception.

SOCIAL COMPLICATIONS OF ALCOHOL ABUSE

The social consequences of excessive drinking become more evident as alcohol increasingly monopolises the drinker's life.

1. Family Problems

Marital conflict and divorce are common, with both the spouse and children at risk of being subjected to violence or neglect. Consequently, the development of behavioural problems in these children is commonplace. Financial hardship and social deprivation often result from the reduced earning power of the drinker, as well as from a large part of the family budget being used to pay for alcohol.

Table 11.1 The physical complications of alcohol abuse

Hepatic	Fatty infiltration (accumulation of triglycerides in liver cells) Alcoholic hepatitis Cirrhosis — ascites, haemorrhage, portosystemic encephalopathy, hepatocellular carcinoma
Gastrointestinal	Oesophagitis, gastritis, peptic ulceration Gastrointestinal haemorrhage secondary to oesophageal varices, erosions, Mallory-Weiss tears Pancreatitis Malabsorption from small intestine, diarrhoea
Cardiovascular	Congestive cardiac failure, alcoholic cardiomyopathy Hypertension
Respiratory	Bronchitis (heavy drinkers are often heavy smokers) Pneumonia (aspiration of vomitus) Tuberculosis (associated with malnourishment and vagrancy)
Central nervous system	Cortical and subcortical dementia Peripheral neuropathy (mainly sensory) Optic atrophy, retrobulbar neuritis Epilepsy, cerebrovascular accidents
Metabolic	Hyperlipidaemia, hyperuricaemia, ketoacidosis Demineralisation of bone Dehydration/overhydration
Endocrine	Hypoglycaemia, diabetes mellitus, Cushingoid syndrome Testicular atrophy, gynaecomastia
Neoplasia	Oropharynx, larynx, bronchus, oesophagus, pancreas, liver, rectum (increased risk for all types)
Nutritional	Vitamin deficiency (A, B, C, D, K) Malnutrition, obesity
Haematological	Iron/folate/B_{12} deficiency anaemias, haemolytic anaemia, leucopenia, thrombocytopenia
Musculoskeletal	Myopathy (acute muscle necrosis with myoglobinuria may occur) Dupuytren's contracture
Cutaneous	Spider naevi, liver palms, rosacea
Miscellaneous	Trauma and burns, subdural haematoma Hypothermia Fetal alcohol syndrome

2. Accidents

Accidents at work and at home are three times more common among heavy drinkers than in the general population. In the UK, one in three drivers killed in road accidents have blood alcohol levels above the statutory limit of 80 mg/100 ml.

3. Criminal Acts

Criminal acts are strongly associated with alcohol abuse. These include a wide range of offences committed under the influence of alcohol, as well as stealing in order to finance the habit. There are approximately 250 000 arrests annually in the UK for either drunk and disorderly behaviour or drink-driving offences. Half of all violent crimes are alcohol-related and 40% of the prison population admit to excessive drinking.

4. Employment

Employment records of heavy drinkers show that they have over twice as many days off work as do their abstinent workmates. Not surprisingly, they are more likely to be dismissed for poor time-keeping and repeated absenteeism, as well as being prone to frequent job changes.

5. Vagrancy

It is estimated that 30% of homeless men are dependent on alcohol.

THE MANAGEMENT OF ALCOHOL ABUSE

Detection of the Problem Drinker

The early recognition of alcohol abuse is of paramount importance in preventing the development of those drink-related problems outlined above, as well as the dependence syndrome. Those at risk frequently conceal their drinking behaviour, so that the clinician must be aware of the various signs and symptoms which are indicative of alcohol abuse. Although there is no substitute for careful **history-taking**, thorough **physical examination** and a high degree of awareness, several **question- naires** have also been developed to aid the identification of alcohol abuse among general and psychiatric hospital patients. These include the MAST (Michigan alcoholism screening test) and CAGE questionnaires, the latter being particularly easy to use as it consists of only four items (Table 11.2). Both claim a 60–75% rate of detection, but they obviously rely upon honest replies, which may not be forthcoming.

Table 11.2 The CAGE questionnaire

---

1. Have you ever felt you ought to cut down your drinking?

2. Have people annoyed you by criticising your drinking?

3. Have you ever felt bad or guilty about your drinking?

4. Have you ever had a drink first thing in the morning to steady your nerves or get rid of a hangover (eye opener)?

Laboratory investigations can be helpful in confirming suspected alcohol abuse, although surprisingly, estimations of **blood** and **urine alcohol levels** are under-used in clinical practice. Other biochemical and haematological tests may be indicative, but not diagnostic, of excessive drinking. The most sensitive indices are elevation of serum gamma glutamyl transpeptidase (**gamma GT**) levels and a raised mean corpuscular red cell volume (**MCV**) in the absence of anaemia. In combination, such results are strongly suggestive of excessive alcohol intake.

A 44-year-old business executive attended his general practitioner with a minor injury to his wrist, having fallen at home. The doctor noted the man's florid facial appearance, and that his breath smelt strongly of peppermint. He had not been seen at the surgery for several years, but his wife was well known to the practice as she was a regular attender. The general practitioner was surprised to learn that the couple had separated a month beforehand, since his spouse had mentioned nothing about marital difficulties during any of her recent consultations. When asked about his alcohol intake the man laughed nervously and replied 'Well I like a drink, but then who doesn't?' When pressed about the actual amount he drank, he became quite angry, retorting that he resented the implication that he was drinking heavily, and stormed out of the surgery.

He returned to see the doctor 4 days later in a highly agitated state, asking for something to calm his nerves. He had received notice from his company that they were terminating his employment for persistent absenteeism and poor time-keeping. On this occasion he admitted to the doctor that he had been drinking heavily for the past 3 years, which he attributed to stress at home and at work. More recently, he had been consuming up to half a bottle of whisky a day, and had needed to drink in the mornings to steady his nerves. The loss of his job, in addition to the breakdown of his marriage, had made him realise that there was little point in carrying on with the deception, and he now accepted that he needed help.

Treatment of Alcohol Abuse

Treatment needs to be considered in terms of both **general** and **specific measures**, the latter dealing with physical, psychiatric and social complications.

GENERAL MEASURES

The importance of comprehensive history-taking and physical examination has already been emphasised. In particular, these are necessary to determine the duration of alcohol abuse, the degree of dependence and the extent of related disabilities. Before entering into any form of therapy, the individual's **motivation** and level of **insight** into the nature of his problems need to be assessed. Denial is often evident and it may be necessary to speak to other family members to determine the true facts. Attending for 'medical help' is not in itself indicative of a desire to stop drinking, as the subject may have been pressured into doing so by an employer or spouse. Similarly, in those individuals whose problem is discovered indirectly, there is little point in starting a programme of treatment if they are clearly unwilling to stop drinking. However, previous unsuccessful but genuine attempts to abstain should not deter the doctor from offering help. Motivation is not an 'all or none' phenomenon, and many drinkers may need several attempts at giving up before they finally succeed.

Once a commitment to stop drinking has been made, the establishment of a **good rapport** between subject and therapist is the foundation of a successful outcome to treatment. Problems should be listened to sympathetically and support offered in order to gain trust. There is little to be achieved by forcing individuals to acknowledge that they are 'alcoholics'. Similarly, emotional statements such as 'you are one drink away from complete ruination' can be antitherapeutic and may induce some drinkers to turn it into a self-fulfilling prophecy.

Admission to hospital is required where (1) outpatient treatment has failed or is unsuitable because of poor family or community support; (2) severe withdrawal symptoms are present; or (3) significant physical or psychological complications have developed. Inpatient care is frequently undertaken on general psychiatric wards, but is sometimes available in **alcohol treatment units** where specialised services are centralised and run by highly trained counsellors in a multidisciplinary setting. Many employ group therapy run on a psychosocial model, incorporating the philosophy of Alcoholics Anonymous (AA) (*see later*).

Formulation of a management plan while still in hospital must include the establishment of a **therapeutic contract** which applies firm boundaries to behaviour. It is essential that both patient and doctor adhere strictly to its terms, because of the highly manipulative tendencies which many problem drinkers develop. Contracts are tailored to the individual's particular needs, as well as to the style of the unit, but must include a commitment to abstain from drinking, without which other aspects of therapy are futile. Further conditions may include an undertaking to attend all aspects of the ward treatment programme, and agreeing to participate in communal activities.

The setting of **short-term realistic goals** maximises the chance of a successful outcome. For example, suggesting that the subject abstains from alcohol for 2 weeks in the first instance is more likely to engender a favourable prognosis than stating at the outset 'you must never drink again for the rest of your life'. Others may find the AA philosophy of 'one day at a time' more acceptable (*see later*). Appropriate reinforcers can be offered, such as demonstrating the improvement in physical health or by comparing the results of liver function tests before and after the period of abstention. Further rewards may be negotiated, such as gaining a commitment from a spouse to stay with their partner while they remain drink-free. Once the initial goals have been achieved, the period of abstention can be extended by offering new incentives.

Additional strategies include encouraging the individual to draw up a **balance sheet** which lists the benefits versus the disadvantages of continued drinking. **Alterations in life-style** may help to minimise those cues which lead to drinking. For example, going home via an alternative route will avoid the pub, where meeting with work colleagues might otherwise result in 'round buying'. Similarly, a man in a high-risk occupation with easy access to alcohol is unlikely to succeed in his attempt to stop drinking unless he changes his job. Nevertheless, there is no guarantee that a change of occupation will ensure that abstinence is maintained. Alcohol is easily accessible from other sources, and if the subject wishes to drink, he will go to any lengths to obtain it. Consequently, major life decisions of this nature can only be undertaken after the drinker has maintained his sobriety for many months. By then, he will have had sufficient opportunity to evaluate fully the likely effects of his actions, and to be certain that they will truly be of benefit to himself or his family.

SPECIFIC MEASURES

Physical treatments

Drugs are used in **detoxification** to control simple withdrawal symptoms and prevent delirium tremens or fits (*see* regimen outlined on p. 201). Other drugs may also be administered as a form of **aversion therapy** to prevent a relapse into drinking after abstinence. **Disulfiram** (Antabuse) can be taken in tablet form daily. If alcohol is then consumed, a reaction occurs producing acetaldehyde, which in turn causes the release of histamine in the body. Nausea, vomiting, headache, fainting, abdominal cramps and flushing of the face may then result, which are sufficiently unpleasant to deter further drinking. The limitation of this form of treatment is that success depends upon the subject's motivation to take the medication regularly. Unfortunately, a few individuals have been known to 'drink through' their Antabuse treatment with disastrous consequences.

Psychological treatments

It is necessary to identify and treat any **psychiatric illness**, such as depression or schizophrenia, where alcohol may have been used as a self-remedy to alleviate symptoms.

Various forms of **psychotherapy** are used in the management of alcohol abuse. Brief counselling sessions, group work and individual supportive and dynamic psychotherapy (*see* Chapter 13) are all advocated. Empathy, warmth and sincerity are important components of all these treatments.

Alcoholics Anonymous is probably the most well-known form of group therapy and was started in Ohio, USA in 1935 by a stockbroker (Bill W), and a surgeon (Dr Bob) who was himself a reformed drinker. The philosophy of AA has now spread worldwide and promotes a policy of **total abstinence** from alcohol, while encouraging members to adopt an approach of 'one day at a time' in order to overcome their problems. Simple advice and mutual support are offered at group meetings, and although the effectiveness of this form of treatment has not been scientifically evaluated (because few records are kept), AA is probably helpful to many of its large following. Al-Anon provides support for the families of problem drinkers.

Behavioural techniques have been employed, with limited success, to modify drinking habits by teaching individuals to take smaller sips and drink more slowly. 'Drinkwatchers' is an organisation which helps members to control their drinking *before* they become seriously dependent.

Social treatments

It is relatively easy to detoxify patients in hospital, mainly because they are removed from the stressors which induced them to drink in the first place. However, despite effecting changes in life-style and setting realistic goals, there remains a high risk of relapse when these individuals are discharged back into the community. For this reason, the involvement of **the family** should be encouraged, not only to provide information about drinking which the subject does not reveal, but also to support their relatives through the burden of abstinence and possible periods of relapse. Both **professional care givers** (such as the general practitioner, field social worker and community psychiatric nurse) and the family can enhance self-esteem by conveying a sense of hope and encouraging the individual to believe in his ability to control his own destiny.

Outside agencies can provide additional support to facilitate successful rehabilitation. **Councils on Alcoholism** are voluntary organisations which attempt to coordinate available services to help the problem drinker.

They also offer free counselling and social activities for the subject and his family. **Hostels** not only provide shelter for the itinerant drinker, but can also function as 'half-way houses' for those recently discharged from inpatient care. Most offer a therapeutic programme and counselling service (often run by a reformed drinker) and demand abstinence as a prerequisite of residence. **Probation officers** have an important role to play in the rehabilitation of drinkers who break the law. The probation service runs detoxification centres in several large cities in the UK. Alcohol treatment units (*see* p. 210) often provide 'drop-in' facilities and **day centre** care.

Prognosis and Evaluation of Treatment

Treatment is most successful where the individual is highly motivated, has adequate social and family support and is entering therapy for the first time. Although a policy of total abstinence is advocated by most authorities, there is some research which suggests that such aims may be unrealistic, and that controlled drinking is a more feasible approach. However, the findings of a recent study suggest that severely dependent drinkers do better with abstinence-orientated treatment than with therapy aimed at controlling intake. The latter may be feasible in some young drinkers with a short history of heavy consumption, few alcohol-related problems and no evidence of dependence.

Prevention

Prevention is the most important element in any overall strategy which attempts to deal with alcohol abuse. **Political measures**, such as increasing the cost of drink in relation to disposable income, are of course unpopular but, nevertheless, have been shown to be effective in reducing consumption. The same consideration applies to legislative restrictions on advertising alcohol and the availability of retail outlets. Cultural attitudes towards alcohol remain entrenched, so that any changes in the pattern of drinking and an appreciation of its dangers are only likely to be achieved slowly. **Health education** in schools and through the media may go some way towards effecting these goals.

OTHER COMMONLY ABUSED DRUGS

Drugs other than alcohol which are commonly abused come from three major sources: those obtained illicitly through **drug dealers**; those obtained from **doctors** ostensibly for therapeutic reasons; and drugs bought **over the counter** from pharmacies or shops. More recently, organic solvents contained in a variety of products (glues, paints, dry-cleaning

214 Student Psychiatry Today

fluids) have become increasingly abused, as inhalation of their vapour produces effects similar to those of alcohol or anaesthetics.

Drugs which are supplied illicitly are mostly those which are controlled under the **Misuse of Drugs Act**, making it illegal to supply or possess them without a certified prescription, or to produce, import or export them without authority. They include heroin, morphine, cocaine, cannabis, amphetamines, barbiturates and LSD.

Aetiology of Drug Abuse and Dependence

There is no single cause of drug abuse and dependence, but it would seem to involve an interaction between the individual, the environment and the effects of the drug.

INDIVIDUAL FACTORS

No clear association exists between drug abuse and any particular personality type. However, those who display **delinquent behaviour** and a **lack of coping resources** to deal with stress are perhaps most vulnerable. As with alcohol, the abuse of other drugs may occur in the setting of a psychiatric or physical disorder as a form of self-medication.

ENVIRONMENTAL FACTORS

In many **cultures**, the use of certain drugs for social and recreational purposes is widely accepted (e.g. cannabis in the West Indies and opium in the Far East). Consequently, if there are a large number of users, a proportion will inevitably become dependent. **Availability** and **peer group pressure** are important factors in the spread of abuse among young people who experiment with drugs in societies where they are not condoned.

Access to drugs by professional personnel, such as doctors, nurses and pharmacists, may lead to them abusing and becoming dependent on the substances they handle or administer. Finally, drug dependence can be caused **iatrogenically** by doctors who irresponsibly prescribe potentially addictive medicines to their patients in excessive quantities.

EFFECTS OF THE DRUG

Although social and individual factors are important in establishing drug abuse, the development of dependence is largely reliant upon the **pharmacological properties** of the substance. For example, heroin produces strong physical and psychological dependence, whereas these do not occur with LSD.

Conditioned learning is also postulated as facilitating the development of psychological dependence which may result from the pleasurable effects of a drug positively reinforcing its further abuse. Environmental cues, such as returning to a place where drugs are regularly taken, can provoke craving by similar means. Finally, the avoidance of withdrawal symptoms is a potent reinforcement to further drug taking, and hence the development of physical dependence.

Individuals often take several different substances at one time. Details of drugs which are commonly abused can be considered in terms of their effect on the central nervous system — depressant, stimulant and hallucinogenic. Solvent and analgesic abuse are considered separately.

CENTRAL NERVOUS SYSTEM DEPRESSANTS

1. The Opioids

This group contains both naturally occurring compounds derived from the opium poppy (**opiates**) and a number of synthetic derivatives. The fluid or 'milk' of the poppy is dried to make **opium**, the active components of which include **morphine** and **codeine**. **Heroin** (diamorphine) was first synthesised from morphine in 1874 in an attempt to find a non-addictive substitute for opium! It is approximately twice as potent as the parent compound. Other synthetic derivatives include the analgesics **pethidine**, **dipipanone**, **methadone** and **dextropropoxyphene**.

PREVALENCE

Heroin use and dependence exceeds that of all other opioids. Much of the street heroin in the UK comes from India and Pakistan. There were over 10 000 registered addicts in 1983, but the total number of regular users is probably five times this figure.

METHODS OF ADMINISTRATION

Heroin powder can be taken orally, or dissolved in water and injected either into a vein (mainlining) or subcutaneously (skin popping). It may also be smoked (chasing the dragon) or sniffed up the nose (snorting). The most rapid and intense effect is obtained intravenously. To increase their profits, drug dealers frequently 'cut' the drug with a variety of impurities to increase its bulk. These include quinine, glucose, strychnine, flour and talc.

EFFECTS

The depressant effects of opioids result in bradycardia, suppression of the cough reflex, respiratory depression and constipation. Peripheral vaso-dilatation leads to itching, increased perspiration and a sensation of great warmth, with resultant lowering of body temperature. Pupillary constriction occurs, and both appetite and sexual energy are diminished, with amenorrhoea a common finding in females who inject opioids intra-venously. (The physical complications of intravenous drug use are discussed on p. 227.)

Initial use of heroin can be unpleasant due to stimulation of the vomiting centre in the brain stem. With repeated doses this effect disappears and is replaced by a 'buzz' or 'rush', which is intensely pleasurable and has been likened to orgasm. Opioids induce a sense of peace and tranquillity and a relaxed detachment from the outside world. **Tolerance** and **dependence** readily develop, so that when the pleasurable effects become less pronounced, drug taking is motivated towards the prevention of withdrawal symptoms. At higher dosages, sedation occurs and can eventually progress to drowsiness, coma and death. Overdosage may be caused by the concurrent use of other depressant drugs, or by addicts who stop taking heroin for a time and then resume at a dosage to which they are no longer tolerant.

Chronic use of the drug results in general malaise, apathy and a persistent tremor. Signs of poor nutrition, self-neglect and infection may also be evident (*see* p. 227). Constipation can become so serious that hospitalisation is sometimes necessary to restore bowel function. Not all heroin users become dependent, however, and some limit their experience of the drug to occasional use only.

WITHDRAWAL SYMPTOMS

Once dependence is established, sudden cessation of the drug produces a **withdrawal syndrome** which begins within a few hours of the last dose. Initially, flu-like symptoms develop, including muscle aches, shaking, chills, rhinorrhoea, lacrimation, sweating and yawning. Abdominal cramps, diarrhoea, pupillary dilatation and tachycardia occur later, together with piloerection (goose flesh). This phenomenon gives rise to the term 'cold turkey' used in the USA because it graphically describes the appearance and feel of the skin of addicts who are undergoing withdrawal. The effects are due to autonomic overactivity and reach a peak 24–48 hours after the last dose, before subsiding completely within 7–10 days.

2. Barbiturates

Barbiturates used to be commonly prescribed as either sedatives to induce relaxation or as hypnotics to help sleep. They have now been largely superseded by the benzodiazepines, but a few older patients continue to receive them from their doctors, and they are still used in the treatment of epilepsy.

PREVALENCE

The availability and use of barbiturates has declined since the mid-1970s, and the number of abusers is now probably less than 10 000.

METHODS OF ADMINISTRATION

Barbiturates mainly come in powder form which may be taken orally, or alternatively dissolved in water and then injected intramuscularly or intravenously.

EFFECTS

Small doses induce relaxation, but larger amounts cause sedation in which reaction time is seriously affected, the speech is slurred and body movements become uncoordinated. There is a cumulative effect with alcohol, and overdosage may lead to coma and eventual death.

Prolonged heavy dosages produce an intoxicated state with persistent drowsiness, poor concentration and judgment, motor incoordination, personality changes and lability of mood tending towards depression. Because barbiturates suppress respiration and the cough reflex, heavy users are more prone to the development of chest infections; hypothermia and bradycardia are additional complications.

WITHDRAWAL SYMPTOMS

As with heroin, long-term barbiturate abuse leads to **tolerance** (due to hepatic enzyme induction) and the development of both physical and psychological **dependence**. Withdrawal symptoms are similar to those which occur with alcohol and include anxiety, restlessness, tremor, muscle twitching, marked insomnia and vivid unpleasant dreams. Vomiting may be severe, and sudden withdrawal after high dosages can cause confusion and seizures. Consequently, any attempt to reduce the dosage must be undertaken slowly in hospital to prevent the development of fits. The prophylactic use of an anticonvulsant drug may also be advisable.

3. Benzodiazepines

Benodiazepines, including **diazepam** (Valium), **chlordiazepoxide** (Librium) and **lorazepam** (Ativan) are the most commonly prescribed drugs in the UK. Also known as minor tranquillisers, they are used as sedatives in the management of anxiety and as hypnotics to induce sleep (*see* Chapter 12).

PREVALENCE AND METHOD OF ADMINISTRATION

In the early 1980s, it was estimated that as many as one million people in the UK were regularly taking these drugs (particularly middle-aged women), but numbers now seem to be falling as doctors become increasingly aware of their dangers. They are not controlled under the Misuse of Drugs Act, so that they are still freely prescribed and hence widely abused. They are almost exclusively taken by mouth, with little evidence of parenteral misuse.

EFFECTS

In addition to reducing tension, they generally depress mental activity and alertness. When taken on their own they produce little euphoria, so that they have not become popular for recreational purposes. They are very safe in overdose, but in combination with alcohol can be lethal.

WITHDRAWAL SYMPTOMS

Physical and psychological **dependence** can develop with benzodiazepines, especially if they have been prescribed for a long time. Withdrawal symptoms, such as anxiety, insomnia, dizziness, palpitations, loss of appetite and hypersensitivity to noise or touch, are often seen following abrupt cessation of medication taken in normal dosage for longer than 3–4 months. Many of these symptoms (such as anxiety and insomnia) resemble the original complaints for which the drug was prescribed, thereby encouraging the assumption that medication is still necessary. Convulsions and confusion may occur after sudden withdrawal from very high doses. Most symptoms subside within 5–6 weeks, but psychological dependence can persist for much longer.

Planned withdrawal can usually be supervised by the general practitioner or in outpatients over a period of 2–4 months, gradually reducing the dosage at weekly intervals to minimise discomfort. Inpatient care ought to be considered in those withdrawing from very high dosages, or where there is a past history of convulsions. Supportive measures should be offered, such as help in developing alternative means of coping with stress (*see* p. 276). A number of self-help organisations (such as TRANX) have recently been established, which provide a counselling service and offer support through regular group meetings to those dependent on, and withdrawing from, benzodiazepines.

CENTRAL NERVOUS SYSTEM STIMULANTS

1. Amphetamines and Related Drugs

Amphetamines are synthetic compounds which were widely prescribed in the 1950s and 1960s to elevate mood and as appetite suppressants. When the problems associated with their administration became apparent, their medical use declined and is now limited to the treatment of narcolepsy and hyperkinetic children (*see* pp. 389 and 326). Other drugs, such as **methylphenidate** (Ritalin) and **diethylpropion** (Tenuate Dospan, Apisate) have amphetamine-like properties but are less powerful. The latter are still prescribed as appetite suppressants, although they are now controlled under the Misuse of Drugs Act.

PREVALENCE AND METHODS OF ADMINISTRATION

Amphetamine powders are comparatively simple to manufacture, and therefore are readily available to abusers. They may be taken orally, sniffed up the nose, or dissolved in water and then injected intravenously.

EFFECTS

Amphetamines produce a number of physical effects which include tachycardia, dilated pupils and exaggerated reflexes. There is also a 'rush' that is described as a sense of enhanced mental capacity, accompanied by euphoria and excitement. Other effects include increased energy and confidence, heightened concentration, a reduced need for food or sleep, and restlessness. These make **psychological dependence** a common problem, although physical dependence (the development of a withdrawal syndrome) does not occur. Many addicts combine amphetamines with opioids in a drug 'cocktail' which is said to enhance the latter's effect.

The actions of the drug last for 3–6 hours, and as they diminish, the user experiences an unpleasant sensation of tiredness and depression, known as 'crashing'. Amphetamines are either taken intermittently and limited to specific occasions, or used continuously for several days at a time (or even longer) to maintain the effect. Eventual cessation is followed by prolonged deep sleep, and on awakening, feelings of apathy, lethargy and depression are increased and may be accompanied by intense hunger.

The development of **tolerance** leads to an escalation in dosage in order to maintain the desired effect. At this stage, the compulsive user is often anxious, irritable and suspicious. An **amphetamine psychosis** may also develop, in which paranoid delusions and hallucinations (which may be tactile, visual or auditory) occur. The illness is sometimes indistinguishable from acute schizophrenia, but it usually abates as the effects of the drug wear off.

2. Cocaine

Cocaine is derived from the leaves of the coca shrub which is found throughout South America, and many of its psychoactive properties are similar to those of amphetamines.

PREVALENCE AND METHODS OF ADMINISTRATION

Although its use was previously restricted to relatively affluent sections of the community, cocaine is now much more widely abused because of increased availability and a dramatic fall in price. It is usually taken by 'snorting', i.e. sniffing up the nose through a tube. Occasionally, it is injected intravenously and an extract may also be smoked (freebasing). More recently, a highly purified form has become available, known as **crack**, which is inexpensive and highly addictive.

EFFECTS

After 'snorting', the effects develop quickly and reach a peak in about 20 minutes, following which they rapidly subside. An increase in energy and sense of well-being are usually experienced, along with elevation of mood and a decreased need for food or sleep, so that 'cocaine parties' have become a popular social venue for taking the drug. In addition, there is an increase in blood pressure and heart rate, a rise in body temperature and pupillary dilatation. Disorders of cardiac conduction have also been described. Repeated dosing every half-hour or so is necessary to maintain the effect. Restlessness, irritability and insomnia can occur with regular use, and may be accompanied by nausea and weight loss.

Occasionally, **tactile hallucinations** are experienced, characteristically of insects crawling on the body ('cocaine bug'). Rarely, a **paranoid psychosis** develops, although symptoms usually disappear once the drug is stopped. **Psychological dependence** may well be a problem, but tolerance and withdrawal symptoms do not seem to occur. Perforation of the nasal septum is a complication of habitual 'snorting'.

3. Cannabis

This drug is derived from the hemp plant *Cannabis sativa* which grows readily in most parts of the world. **Marijuana** is made from a dried mixture of the crushed leaves and flowering tops of the plant. **Hashish** is a derivative of a clear sticky resin produced by the plant, which is then dried and compressed into blocks. It is four to eight times more potent than marijuana. The active component of both forms of the drug is **tetrahydrocannabinol**.

PREVALENCE AND METHODS OF ADMINISTRATION

Cannabis is widely taken for recreational purposes on a regular or intermittent basis, making it the most commonly abused illicit drug in the UK and North America. Supplies imported into Europe come from Africa, Pakistan, India, the Middle East and South America.

Both marijuana and hashish may be smoked on their own or mixed with tobacco, or taken by mouth in combination with various foods and drink. Smoking produces a rapid and easily controlled effect, so that it is the most popular route of administration.

EFFECTS

The effects of cannabis are highly variable and depend on the dose and route of administration, as well as the individual's personality and previous experience of the drug. Personal expectations and the environmental setting in which it is taken also exert an influence. In general, the effects usually begin within minutes and last for a few hours, and include a sense of relaxation, sociability and well-being. Mood changes are variable, ranging from euphoria and hilarity at one extreme to the exaggeration of pre-existing unpleasant states (such as depression) at the other.

Colours, sounds and tastes are often experienced more vividly, and time seems to pass more slowly. Motor performance and reaction time may be impaired, which most importantly affects driving. Physical effects include tachycardia, hypotension, lowering of body temperature, increased appetite, reduced intraocular pressure, coughing and conjunctival irritation. Some authorities propose that the drug can either produce a transient **psychotic episode** or exacerbate a pre-existing tendency to this type of illness. However, the evidence for this is inconclusive.

Although chronic cannabis abuse has not definitely been shown to cause long-term health problems, a number of conditions have been implicated as resulting from its use. These include respiratory disorders (which may arise from concurrent tobacco smoking), cerebral atrophy, reduced spermatogenesis and fetal abnormalities. An **amotivational syndrome** has been described which involves loss of drive and apathy. 'Flashback' phenomena may also occur (*see below*).

Psychological dependence sometimes develops, as does **tolerance** to certain effects of the drug, notably the euphoria and sense of well-being. No definite withdrawal syndrome has been observed.

LYSERGIC ACID DIETHYLAMIDE (LSD) AND OTHER HALLUCINOGENS

LSD is a synthetic compound belonging to a group known as **psychedelics** or **hallucinogens**, which also include **phencyclidine** (known commonly as 'angel dust' or PCP), **dimethyltryptamine** (DMT) and **psilocybin** (found in certain mushrooms). All hallucinogens are characterised by their ability to produce distinctive alterations in thought, feeling, behaviour and the way in which the world is perceived.

PREVALENCE AND METHOD OF ADMINISTRATION

LSD became popular in the early 1960s, and although its widespread use has since declined, it is still taken regularly by certain sections of the drug subculture.

In its pure form it is a white powder, and because only minute amounts are necessary to produce psychological effects, it is generally mixed with other substances and then taken by mouth.

EFFECTS

Psychoactive effects (popularly known as a **trip**) begin within an hour of taking the drug, reaching maximum effect 2–6 hours later. Symptoms begin to resolve after 10–12 hours, although fatigue and tension may persist for much longer. As with cannabis, experiences produced by LSD depend not only upon the dose, but also the user's mood, expectations and surroundings.

Perception is often heightened, so that colours and sounds seem more intense. Distortions of real objects (**illusions**) are common, so that things seem to move in a wave-like fashion or dissolve away, but true hallucinations are rare. The user may attach great importance to his thoughts, and experiences a sense of increased self-confidence, clarity and enlightenment. Feelings of unreality and mysticism frequently occur, such as seeming to be outside one's own body.

Mood is highly variable, ranging from extreme elation to depression and panic. The latter may be experienced as part of a 'bad trip', in which sensations of breathlessness, paralysis and impending doom predominate. This reaction is more likely if the user feels insecure, anxious or takes the drug unsupervised in an unfamiliar setting. Suicide resulting from the effects of a 'bad trip' is rare, and death from overdose has not been reported.

Physical effects of LSD include pupillary dilatation, increase in body temperature and blood pressure, tachycardia, and occasionally nausea and vomiting.

Physical dependence does not develop, and for several days after taking the drug, further doses are less effective, so that psychological dependence is not marked either. However, an interesting psychological phenomenon, known as **flashback**, may develop, in which there is a recurrence of the drug experience some length of time after LSD was last taken, often creating a feeling of disorientation and distress. Both 'bad trips' and 'flashbacks' tend to be transient and usually respond well to simple reassurance, although severe cases may require sedation with a drug such as diazepam or haloperidol.

Hallucinogenic ('Magic') Mushrooms

Several species grow wild in the UK, the **Liberty cap** (*Psilocybe semilanceata*) being the most common variety. They contain **psilocybin** which, when ingested in sufficient quantity, produces an hallucinogenic experience similar to that with LSD, although of milder intensity and shorter duration.

Phencyclidine (PCP or 'Angel Dust')

The use of phencyclidine in the UK is still relatively infrequent, although it is widely abused in the USA. It may be taken orally, injected or inhaled, and is often mixed with other illicit substances. Common effects of the drug include intoxication, aggressiveness, agitation and a psychotic reaction producing delusions and hallucinations. Numbness and paralysis, elevation of the blood pressure, convulsions and stupor can all occur, and overdosage may result in death. **Physical dependence** sometimes develops and withdrawal symptoms, consisting of abdominal cramps, depression and craving for the drug, have been described.

SOLVENT ABUSE

This takes the form of the inhalation of chemical fumes from a wide variety of common domestic substances, including glues, plastic cements, paint thinners, petrol, hair lacquer, lighter refills and typewriter correcting fluid, in order to produce an intoxicating effect. Most substances which are used have either **toluene** or **acetone** as the main volatile constituent. Fluorinated hydrocarbons contained in aerosol propellants are particularly dangerous, as they may cause spasm of the larynx, although all substances carry the risk of death through inhalation of vomit or asphyxiation.

PREVALENCE

The deliberate inhalation of gasoline fumes was first reported in the USA in the 1950s, and was followed a decade later by **glue sniffing**. By the early 1970s the problem had spread to the UK.

Solvent abuse is primarily a disorder of children and adolescents with an age range between 7 and 18 years; boys outnumber girls by 10 to 1. Glue sniffers fall into two categories; the larger involves intermittent abuse within a group setting and is frequently associated with adolescent rebellion. Members of this category tend to abandon the practice after a relatively short time, and in many cases their parents will have been totally unaware of their behaviour. Physical or psychological problems rarely develop. The second smaller group comprises those who persist with the habit and regularly abuse solvents over a period of months or years. They often conduct their sniffing alone and tend to use methods which can result in suffocation. There may be a history of truancy, parental alcoholism and family discord.

METHODS OF ADMINISTRATION

The substance is either applied to a cloth or rag and held over the mouth and nose, or inhaled directly from the container. Alternatively, the solvent may be inhaled from a plastic bag or beer can. To prolong the effect, additional bags are sometimes placed over the head, often with disastrous consequences.

EFFECTS

Initial effects, notably euphoria and excitement, are similar to those of alcohol intoxication. Continued inhalation causes the development of further symptoms such as dizziness, slurred speech, unsteady gait, diplopia, disorientation, drowsiness and perceptual abnormalities. Feelings of disinhibition can result in impulsive and destructive behaviour.

Signs of chronic solvent abuse are indicated by the presence of:

1. a **rash** around the nose and mouth outlining where glue inhaled from a bag has come into contact with the skin
2. a persistent **cough** resulting from excessive oral and nasal secretions
3. halitosis or the **smell** of solvent on the breath
4. **poor general health** associated with nausea, anorexia and weight loss
5. **listlessness** and **apathy** resulting in poor performance at school, college or work.

Toxic damage to the liver, kidney, myocardium and central nervous system has been reported following chronic inhalation of substances containing toluene or carbon tetrachloride. Tolerance to the effects of solvents can occur and withdrawal symptoms, in the form of abdominal cramps, aching limbs, nausea and fatigue, have also been described.

Solvent abuse among preadolescent and older children often reflects underlying family conflicts and difficulties. In these cases, family and marital work or individual psychotherapy may be indicated.

ANALGESIC ABUSE

The consumption of non-prescribed pain-killing drugs, such as **aspirin** and **paracetamol**, has risen progressively since the late 1940s. When abused, these analgesics are frequently taken in the form of compound powders which also contain caffeine or codeine (both of which produce psychological effects). Inappropriate indications for use include insomnia, agitation and depression. Although physical dependence does not occur, the development of psychological dependence to these drugs is evident from users continuing to consume them despite warnings about the medical risks. Analgesic abuse can produce kidney or liver damage, while overdosage may be fatal.

THE MANAGEMENT OF DRUG ABUSE AND DEPENDENCE

Diagnosis and Assessment

The early **detection** of drug abuse is essential to maximise the chances of subsequent treatment being effective. However, not all patients who seek help are genuine in their intentions, in that some merely wish to obtain an additional supply of drugs for personal use or re-sale. Therefore, doctors who manage such cases should, wherever possible, attempt to verify the information they are given by using independent sources. Since it is a legal requirement for physicians to inform the Home Office of individuals suspected or known to be addicted to certain drugs (opioids and cocaine), details of previous notification may be helpful.

In addition to those who present directly for help, drug abuse or dependence can be detected in many other ways. For example, regular attenders at general practitioners or casualty departments, who request strong analgesics for inappropriate reasons or simulated complaints, should give cause for suspicion. Similarly, psychiatric patients who present with unexplained disturbed behaviour may prove to have a positive blood or urine drug screen.

Assessment should commence by taking a full **drug history** inquiring into:

1. the **type of drug** used: some substances are more likely than others to produce physical dependence, or may be more dangerous in overdosage
2. **dosage and duration of use**: indicate the degree of tolerance/dependence and likely outcome of treatment; long-standing heavy abuse is often associated with a poor prognosis
3. **pattern of use**: regular (as opposed to intermittent) administration is indicative of dependence; taking a drug parenterally, rather than orally, is more likely to lead to physical complications and the development of dependence; multiple drug-taking is associated with a poor response to treatment and an increased risk of death from drug interactions
4. periods of **abstinence** and any evidence of **withdrawal symptoms**, which indicate physical dependence.

Further questioning should elicit whether there are any **psychological** or **social complications** arising from drug abuse. Mild depression and anxiety are common, although certain drugs may cause more serious psychiatric conditions (*see above*). Insomnia, poor concentration, apathy and reduced libido are other frequently encountered complaints.

Efficiency at work is commonly affected and the general lack of interest in non-drug-related activities may result in dismissal or resignation. This often occurs at a time when the habit is a severe drain on financial resources, so that the abuser might be forced to resort to crime, prostitution or drug dealing as an alternative means of income. Relationships frequently suffer, and the addict may slip into a squalid existence where he is shunned by family and friends, who are replaced by members of the drug subculture. However, deterioration of this type is not inevitable, and many regular drug users maintain an otherwise normal life-style.

Because corroborative evidence of drug abuse should be sought, thorough **physical examination** of the patient assumes particular importance. The skin may show evidence of needle tracks, thrombosed veins or abscesses in those who inject drugs, the commonest sites being the ante-cubital fossae, axillae and groins. Other physical complications include serum hepatitis, generalised infections and the acquired immune deficiency syndrome (AIDS).

Diagnosis of illicit drug abuse by **urine** or **blood testing** is of limited value, in that the estimations are qualitative but not quantitative. They can therefore confirm the presence or absence of a drug within the body, but not how much has been taken. Heroin is particularly difficult to detect because it is rapidly metabolised, although impurities with which it is 'cut' or diluted (such as quinine) may provide indirect evidence of its use. Cannabis is fat-soluble, and can be excreted in the urine 2–3 months after the last exposure in very heavy users. **Liver function tests** are helpful in assessing the degree of hepatic damage.

Assessment of **motivation** is important, not only to determine the likely efficacy of treatment, but also to establish whether the individual is asking for help in giving up drugs completely or merely to control his intake.

General Principles of Treatment

Because illicit drug-taking frequently involves the abuse of several different substances, certain general therapeutic principles need to be considered.

The treatment of drug dependence is governed by several factors, including the type of drug abused, the patient's needs and motivation, and the facilities available. Although **total withdrawal** from drugs is preferable, in practice this cannot always be achieved and **maintenance therapy** needs to be considered. This aims to reduce the intake of the substance to the lowest level which the subject finds tolerable. The degree of dependence varies widely among users, so that some will find it much easier than others to reduce or stop completely.

Both inpatient and outpatient facilities exist for the management of withdrawal and the provision of maintenance therapy. Withdrawal from certain drugs, such as benzodiazepines or amphetamines, can often be achieved on an outpatient basis, and this mode of treatment may also be suited to any short-term drug taker with a regular job and stable home environment. With substances that produce strong physical dependence, such as opioids and barbiturates, inpatient supervision of withdrawal might be necessary. Similarly, long-term abusers and those with an unstable life-style may also benefit from admission to an in-patient unit. Unfortunately, in many areas few facilities exist to manage the problems of drug abuse and supervision of care is often left to the general practitioner.

Management of Opioid Withdrawal

The strong physical dependence which opioids induce, combined with a tendency for users to develop serious physical complications, present special problems of management which warrant separate consideration.

Withdrawal from opioids, notably heroin, is most successfully accomplished by substituting oral **methadone**, often provided at a **drug dependency unit**. The main advantage of this approach is that, because it is also an opioid, it minimises the development of withdrawal symptoms and yet does not possess the euphoriant properties of heroin. Consequently, the individual is maintained in a 'normal' state. Further benefits are that it is effective orally and each dose lasts for relatively long periods. Depending upon the amount of heroin being taken, 20–40 mg of methadone linctus are substituted daily, followed by a gradual reduction over the next 4 weeks. In practice, this approach is fraught with difficulties, as many addicts will accept methadone, while continuing to obtain illicit supplies of other drugs.

Where total withdrawal is not possible, maintaining the subject on methadone linctus has a number of advantages over continued intravenous use:

1. it avoids the dangers of injecting powder or crushed tablets (*see* p. 227)
2. the amount of the drug can be adjusted more easily to achieve the minimum maintenance dose
3. it provides the user with a legitimate supply of medication, making it easier to withdraw him from drugs, and reducing the likelihood of further illicit supplies being sought
4. it maintains contact with professional services so that medical, psychological and social problems can be dealt with when they arise.

Psychological treatment is often provided in the form of **group therapy** during admission for detoxification. It attempts to help individuals acquire insight into those aspects of their personality and relationships which lead to them abusing drugs, and to find more appropriate ways of dealing with their problems and difficulties. The therapeutic regimen is often strict, and breaking the initial contract by further abuse of drugs results in eviction from the programme. In some areas, Narcotics Anonymous groups have been established which adopt a similar philosophy to AA (*see* p. 212). Help is also provided for relatives (Families Anon), in order to share their problems with other affected families and to learn more about drug abuse from films and lectures.

Long-term **rehabilitation** may involve the individual residing temporarily in a community with other former addicts. This provides an opportunity to learn new social and living skills, thereby increasing the likelihood of remaining drug-free in the future.

Prognosis

The long-term follow-up of opiate addicts shows a significant rate of mortality; 2–3% die annually, usually from infections, suicide or accidental overdose. Of those that survive, there is a tendency towards adopting a more stable life-style by establishing new relationships with non-addicts and choosing a different cultural environment. One study showed that 25% of opiate addicts had become abstinent at 5-year follow-up, this increasing to 40% after 10 years.

Prevention of Drug Abuse

Political measures to prevent drug-trafficking and dealing have been implemented worldwide, but appear to have had only limited success in restricting supplies. Consequently, the need to **educate** children and other young people about the dangers of illicit drugs assumes greater importance. Because experimentation with drugs is often facilitated by peer pressure, assertiveness training, which teaches young people how to say 'no' when offered them, may prove to be an effective preventive measure.

OTHER FORMS OF ADDICTION

Nicotine Dependence

Addiction to smoking is largely psychological, but heavy smokers may demonstrate physical dependence on nicotine. The latter has the capacity both to increase cerebral arousal and relax skeletal muscle, so that tobacco use is reinforced by situations which cause high levels of either boredom or stress. Nicotine withdrawal is identified by intense craving, feelings of anxiety and depression, restlessness and difficulty in concentration. Physical effects include bradycardia, hypotension, constipation and sleep disturbance.

Efforts to stop smoking are nearly always motivated by the associated health risk. Individual treatments using hypnosis, cognitive therapy, tobacco substitutes and nicotine chewing gum may be successful in the short term, but the rate of relapse is high. Increasing the cost of tobacco has some impact on the total annual consumption, although encouraging people to switch to low-tar brands of cigarettes is difficult, because tar levels correlate highly with nicotine content.

Pathological Gambling

Gambling exists in virtually every society throughout the world, but only in a minority of cases does it lead to personal and social problems. Pathological gambling can be identified by a number of features:

1. the gambler, or more usually a member of his family, becomes concerned that the amount of gambling is excessive
2. the subject describes a feeling of tension which is relieved by gambling
3. the individual is intermittently or continuously preoccupied with thoughts of gambling, leading to an overpowering urge to gamble
4. an inability to stop gambling once started, despite being aware of the adverse consequences of such behaviour
5. interference with the psychological, social or economic functioning of the gambler and/or his family.

Effective management depends upon the establishment of a trusting relationship between therapist and gambler, and the involvement of the partner at an early stage of treatment. Any associated psychiatric disorder should be treated, and counselling offered to deal with practical problems such as debts. A behavioural assessment to identify cues which lead to gambling may be useful, following which behavioural modification can be attempted (*see* Chapter 13). Psychotherapy might be of benefit where pathological gambling has arisen as a result of relationship or intrapersonal problems. Long-term support is usually necessary, and help may be derived from organisations such as Gamblers Anonymous.

SUMMARY

1. A **drug** is any substance that is taken into a living organism and modifies one or more of its functions. **Drug abuse** is persistent or occasional excessive use of a drug which is out of keeping with accepted medical practice. **Tolerance** develops when the user has to increase the

dose of a drug to achieve the original effect. Dependence describes a need to take the drug following its repeated administration and is of two types. With **physical dependence**, a specific group of unpleasant withdrawal symptoms occur after the individual stops the drug, whereas **psychological dependence** involves craving for the drug in order to experience its psychic effects or to avoid the discomfort of its absence.

2. **Alcohol abuse** is widespread and can result in physical, psychological and social problems. In the UK, it is estimated that approximately half a million people are dependent on alcohol, although the number with alcohol-related problems is considerably higher. In all age groups, abuse of alcohol is more prevalent among men. Certain occupational groups (such as barworkers, doctors, journalists, entertainers, merchant seamen) are at increased risk of abusing alcohol. The issue of whether alcohol abuse is an 'illness' or a result of moral weakness remains unresolved, although its causation is probably multifactorial.

3. The establishment of dependence is marked by features of the **alcohol dependence syndrome**. Withdrawal symptoms can be considered in terms of simple withdrawal phenomena, withdrawal fits and delirium tremens. The latter is an example of an acute organic reaction in which confusion, hyperarousal and perceptual abnormalities are often marked. Accompanying physical complications include dehydration, electrolyte imbalance and infection. Management usually involves hospitalisation, sedation, vitamin supplementation, rehydration and antibiotic therapy. Despite treatment, delirium tremens has a mortality rate of approximately 10%.

4. **Psychological impairment** associated with alcohol abuse can result from intoxication, alcoholic dementia or Wernicke–Korsakoff syndrome. Alcoholic dementia causes a global impairment of cerebral function usually after several years of heavy drinking. Wernicke's encephalopathy is the acute reaction to severe vitamin B_1 deficiency and may present with clouding of consciousness, ataxia, nystagmus, peripheral neuropathy and ophthalmoplegia. Over 80% of untreated cases progress to the chronic phase of Korsakoff's psychosis, which causes a specific defect of short-term memory resulting in both anterograde and retrograde amnesia, often accompanied by confabulation. Alcohol-induced **psychiatric disorders** include alcoholic hallucinosis (auditory hallucinations in a setting of clear consciousness), paranoid states, depression, personality deterioration, morbid jealousy and sexual dysfunction. **Physical complications** of alcohol abuse include cirrhosis, gastritis, peptic ulceration, pancreatitis, cardio-respiratory disease, neoplasia, infections, vitamin deficiency, fits and peripheral neuropathy. Babies born to women who drink heavily during pregnancy are at risk of developing the fetal alcohol syndrome. **Social complications** include problems within the family and at work, accident proneness, criminal behaviour and vagrancy.

5. The early recognition of alcohol abuse is the cornerstone to effective **management**. A high degree of awareness, in conjunction with careful

history-taking and thorough physical examination, is the most effective method of detection, although standardised questionnaires are also used. Laboratory investigations are sometimes helpful in establishing the diagnosis. Assessment should aim to determine the duration of abuse, the degree of dependence, the extent of related disabilities and the level of motivation to stop drinking.

6. During detoxification, sedative drugs are usually prescribed to control and minimise the unpleasant effects of withdrawal. It is important to establish a therapeutic contract, which must include a commitment to total abstention from alcohol, based upon setting realistic short-term goals. Maintaining abstinence following discharge from hospital is the most difficult aspect of treatment and can be assisted by various physical, psychological and social measures. Alcoholics Anonymous have established group meetings worldwide to provide support and advice to problem drinkers and their families. AA encourages its members to view alcohol abuse as a life-long illness, and to adopt a philosophy of 'one day at a time' in overcoming their problems. Additional support may be provided by Councils on Alcoholism, hostels and day centres for reformed drinkers, and the probation service. Disulfiram is sometimes used as a form of aversion therapy to prevent a relapse into drinking following abstinence. **Prevention** is the most important element in dealing with alcohol abuse; political and educative measures appear to have met with only limited success.

7. **Drugs** other than alcohol which are commonly abused come from three major sources: those obtained illicitly from drug dealers, those obtained from doctors (initially for therapeutic reasons), and those bought over the counter from shops and pharmacies. The development of drug **abuse** and **dependence** involves an interaction between the individual, the environment and the effects of the drug.

8. **Heroin**, a central nervous system depressant, is the most commonly abused opioid drug, being taken both orally and parenterally. Dependence develops readily, and sudden cessation of the drug produces a severe withdrawal syndrome. Chronic abuse is associated with apathy, self-neglect and the risk of infection with intravenous administration. **Barbiturate** abuse has declined in recent years. Physical dependence develops, and withdrawal symptoms are similar to those which occur with alcohol. **Benzodiazepines** are widely prescribed and dependence can develop at therapeutic dosages. Withdrawing people from these drugs can be extremely difficult, often because of persistent psychological dependence.

9. The stimulant effects of **amphetamines** induce strong psychological (but not physical) dependence. An amphetamine psychosis sometimes develops, features of which may be indistinguishable from acute schizophrenia. The effects of **cocaine** are similar to those of amphetamine, and can cause tactile hallucinations ('cocaine bug') or a paranoid

psychosis. **Cannabis** is widely abused and its effects are variable, depending upon the expectations and personality of the user, as well as the environment in which it is taken. Transient psychotic episodes sometimes occur and an 'amotivational syndrome' has been described.

10. **LSD** is an hallucinogen which produces variable changes in mood and perception. 'Flashback' phenomena sometimes occur. **Solvent abuse** involves the inhalation of chemical fumes to produce an intoxicating effect. Glue sniffing is mainly prevalent among children and adolescents. Initial effects are similar to those of alcohol intoxication, but chronic abuse can result in physical complications which may be fatal. The inappropriate use of minor **analgesics** is widespread, and significant abuse can cause liver or kidney damage.

11. **Assessment** should include information about the type(s) of drug used, its dosage and duration, the pattern of use and method of administration, the degree of dependence and any related disabilities. Corroborative evidence of drug abuse may be sought by physical examination and urine or blood testing. Total abstinence should always be the aim of **treatment**, but when this cannot be achieved, maintenance therapy may need to be considered. Withdrawal from heroin is best carried out under specialist care, through substitution with oral methadone which should then be gradually reduced over the course of a few weeks. Psychological treatment is often provided in the form of group therapy. Long-term rehabilitation may involve the individual residing in a community with other reformed addicts to learn new social and living skills in order to help maintain abstinence. Around 2–3% of opiate addicts die annually, but those that survive tend to 'mature out' and eventually achieve a more stable abstinent life-style.

REFERENCES AND FURTHER READING

Department of Health and Social Security (1984). *Guidelines of Good Clinical Practice in the Treatment of Drug Misuse.* Report of the Medical Working Party on drug dependence. London: DHSS.

Edwards, G., Gross, M. M. (1976). Alcohol dependence: provisional description of a clinical syndrome. *British Medical Journal*; **1**: 1058-61.

Foy, D. W., Nunn, L. B., Rychtarik, R. G. (1984). Broad-spectrum behavioural treatment for chronic alcoholics: effects of training controlled drinking skills. *Journal of Consulting and Clinical Psychology*; **52**: 218–30.

Grantham, P. (1987). Benzodiazepine abuse. *British Journal of Hospital Medicine*; **37**: 292–300.

Herzberg, J. L. Wolkind, S. N. (1983). Solvent sniffing in perspective. *British Journal of Hospital Medicine*; **29**: 72–76.

Higgitt, A. C., Lader, M. H., Fonagy, P. (1985). Clinical management of benzodiazepine dependence. *British Journal of Psychiatry*; **291**: 688–90.

King, M. (1986). At risk drinking among general practice attenders: prevalence, characteristics and alcohol-related problems. *British Journal of Psychiatry*; **148**: 533–40.

Paton, A., Saunders, J. B. (1981). ABC of alcohol: asking the right questions. *British Medical Journal*; **283**: 1458–59.

Perkin, G. D. (1983). Wernicke–Korsakoff syndrome. *British Journal of Hospital Medicine*; **30**: 331–34.

Ron, M. A. (1986). Volatile substance abuse: a review of possible long-term neurological, intellectual and psychiatric sequelae. *British Journal of Psychiatry*; **148**: 235–46.

Special Committee of the Royal College of Psychiatrists (1986). *Alcohol: our favourite drug*. London: Tavistock.

Thorley, A. (1986). Drug problems. In *Essentials of Postgraduate Psychiatry* (Hill, P., Murray, R., Thorley, A., eds.) pp. 279–310. London: Grune and Stratton.

World Health Organisation (1952). *Expert Committee on Mental Health, Alcoholism Subcommittee, second report*. Geneva: Technical report series no. 48.

12

DRUG TREATMENTS IN PSYCHIATRY

Drugs which act upon the mind are referred to as **psychotropic** compounds, and in order to exert their effect, they must enter the brain in sufficient amounts. Most of them can be taken orally, following which they are **absorbed** into the bloodstream through the gut wall. Passage to the liver via the hepatic portal system inactivates a large proportion of the drug through **first pass metabolism**, which is avoided when they are given intramuscularly or intravenously. Parenteral administration therefore allows much more of the active compound to reach the general circulation and hence the brain. Consequently, a 50 mg dose given intramuscularly is more potent than an equivalent amount given by mouth. Once in the bloodstream, much of the drug is attached to **plasma protein**, so that only the unbound fraction remains active and is able to cross lipid soluble membranes in the brain and fat stores. Further metabolism occurs in the liver, following which the compound and its metabolites are largely **excreted** through the kidneys. Patients with renal impairment may therefore experience toxic effects at otherwise therapeutic dosages.

The clinical properties of a drug depend upon the route of administration, the rate of absorption and excretion, the degree of metabolism and the extent of plasma protein binding. These factors vary from person to person, so that two people of similar age, build and sex may have widely different responses to the same dosage. Giving two or more psychotropic compounds concurrently may also influence their actions. For example, one drug can block absorption of another, increase its rate of breakdown by hepatic enzyme induction, or potentiate its activity by competitive plasma protein binding.

General Principles of Drug Treatment in Psychiatry

The rationale for prescribing any drug must be based upon its potential benefits outweighing any adverse effects which are likely to occur. Particular factors to be borne in mind before commencing treatment are potentially dangerous side-effects and interactions with other drugs or foods, the hazards of prescribing to certain groups of patients (especially

235

the elderly, pregnant women, breast-feeding mothers and those who are a suicide risk), the cost of the drug and the patient's likely compliance with treatment. In order to minimise the adverse consequences of drug use, the doctor needs to familiarise himself with the actions and side-effects of a small number of compounds in each therapeutic group. Furthermore, he should aim to give the drug at the lowest dose and for the shortest time possible in order to achieve the desired therapeutic effect. Where treatment appears to have failed, the clinician will need to review the diagnosis (is it correct?), the drug dosage and duration (is it adequate?) and the subject's compliance with the medication (about 30% of all patients fail to take the drugs prescribed for them).

1. HYPNOTICS AND ANXIOLYTICS

Since the mid-1960s, benzodiazepines have replaced barbiturates as the most commonly used hypnotics and anxiolytics. A **hypnotic** is a drug which induces sleep, while an **anxiolytic** is used to lower arousal in anxiety states. In practice, the division is somewhat arbitrary, since many compounds possess both properties. Beta-blockers, such as propranolol, also have a use in the management of anxiety.

(a) Benzodiazepines

PHARMACOLOGY AND MODE OF ACTION

Benzodiazepines are well absorbed orally and are highly lipid soluble. They bind to specific receptors on neurones in the cerebral cortex, midbrain and limbic system, facilitating the effects of the inhibitory neurotransmitter **GABA** (gamma-aminobutyric acid).

INDICATIONS FOR USE

   (i) To relieve anxiety and insomnia.
  (ii) In the treatment of delirium tremens and other withdrawal syndromes (*see* p. 201).
 (iii) To facilitate abreaction (*see* p. 284).
 (iv) For premedication and minor operative techniques.
  (v) For treating epileptic fits.
 (vi) To relieve muscle spasticity.
(vii) As an adjunct to certain forms of behaviour therapy (*see* p. 63).

Table 12.1 Profile of some commonly used benzodiazepines

Generic name	Trade name	Half-life	Half-life of metabolite
Triazolam	Halcion	2–4 h	3–6 h
Temazepam	Euhypnos	5–9 h	None
Lorazepam	Ativan	10–20 h	None
Nitrazepam	Mogadon	20–40 h	None
Chlordiazepoxide	Librium	10–20 h	10–30 h
Diazepam	Valium	20–45 h	50–100 h

ADMINISTRATION

Because of the risk of developing dependence (*see* Chapter 11), if used at all these drugs should only be given for short periods in low dosage.

CHOICE OF DRUG

Several benzodiazepines are available, and although they have similar properties and side-effects, their duration of action varies considerably and is the main factor in determining the choice of drug. Numerous active metabolites are produced, often with half-lives exceeding those of the parent compounds (Table 12.1).

Short-acting compounds are useful as hypnotics where daytime sedation is undesirable, although tolerance to this effect develops with chronic use. Where an anxiolytic effect is required the following day, long-acting benzodiazepines can be given before sleep.

SIDE-EFFECTS

These include drowsiness, dizziness, ataxia, impaired coordination (affecting motor skills such as driving), release of aggressive behaviour and confusion. Respiratory depression may be problematic in those with impaired lung function, and since the drug is secreted in breast milk, it should not be given during lactation to avoid causing lethargy and weight loss in the neonate. The problems of dependence and withdrawal are dealt with in Chapter 11.

TOXICITY AND DRUG INTERACTIONS

Benzodiazepines have few toxic effects and are relatively safe in overdosage, but can potentiate the actions of other CNS depressants, such as alcohol or barbiturates.

(b) Beta-blockers

MODE OF ACTION AND USE

These drugs are used to relieve certain somatic manifestations of anxiety, such as tremor and palpitations, by blocking peripheral adrenergic receptors. **Propanolol** is one of the most commonly used beta-blockers and this group of compounds is also employed to treat angina and hypertension.

SIDE-EFFECTS

Unwanted effects include bradycardia, tinnitus, purpura and rashes, insomnia, nightmares and nausea. They may precipitate cardiac failure in susceptible individuals and should not be given to people with low blood pressure or heart block. Beta-blockers are also contraindicated in those with a history of asthma (since they induce bronchospasm) or diabetes (as they can mask the signs of hypoglycaemia).

(c) Buspirone

MODE OF ACTION AND USE

Buspirone (BuSpar) is a recently introduced anxiolytic, which has a unique chemical structure, and acts in a different way from the benzodiazepines, most probably by increasing the inhibitory actions of 5HT in the brain. The anxiolytic effect is not immediate, but becomes apparent over a week or so. Other important differences from the benzodiazepines include:

1. a lack of clinically significant sedation at normal dosages
2. little observable interaction with alcohol
3. absence of dependence with long-term use, so that discontinuation is unlikely to be followed by withdrawal symptoms
4. absence of anticonvulsant or muscle relaxant properties.

SIDE EFFECTS

Unwanted effects appear to be minimal, although at the time of writing, clinical experience of the drug is limited. Buspirone should not be used in patients with severe hepatic or renal impairment, epilepsy and those taking monoamine oxidase inhibitors. It is also contraindicated in pregnancy and breast-feeding mothers.

(d) Other Hypnotics

Barbiturates are now mainly used illicitly, but are still occasionally prescribed to elderly patients who have been taking them for years as sleeping tablets, and have not been successfully weaned onto safer medication. Amylobarbitone is sometimes used for the purposes of abreaction (*see* p. 284). Side-effects, dependence and withdrawal symptoms are discussed in Chapter 11.

Chlormethiazole (Heminevrin) is a derivative of vitamin B_1 (thiamine). Its short half-life makes it a popular hypnotic for use in the elderly. Because of its anticonvulsant properties, it is often prescribed to minimise or prevent alcohol withdrawal symptoms. Side-effects include gastrointestinal upset, nasal congestion and conjunctival irritation. Since tolerance and dependence occur with habitual use, long-term administration of the drug should be avoided.

Chloral hydrate has few side-effects and consequently is safe for use in the elderly insomniac, although tolerance to its hypnotic actions develops after a few weeks.

Paraldehyde is renowned for its pungent odour, and because it is a gastric irritant, it is usually given intramuscularly. It is metabolised in the liver, but excreted in the sweat and breath.

Phenothiazines and **tricyclic antidepressants** are sometimes prescribed for their anxiolytic and hypnotic effects. They are discussed later in this chapter.

2. ANTIDEPRESSANTS

This group of drugs has been in use since the late 1950s, and currently there are more than 30 different compounds to choose from. They probably exert their effect by increasing levels of cerebral amines (*see* p. 87) and can be broadly classified into three groups: monoamine reuptake inhibitors (**MARIs**), monoamine oxidase inhibitors (**MAOIs**), and other antidepressants which have a different mode of action (*see also* Chapter 5).

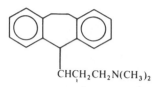

CHCH$_2$CH$_2$N(CH$_3$)$_2$

Amitriptyline

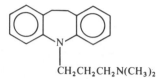

CH$_2$CH$_2$CH$_2$N(CH$_3$)$_2$

Imipramine

Fig. 12.1. Chemical structure of two tricyclic monoamine reuptake inhibitor antidepressants

(a) Monoamine Reuptake Inhibitors (MARIs)

The majority of compounds in this group are **tricyclic antidepressants**, so-called because of their three-ringed molecular structure (Fig. 12.1).

PHARMACOLOGY AND MODE OF ACTION

They are well absorbed by mouth, and although parenteral preparations are available, they have no therapeutic advantage and are rarely used. MARIs act by increasing the availability of the biogenic amine neurotransmitters noradrenaline and 5-hydroxytryptamine (5-HT) in the synaptic cleft through blocking their reuptake into the presynaptic neurone. Because MARIs have a long half-life, they are therapeutically effective if given once a day. They should only be given in divided doses to minimise unwanted effects. The more times a patient has to remember to take his medication, the less likely he is to do so. Absorption and metabolism vary widely among individuals, so that dosage should be adjusted according to clinical response.

The onset of their antidepressant action is relatively slow and variable, 2–4 weeks elapsing before any noticeable improvement in mood occurs. However, unwanted actions can develop after the first dose, so that a 'lag period' is created during which the individual may experience unpleasant drug-related symptoms but no therapeutic benefit.

MARI drugs can be classified into:

(i)   tertiary amines: preferentially block reuptake of 5-HT (**amitriptyline, imipramine, trimipramine** and **clomipramine**)
(ii) secondary amines: selectively block reuptake of noradrenaline (**desipramine, nortriptyline** and **protriptyline**); these are also produced by the metabolic demethylation of tertiary compounds
(iii) amitriptyline derivatives: **dothiepin** and **doxepin**.

INDICATIONS FOR USE

(i) First line drug treatment of depressive illness.
(ii) Prevention of relapse in recurrent depression.
(iii) Obsessional and phobic disorders with a significant depressive component.
(iv) Childhood enuresis (*see* Chapter 16).
(v) The management of chronic pain, especially where there is no demonstrable organic pathology to account for symptoms.

SIDE-EFFECTS AND TOXICITY

There are numerous unwanted actions associated with the use of these drugs, the majority of which arise from anticholinergic effects and the blockade of amine reuptake in peripheral tissues (particularly the heart). These are shown in Table 12.2.

MARI antidepressants can be fatal in overdosage, with death resulting from respiratory depression or their cardiotoxic effects (notably arrhythmias). Consequently, they should be prescribed with caution to all patients, especially those who pose a serious suicidal risk. The risk can be minimised by assessing the patient at frequent intervals, only giving medication to cover the period until he is seen again, and by entrusting the handling of the tablets to a relative or friend. Tricyclic antidepressants should also be prescribed with caution in the elderly, because a normal therapeutic dose for a young adult may prove to be toxic in an older person, in whom side-effects can be especially troublesome.

CONTRAINDICATIONS

These drugs should never be given to those who have recently suffered a myocardial infarct, are in heart block, or have bone marrow suppression. Relative contraindications include cardiac arrhythmias, liver disease, renal impairment, prostatic hypertrophy, glaucoma and epilepsy.

DRUG INTERACTIONS

When prescribed with phenothiazines, the serum levels of both drugs are increased by competitive reduction of hepatic metabolism. The actions of CNS depressants, including alcohol and barbiturates, are potentiated by MARI compounds. The anticholinergic effect may summate with those of other drugs, such as certain neuroleptics and antiparkinsonian medication.

Table 12.2 Possible side-effects of MARI antidepressants

System	Side-effect
Cardiovascular	Postural hypotension Tachycardia Cardiac arrhythmias Altered conduction producing ECG changes Precipitation of myocardial infarction
Gastrointestinal	Dry mouth Nausea Constipation
Genitourinary	Hesitancy of micturition Urinary retention Delayed ejaculation
Ocular	Blurred vision Precipitation of glaucoma
Haematological	Eosinophilia Agranulocytosis (rare)
Endocrine/metabolic	Weight gain Amenorrhoea
Neuropsychiatric	Sedation Tremor Confusion in the elderly Convulsions (uncommon) Precipitation of mania in predisposed individuals
Others	Increased sweating Skin rashes Jaundice (rare)

Hypotensive drugs, e.g. guanethidine, bethanidine and clonidine, are antagonised by MARIs. If a MARI drug is combined with a monoamine oxidase inhibitor (MAOI), severe hypertension can result.

(b) Monoamine Oxidase Inhibitors (MAOIs)

It has been repeatedly shown in clinical trials that MAOIs are less effective than MARIs in treating most cases of depressive illness, and consequently, they are generally regarded as a second line of anti-depressant therapy. However, there are other indications for their use (*see below*).

PHARMACOLOGY AND MODE OF ACTION

These compounds increase the level of biogenic amine neurotransmitters by blocking monoamine oxidase enzymes, which are involved in their intracellular degradation. MAOIs are classified as either derivatives of hydrazine, which are potentially hepatotoxic (e.g. phenelzine, isocarboxazid, iproniazid), or non-hydrazines (e.g. tranylcypromine, which has amphetamine-like actions). They are absorbed by mouth and the hydrazine derivatives are metabolised by acetylation in the liver.

INDICATIONS FOR USE

(i) Treatment of 'atypical' depression (e.g. if symptoms of anxiety predominate, or where there is increased appetite and sleep).
(ii) Treatment of 'resistant' depression which has failed to respond to MARI antidepressants and/or ECT.
(iii) Treatment of phobic anxiety states.

SIDE-EFFECTS AND TOXICITY

Anticholinergic effects include dry mouth, nausea, blurred vision, hesitancy of micturition, constipation and sweating. Other unwanted actions are weight gain, postural hypotension, ankle oedema, drowsiness, confusion, tremor and paraesthesiae in the extremities. Hepatocellular jaundice occurs rarely with hydrazine derivatives.

In overdosage, MAOIs may produce a state of over-arousal characterised by agitation, increased reflexes, hyperpyrexia and labile blood pressure, leading to convulsions.

CONTRAINDICATIONS

Patients with liver disease or cardiac failure should not be given these drugs.

DRUG AND FOOD INTERACTIONS

MAOIs can interact dangerously with certain foods containing tyramine or with sympathomimetic amines. Inhibition of the enzyme monoamine oxidase prevents the normal metabolism of these substances in the gut and liver. Consequently, pressor amines are able to enter the circulation and cause prolonged release of noradrenaline, resulting in a **hypertensive crisis** characterised by a pounding headache, palpitations, flushing, hyperpyrexia, convulsions and possible cerebral haemorrhage. Foods containing tyramine include certain wines and cheeses, yeast extracts, pickled or smoked fish, pâté and 'hung' game. Sympathomimetic amines are contained in many drugs available without prescription, such as antihistamines, cold remedies and cough mixtures, as well as certain local anaesthetics.

Patients receiving MAOIs should carry a treatment card which warns of these possible interactions, and advises other doctors or dentists against prescribing potentially dangerous drugs.

Dangerous interactions can also occur between MAOIs and certain opioids (notably morphine and pethidine), central nervous system depressants (i.e. alcohol and barbiturates), hypoglycaemic agents (oral compounds or insulin) and hypotensive drugs (methyldopa or guanethidine). Although MARI drugs can interact adversely with MAOIs, they are sometimes given in combination, particularly where a depressive illness has been resistant to treatment by each alone.

(c) Other Antidepressants

The unpleasant side-effects and toxicity in overdosage of many well-established antidepressant drugs has led to a search for safer 'second generation' compounds with minimal unwanted effects. Some of these (such as **lofepramine**) are MARI antidepressants, while others (e.g. mianserin) have different modes of action.

Tetracyclic antidepressants have a four-ringed nucleus. One such drug, **mianserin**, acts by blocking presynaptic alpha-2 receptors which normally inhibit noradrenaline release at the synapse. Although it is relatively safe in overdosage, its use has been associated with the development of serious blood dyscrasias. **Maprotiline** is a MARI drug with few unwanted effects, apart from skin rashes and a tendency to lower the epileptic threshold. **Viloxazine** is a bicyclic compound with minimal cardiovascular and anticholinergic actions, although it is liable to cause nausea and headaches.

L-tryptophan is an aminoacid which is a precursor of 5-hydroxytryptamine. Although claimed to have antidepressant actions of its own, it is mainly used as an adjunct to MAOI therapy in resistant cases of depression.

Choice of Antidepressant Drug

This depends on many factors, including the age and state of health of the patient, features of the depressive illness (especially the risk of suicide),

Table 12.3 Profile of antidepressant drugs in clinical use

Drug			Side-effects	
Generic name	Trade name	Group	Sedative	Anticholinergic
Amitriptyline	Tryptizol	MARI	Strong	Strong
Trimipramine	Surmontil	MARI	Strong	Strong
Dothiepin	Prothiaden	MARI	Strong	Moderate
Doxepin	Sinequan	MARI	Strong	Moderate
Maprotiline	Ludiomil	MARI	Strong	Mild
Mianserin	Bolvidon	Presynaptic alpha-2 receptor blocker	Strong	Mild
Imipramine	Tofranil	MARI	Moderate	Moderate
Clomipramine	Anafranil	MARI	Moderate	Moderate
Nortriptyline	Aventyl	MARI	Mild	Moderate
Desipramine	Pertofran	MARI	Mild	Mild
Lofepramine	Gamanil	MARI	Mild	Mild
Viloxazine	Vivalan	MARI	Mild	Mild
Protriptyline	Concordin	MARI	None	Moderate
Isocarboxazid	Marplan	MAOI	Moderate	Moderate
Iproniazid	Marsilid	MAOI	Mild	Moderate
Phenelzine	Nardil	MAOI	Mild	Moderate
Tranylcypromine	Parnate	MAOI	None	Moderate

unwanted effects, the cost of the drug and the personal preference of the doctor.

In those with clear-cut biological features of depression, a MARI drug is usually the first choice of treatment. Where anxiety or agitation are predominant symptoms, one of the more sedative compounds should be prescribed. On the other hand, evidence of retardation would indicate giving a drug with alerting or less sedating properties (Table 12.3). In elderly patients, where cardiotoxicity is a potential risk, it may be safer to prescribe one of the newer antidepressants, such as lofepramine or mianserin. This principle might also apply to those who experience intolerable side-effects with well-established compounds, such as amitriptyline or imipramine, and where there is a clear danger of suicide. However, it should be noted that the newer antidepressants are considerably more expensive than the original drugs, and many of their side-effects are still being evaluated. Since the therapeutic effect can take up to 4 weeks to develop, MARIs need to be taken for at least 5–6 weeks before a course of treatment is said to be unsuccessful. Antidepressant treatment should continue for at least 6 months following the resolution of symptoms, to minimise the risk of relapse.

If treatment fails with a MARI drug, the doctor should first establish whether or not the patient is complying with medication, and if the drug has been given in a therapeutically effective dosage for a sufficient length of time. If so, some clinicians would consider giving an MAOI or administering ECT (*see* Chapter 5).

3. LITHIUM

Lithium is a chemical element which has been used in the past to treat gout and hypertension. Since the mid-1960s, however, lithium salts have become established in the treatment and prophylaxis of affective disorders (*see also* Chapter 5).

PHARMACOLOGY AND MODE OF ACTION

Lithium is well absorbed by mouth and distributed throughout the body tissues, peak plasma levels being reached in approximately 2 hours. It is not metabolised and is therefore excreted unchanged, mainly via the kidney (minimal quantities also appearing in sweat and saliva). Sodium and lithium are competitively reabsorbed at the proximal renal tubule. Consequently, thiazide diuretics which increase sodium excretion will also increase serum lithium levels, in some cases leading to toxicity. Dehydration and a low salt diet can produce a similar effect. The mode of action of lithium in the treatment and prevention of affective disorders is not clearly understood, although it is possibly due to interference with ionic transfer across cell membranes.

INDICATIONS FOR USE

(a) Treatment of mania and hypomania.
(b) Prophylaxis of recurrent affective disorder (bipolar or unipolar).
(c) In combination with other drugs in the treatment of resistant depression.
(d) Treatment of schizoaffective disorders (often as an adjunct to neuroleptics).
(e) Treatment of recurrent behavioural disturbances in certain individuals.

ADMINISTRATION

Before commencing treatment with lithium, it must be established that the patient has adequate renal function to enable excretion of the drug. In addition, thyroid function tests should be performed, since therapeutic doses of lithium can produce hypothyroidism. Steady serum levels are best achieved by giving the drug once or twice daily.

Lithium has a narrow therapeutic range, outside of which the drug is either toxic or ineffective. Therefore, it is important that regular estimations are made of serum levels. As these reach a peak about 2 hours after ingestion, it is advisable to measure the serum lithium concentration when a steady state has been achieved, that is about 12 hours after the last dose. For the treatment of acute mania or hypomania, serum levels of approximately 1.0–1.2 mmol/l are required, whereas prophylactic levels can be somewhat lower, i.e. 0.6–1.0 mmol/l. Initially, blood tests will need to be repeated weekly, but once a stable level has been achieved, the interval between estimations can be extended to once a month and then every 8–12 weeks. Thyroid and renal function tests should be performed every 6 months.

SIDE-EFFECTS AND TOXICITY

These can be conveniently divided into early and long-term effects. **Early side-effects** tend to be transient, relatively harmless and are usually related to peak serum levels prior to stabilisation of therapy. They include nausea and vomiting, diarrhoea, dry mouth and thirst, stuffy nose, a metallic taste, drowsiness, fatigue, a fine tremor (mainly of the hands) and a mild diuresis.

Long-term side-effects are often more troublesome. **Polyuria** and **polydipsia** (features of nephrogenic diabetes insipidus) may persist throughout treatment in about 10% of patients, and result from lithium rendering the distal renal tubule less sensitive to the actions of antidiuretic hormone (ADH). **Hypothyroidism** occurs in approximately 10% of all patients on long-term lithium therapy, particularly women. This may be treated with thyroxine, but as with nephrogenic diabetes insipidus, it is reversible once treatment is stopped.

Irreversible **renal damage** has been reported in some patients on maintenance therapy, although this finding is not universally attributed to the drug. Other possible long-term effects include leucocytosis, weight gain, oedema, exacerbation of psoriasis and acne, cardiac arrhythmias and minor ECG changes, mild memory impairment, osteoporosis and muscle weakness.

Signs of **lithium toxicity** begin to appear with plasma levels above 2.0

mmol/l. These include diarrhoea and vomiting, slurred speech, coarse tremor, ataxia, motor incoordination, drowsiness and confusion. If action is not taken at this stage, muscle twitching, nystagmus and convulsions may develop, leading to coma and eventual death. Initial treatment consists of stopping the drug and giving a high fluid intake, supplemented with extra sodium. However, if lithium levels remain high, intravenous mannitol, forced alkaline diuresis or renal dialysis may be necessary.

CONTRAINDICATIONS

Lithium therapy should be avoided, if possible, in patients with cardiac or renal disease, hypothyroidism, Addison's disease, psoriasis or severe acne.

Because lithium crosses the placenta, it should not be given during **pregnancy**, particularly in the first 3 months, as an increase in cardiac abnormalities has been reported in babies born to mothers taking the drug. **Breast feeding** is also contraindicated because lithium is excreted in the milk and can cause high neonatal blood levels leading to hypotonia, hypothermia and cyanosis.

DRUG INTERACTIONS

Lithium should not be given to patients taking thiazide diuretics or phenytoin, as toxic lithium levels can result. Although high doses of haloperidol are sometimes given in conjunction with lithium to treat acute mania, this combination has been reported as causing serious neurological impairment, including confusion, tremor, convulsions and coma. Signs of extrapyramidal and cerebellar dysfunction may also be present and the outcome is sometimes fatal. Other investigators have found this drug combination to be entirely safe, but it is probably wise to restrict the dosages of haloperidol and lithium to low levels when they are given together.

Other Drugs Used in the Treatment of Bipolar Affective Disorder

Some patients with bipolar affective illness appear to be resistant to the effects of lithium and their relapse rate is not reduced. This is particularly so of individuals who have severe rapid swings in mood ('rapid cyclers'). Two anticonvulsant drugs, **carbamazepine** and **sodium valproate**, may be effective for this group, and are sometimes given either in combination with lithium or alone.

4. NEUROLEPTICS

These drugs (also known as **major tranquillisers**) induce 'neurolepsis', a state of calm indifference without loss of consciousness. In addition, they possess specific antipsychotic properties and are widely used in the treatment of schizophrenia and other psychoses (*see* p. 145). They are classified according to their chemical structure into a number of groups, namely phenothiazines, thioxanthines, butyrophenones, diphenylbutyl-piperidines and benzamide derivatives. Although they vary in potency and side-effects, they all share the ability to block dopamine receptors to some degree.

(a) Phenothiazines

Chlorpromazine, the standard compound among neuroleptics, was the first member of this group to be synthesised in 1950. There are three categories of phenothiazines in clinical use, which are classified according to the configuration of the side chain attached to the basic nucleus (Fig. 12.2). They are:

(i) aliphatic compounds: **chlorpromazine, promazine**

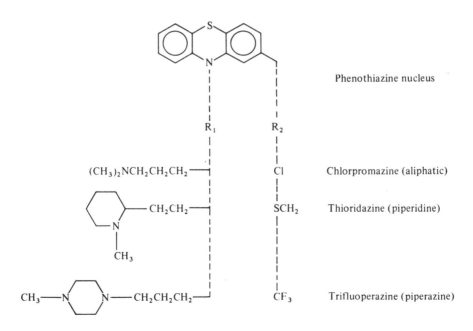

Fig. 12.2 Chemical structure of the phenothiazines

(ii) piperidine compounds: **thioridazine, pipothiazine**
(iii) piperazine compounds: **trifluoperazine, prochlorperazine, fluphenazine.**

PHARMACOLOGY AND MODE OF ACTION

Dopamine receptors in the brain are aggregated into four main systems, all
of which are blocked by phenothiazines. Blockade in the **mesolimbic
pathway** is probably responsible for their antipsychotic activity, whereas
blockade in the **nigrostriatal pathways** accounts for their extrapyramidal
side-effects. Inhibition of prolactin release from the pituitary gland is
suppressed when the **hypothalamic–pituitary pathway** is interrupted, and
leads to hyperprolactinaemia. The **medullary pathway** stimulates the
vomiting centre, blockade of which accounts for the antiemetic activity of
these drugs.

In addition to their ability to block dopamine receptors, phenothiazines
produce complex and variable effects on the autonomic nervous system
due to their anticholinergic, antiadrenergic and antihistaminic actions (*see
below*).

Phenothiazines are well absorbed and effective by mouth, but due to
the effects of first pass metabolism, equivalent parenteral doses are more
potent. Chlorpromazine has a relatively short half-life, but a number of
active metabolites may persist in the body and continue to exert an effect
for several weeks after the drug is discontinued.

INDICATIONS FOR USE

(i)   Treatment of schizophrenia (particularly the 'positive symptoms')
      and prevention of relapse (*see* Chapter 8).
(ii) Treatment of hypomania and mania.
(iii) As an adjunct to other forms of treatment in severe depressive
      illnesses where delusions and/or hallucinations are a clinical
      feature.
(iv) Treatment of other psychoses, such as paranoid or organic states.
(v)   Control of disturbed, agitated or aggressive behaviour.
(vi) As an antiemetic, e.g. in the care of the terminally ill.

SIDE-EFFECTS

The unwanted actions of phenothiazines (and other neuroleptics) are
shown in Tables 12.4 and 12.5.

Table 12.4 Extrapyramidal side-effects associated with phenothiazines and other neuroleptic drugs

Side-effect	Features	Management
Acute dystonia	Involuntary contraction of skeletal muscle; most commonly affects muscles of head and neck, producing an oculogyric crisis, in which the eyes turn upwards, the neck extends and the mouth opens. The muscles of the trunk and limbs may also be involved. Potentially dangerous as respiratory muscles may be affected. Onset usually within 24 h of starting medication, especially in young men	IM or IV injection of anticholinergic drug e.g. 5–10 mg of procyclidine. Start patient on regular oral anticholinergic medication
Akathisia	Motor restlessness, particularly in the legs, which develops within a few weeks of starting treatment. Patient fidgets and is unable to sit still. May be accompanied by psychological tension	Reduce or stop neuroleptic
Pseudoparkinsonism	Muscle rigidity, tremor and bradykinesia. Dribbling may occur. Can be observed in up to 40% of those receiving neuroleptic medication. Onset 6–12 weeks after commencing medication, but may occur earlier	Reduce or stop neuroleptic for a few days. Symptoms may resolve and not reappear on restarting medication. Alternatively, administer anticholinergic drugs
Tardive dyskinesia	Orofacial involuntary movements involving grimacing, chewing, pouting, tongue protrusion and lip-smacking. Occasionally, the whole body may be involved, producing body-rocking, arching of the back, swinging movements of the limbs and shrugging of the shoulders. Onset usually after 2–3 years' treatment, but can	Prevention is the best cure. In maintenance treatment, prescribe the lowest dose of neuroleptic for the minimum period. Early signs should be treated by stopping the neuroleptic. Once established, the condition is difficult to treat and may be irreversible. Anticholinergic drugs are ineffective and possibly worsen the situation.

continued overleaf

Table 12.4 *Continued*

Side-effect	Features	Management
	occur sooner. Possibly due to supersensitivity of dopamine receptors following prolonged blockade with neuroleptics. Risk greatest in elderly females and those with brain damage; more likely with long-term treatment at high dosage (approximately 20% of patients being affected)	GABA-nergic drugs (such as benzodiazepines and sodium valproate), dopamine–depleting compounds (i.e. tetrabenazine) and choline precursors (deanol) have all been used in treatment without clear benefit

(b) Thioxanthines

This group includes **clopenthixol** and **flupenthixol**, which are often administered in the form of depot preparations. Thioxanthines are produced by minor changes in the phenothiazine nucleus, and the indications for their use and unwanted effects are similar to those of the phenothiazines, although no cholestatic jaundice has been reported. Flupenthixol is also alleged to have antidepressant properties in low dosage.

(c) Butyrophenones

These are structurally unrelated to the phenothiazines, but nevertheless block dopamine receptors and have potent antipsychotic actions. They include **haloperidol** and **droperidol**. Indications and unwanted effects are similar to those of the phenothiazines, except that sedation is usually less marked and postural hypotension is uncommon. Extrapyramidal side-effects tend to be pronounced, especially in the elderly.

(d) Diphenylbutylpiperidines

This group includes **pimozide** and **fluspirilene**, which are derivatives of the butyrophenones. They have a longer duration of action than the parent compounds and fewer unwanted effects.

(e) Benzamide Derivatives

The dopamine receptors in the brain are of two types. Blockade of D1 receptors, such as those located in the nigrostriatal pathway, is thought to produce the extrapyramidal symptoms of neuroleptic drugs. On the other hand, antipsychotic action is attributed to D2 receptor blockade.

Table 12.5 Side-effects of neuroleptic drugs (excluding extrapyramidal actions)

System	Side-effect	Cause
Cardiovascular	Postural hypotension with reflex tachycardia	Anti-adrenergic
	Abnormal T waves on ECG	Unknown
Gastrointestinal	Dry mouth Constipation	Anticholinergic
Genitourinary	Urinary hesitancy and retention	Anticholinergic
	Delayed ejaculation	Antiadrenergic
Skin	Reduced sweating	Anticholinergic
	Increased pigmentation	? Catalytic effect of UV light on melanin in presence of phenothiazines
	Rashes and increased photosensitivity	Hypersensitivity reaction
Ocular	Blurred vision Precipitation of glaucoma	Anticholinergic
	Retinal pigmentation (especially thioridazine)	? Catalytic effect of UV light on melanin
Endocrine/metabolic	Weight gain	Unknown ? Hypothalamic effect
	Amenorrhoea and infertility Galactorrhoea	Hyperprolactinaemia
	Gynaecomastia	Unknown
	Hypothermia (especially in the elderly)	Unknown
	Cholestatic jaundice	Hypersensitivity reaction
Haematological	Agranulocytosis	Bone marrow depression due to hypersensitivity reaction
Neuropsychiatric	Sedation	Antihistaminic
	? Depression	Unknown
	Convulsions	Reduced epileptic threshold

continued overleaf

Table 12.5 *Continued*

System	Side-effect	Cause
Others	Nasal congestion	Anti-adrenergic
	Neuroleptic malignant syndrome (rare and sometimes fatal condition involving hyperpyrexia, fluctuating blood pressure, tachycardia, muscle rigidity and coma)	? Excessive dopamine blockade

Benzamide derivatives, such as **sulpiride**, confer a theoretical advantage over other major tranquillisers, in that they selectively block D2 receptors with only minimal activity at D1 sites. Consequently, they should produce antipsychotic actions without the development of extrapyramidal side-effects, although this has yet to be confirmed in practice.

Contraindications and Interactions with other Drugs

Phenothiazines are contraindicated when previous administration has produced severe sensitivity reactions, such as cholestatic jaundice or bone marrow suppression. They should be used with caution in those patients suffering from cardiorespiratory disease, hepatic or renal impairment, Parkinson's disease, hypothyroidism, myasthenia gravis, acute infections, epilepsy, glaucoma, or prostatic hypertrophy.

Neuroleptics potentiate other central nervous system depressants, such as barbiturates, opioids and alcohol. When prescribed together with antidepressant medication, the serum levels of both drugs are increased, so that therapeutic effects may be achieved with smaller doses. Propranolol is sometimes used as an adjunct to antipsychotic treatment, due to its ability to potentiate neuroleptic blood levels.

Choice of Neuroleptic Drug

Of the neuroleptic drugs available, the choice will depend upon the needs of the patient, a consideration of the side-effects of each compound, as well as personal preference. This is discussed more fully under the management of schizophrenia (*see* p. 145), along with the most appropriate route of administration (oral versus parenteral use). The relative potency of these drugs and a comparison of their unwanted effects are shown in Table 12.6.

Table 12.6 Summary of neuroleptic drugs in common use

Drug	Group	Equivalent potency	Side-effects Sedative	Side-effects Anticholinergic	Side-effects Extrapyramidal
Chlorpromazine (Largactil)	Aliphatic phenothiazine	100 mg	+++	++	++
Thioridazine (Melleril)	Piperidine phenothiazine	100 mg	++	+++	+
Trifluoperazine (Stelazine)	Piperazine phenothiazine	5 mg	+	+	+++
Haloperidol (Serenace)	Butyrophenone	5 mg	+	+	+++
Pimozide (Orap)	Diphenylbutyl-piperidine	2 mg	+	+	++
Depot injections *					
Fluphenazine decanoate (Modecate)	Piperazine phenothiazine	25 mg IM fortnightly	++	+	+++
Flupenthixol decanoate (Depixol)	Thioxanthene	40 mg IM fortnightly	+	+	+++
Clopenthixol decanoate (Clopixol)	Thioxanthene	200 mg IM fortnightly	+	+	+++

* Doses shown are equivalent to 100 mg of oral chlorpromazine given daily.

In acute psychoses, a typical starting dose of oral chlorpromazine for a 70 kg man would be 400 mg daily in divided doses (when chlorpromazine or other drugs need to be given intramuscularly, dosages should be reduced accordingly). From Table 12.6, it can be seen that this regimen would be equivalent to 20 mg of haloperidol or trifluoperazine daily. In severe cases, medication may be increased until symptoms are controlled, although the development of side-effects usually determines the maximum dose that can be safely given. Where maintenance treatment is indicated, the daily oral dosages can often be reduced considerably or, alternatively, a depot preparation substituted.

5. SYNTHETIC ANTICHOLINERGIC DRUGS

These drugs are used to counteract the extrapyramidal side-effects which occur in association with prescribing antipsychotic medication. They include **procyclidine** (Kemadrin), **orphenadrine** (Disipal), **benzhexol** (Artane) and **benztropine** (Cogentin), and exert their effect by correcting the relative excess of acetylcholine which occurs in the nigrostriatal system after dopamine blockade. Because there are a number of problems associated with their use, they should only be given when the dose of neuroleptic drug has been reduced to the lowest level compatible with therapeutic efficacy. In addition to unwanted anticholinergic effects, they can cause acute organic relations, particularly in the elderly. They also reduce the serum levels of neuroleptics by decreasing their absorption from the gut, and by increasing hepatic metabolism through enzyme induction. High dosages can produce excitement and euphoria, which may result in abuse.

SUMMARY

1. Drugs which act upon the mind are referred to as psychotropic compounds. In keeping with other drugs, their actions will be affected by their rate and mode of absorption, metabolism and excretion, and the extent of binding to plasma proteins. Before a drug is prescribed, its potential benefits must be weighed against any adverse effects, as well as considering dangerous interactions with other compounds.
2. **Benzodiazepines** are widely used as hypnotics and anxiolytics. They are well absorbed orally, and are unlikely to be fatal in overdosage. They facilitate the actions of the inhibitory neurotransmitter GABA. Because of their addictive properties, they should only be prescribed in low dosages for short periods of time. The choice of benzodiazepine is primarily determined by its duration of action. Short-acting compounds are useful as hypnotics, whereas longer acting benzodiazepines can be prescribed if an anxiolytic effect is required the following day. **Beta-blockers** may be helpful in managing the somatic symptoms of anxiety. Other hypnotic drugs which are used include chlormethiazole, chloral hydrate, paraldehyde and (rarely) certain barbiturates.
3. **Antidepressants** probably exert their effect by increasing the levels of biogenic amine neurotransmitters and are classified into monoamine reuptake inhibitors (MARIs), monoamine oxidase inhibitors (MAOIs) and other compounds which have a different mode of action. **MARIs** include the tricyclic antidepressants, which are well absorbed by mouth. They impede the reuptake of noradrenaline and/or 5-hydroxytryptamine (5-HT) from the synaptic cleft. There is a 'lag period' of up to 4 weeks

after commencing treatment before their antidepressant action becomes evident. MARI compounds are often used as the first line drug treatment of depressive illness. Unwanted side-effects are common, and mainly arise from their anticholinergic and cardiotoxic actions. A history of recent myocardial infarction is a contraindication to their use. They should be prescribed with great caution in the elderly, and to those who pose a significant suicidal risk, because of their toxicity in overdosage. **MAOIs** are generally less effective than MARIs in treating depression, although they may be useful in atypical or resistant cases. They are well absorbed by mouth and act by blocking monoamine oxidase enzymes which are involved in the intracellular degradation of biogenic neurotransmitters. As well as causing unwanted anticholinergic effects, MAOIs may interact dangerously with certain foods containing tyramine or with drugs containing sympathomimetic amines to produce a hypertensive crisis. **Second generation antidepressants**, such as mianserin and lofepramine, have fewer anticholinergic and cardiotoxic effects, although their efficacy is not as well proven as with older compounds.

4. **Lithium** is used in the treatment and prophylaxis of affective disorders, although its mode of action is not clearly understood. It is well absorbed by mouth and excreted unchanged, mainly via the kidney. Renal and thyroid function should be checked before commencing treatment with lithium. The drug has a narrow therapeutic range, outside of which it is ineffective or results in toxicity. Regular estimations should be made of serum levels throughout treatment, which may need to be continued indefinitely. Long-term side-effects include polydipsia and polyuria, hypothyroidism and possibly renal damage. Lithium toxicity is potentially fatal, so that therapeutic action should be taken without delay if it is suspected or confirmed. The drug should be avoided in patients with cardiac, renal or thyroid disease, as well as in pregnant women and breast-feeding mothers.

5. **Neuroleptics** (or major tranquillisers) possess specific antipsychotic properties and are widely used in the treatment and prophylaxis of schizophrenia and other psychoses. They are classified according to their chemical structure into a number of groups: phenothiazines, thioxanthenes, butyrophenones, diphenylbutylpiperidines and benzamide derivatives. All neuroleptics share the ability to block dopamine receptors, which is thought to account for their therapeutic actions. The drugs may be administered orally or parenterally. Unwanted effects mainly result from extrapyramidal, anticholinergic and antiadrenergic actions. Synthetic anticholinergic drugs, such as procyclidine, are sometimes given to counteract the extrapyramidal side-effects.

REFERENCES AND FURTHER READING

Catalan, J., Gath, D. H. (1985). Benzodiazepines in general practice: time for a decision. *British Medical Journal*; **290**: 1374–76.

Cookson, J. C. (1985). Drug treatment of bipolar depression and mania. *British Journal of Hospital Medicine*; **34**: 172–75.

Johnson, D. A. W. (1979). Further observations on the duration of depot neuroleptic maintenance therapy in schizophrenia. *British Journal of Psychiatry*; **135**: 524–30.

Johnstone, E. C. (1985). Drug treatment in psychiatry: acute schizophrenia. *British Journal of Hospital Medicine*; **34**: 198–201.

Lader, M. (1986). A practical guide to prescribing hypnotic benzodiazepines. *British Medical Journal*; **293**: 1048–49.

Manchanda, R., Hirsch, S. R. (1986). Low dose maintenance medication for schizophrenia. *British Medical Journal*; **293**: 515–16.

Paykel, E. S., Coppen, A., eds (1979). *Psychopharmacology of Affective Disorders*. Oxford: Oxford University Press.

Quitkin, F. M. (1985). The importance of dosage in prescribing antidepressants. *British Journal of Psychiatry*; **147**: 593–97.

Schou, M. (1986). Lithium treatment: a refresher course. *British Journal of Psychiatry*; **149**: 541–47.

Silverstone, T., Turner, P. (1982). *Drug Treatment in Psychiatry*, 3rd edn. London: Routledge and Kegan Paul.

13 PSYCHOTHERAPY, BEHAVIOUR THERAPY AND OTHER PSYCHOLOGICAL TREATMENTS

Psychotherapy is a term which covers a number of different treatments, all of which use **talking** and **listening** to bring about relief from specific symptoms, or to help people adjust to and cope with the problems of everyday life. **Behavioural treatments** employ somewhat different principles and are discussed later in the chapter.

Talking as a form of therapy has undoubtedly existed for countless generations, but specific concepts of how and why the treatment is effective have only evolved in the last century. Psychotherapy may be conducted with **individuals**, **couples**, **families**, **small groups** of approximately 6–10 people, as well as with **large groups** of 20 or more. In all cases, the relationship which develops between the subject and therapist is important in bringing about change.

In addition to the number of people involved, psychotherapy can be further considered in terms of **duration** of treatment and the **complexity** of the procedure. Some forms are relatively simple and conducted for a brief period of time, while others may last for years and are both intensive and emotionally demanding. Nevertheless, neither duration nor complexity of treatment are necessarily equated with efficacy, and sometimes a sympathetic and carefully taken history is in itself a gratifying and therapeutic experience for the patient.

Irrespective of the above considerations, psychotherapy can be broadly differentiated into supportive or dynamic types. **Supportive psychotherapy** is aimed at reducing anxiety, and carrying or supporting the individual at a time when continuing stress is likely to result in a breakdown of functioning. **Dynamic psychotherapy** fulfils similar functions but, in addition, aims to bring about change by detecting and resolving underlying psychological conflicts which are the root cause of disturbed personal relationships and the unpleasant symptoms which often accompany them. For this reason, it is frequently anxiety-provoking, although it does aim to provide support and comfort when needed.

THERAPEUTIC FACTORS COMMON TO ALL TYPES OF PSYCHOTHERAPY

Psychotherapy affords an opportunity for people to **make sense** of their problems and to discover ways of dealing with them more effectively. Many of those who enter therapy have already tried and failed to overcome their difficulties, which may have had an adverse effect on their morale. A consequence of therapy is therefore an **increase in self-esteem**, and facilitating the **release of emotion** sometimes results in the lowering of arousal and the relief of distress.

SUPPORTIVE PSYCHOTHERAPY

Supportive psychotherapy aims to minimise disabling symptoms by encouraging the ventilation of feelings, demonstrating empathy with the individual's worries and offering advice where appropriate. This is accomplished without necessarily trying to understand the fundamental origins of the presenting difficulties. The majority of people with psychological problems respond to help at this level, and the procedure is commonly used in conjunction with other forms of treatment, such as psychotropic drugs or behaviour therapy.

Even though supportive psychotherapy is frequently given by people without formal training, the technique does have important differences from simply offering advice and support to acquaintances. The element of suggestion is often a potent factor within the therapeutic relationship, so that the influence of the therapist may be far greater than a similar interaction with a relative or friend. For example, suggesting to someone that they will soon feel better may indeed have some therapeutic value, because this is usually what the person wants to believe, so that he is likely to be favourably influenced by such a remark. However, reassurance will only maintain confidence and instil hope for the future provided it is couched in realistic terms.

Supportive psychotherapy should proceed at a comfortable pace, so that the individual has time to consider the implications of any decisions that need to be made. Effecting a solution to a problem is most likely if the person arrives at the answer himself, and the therapist can assist this aim by striving to remain impartial and non-judgemental when offering advice. In this way, an opportunity is created to share ideas or concerns with someone else prior to reaching a decision which is both reasonable and practicable. Failure of the therapist to take heed of these principles can have adverse consequences, as illustrated in the following example:

A 27-year-old woman became tense and miserable after discovering that her husband was having an affair with his secretary. At her request, she was referred by her general practitioner to the local psychiatric unit where she was offered 'supportive psychotherapy'. Due to a number of staff being on sick leave, she was seen by a therapist who, although enthusiastic and caring, was very inexperienced. The woman recounted her story and finally asked what she should do. Unfortunately, the therapist's own marriage had ended a year beforehand, and she herself had failed to acknowledge the intense anger she continued to feel towards her ex-husband, which subsequently affected her judgement and the advice she gave. Empathising with her patient's plight, the therapist advised the woman to tell her husband to leave because of his contemptible behaviour, reassuring her that she would feel much better afterwards. When the patient returned a few weeks later, she was even more distraught than she had been on the first occasion. She had acted on the advice she had been given, but now felt that she had made a terrible mistake. The woman rebuked the therapist for promising that she would feel better, and said it was 'her fault' that her husband was now living with his secretary, leaving her and their two children without financial support.

A number of important points are illustrated in the above case, relating to the manner in which supportive psychotherapy is conducted. Offering advice based on personal experience is a dangerous premise, since it presupposes that the subject has the same attitudes, coping skills and understanding of the problem as the therapist. It would have been far more appropriate to have dealt with the question 'What shall I do?' by responding 'Now that you've found out about the affair, how do you view the future of your marriage?'. This would have given the woman an opportunity to ventilate her feelings and allow the therapist to make some assessment of what *the subject* herself thought she should do. It is possible that the woman did not want her husband to go, or had already considered asking him to leave, but had rejected this option because of unresolved dependency needs or the practical implications of supporting herself. People are more likely to act on decisions they feel they can cope with, rather than on proposals which are beyond their capabilities.

Giving an undertaking that someone will definitely feel better by acting in a particular way is almost certain to undermine confidence and trust should the promise not be fulfilled, as well as having an adverse effect on the therapeutic relationship through the therapist's loss of credibility. It might have been more appropriate to state, 'I understand how angry and hurt you must feel at the moment, but in time, when the shock has passed and you've had a chance to think things over, I'm sure you'll begin to feel better.' The response not only displays a degree of caring and understanding, but is also a reasonable prediction of the likely course of events.

INDIVIDUAL DYNAMIC PSYCHOTHERAPY

Dynamic psychotherapy is practised in a number of forms which differ according to their aims and duration of treatment. In **brief dynamic psychotherapy**, weekly sessions are usually conducted over a period of 3–6 months, during which treatment focuses on the major conflicts which underlie presenting symptoms or personality problems. In **intermediate analytical psychotherapy**, patient and therapist normally meet two or three times per week over a period of 6 months–3 years. The nature of the work undertaken may be very similar to that in **psychoanalysis**. The latter can last for several years, with up to five sessions a week being held, during which time a detailed and intensive exploration is conducted into the patient's behaviour and psychological functioning. The average frequency of individual therapy conducted within the National Health Service in the UK is approximately one session per week for a year.

Analytical Theory and Psychodynamics

The process of **dynamic psychotherapy** is based upon **analytical theory** developed by **Sigmund Freud**. In his dynamic model of mental functioning, Freud saw all aspects of mental life – thoughts, emotions and resultant behaviour – as being influenced by inborn psychological forces, which often come into conflict with each other and also collide with the demands of the environment. These forces exist at varying levels of consciousness: the **conscious** mind containing present awareness, the **preconscious** in which unconscious mental activity is capable of recall, and the **unconscious** containing memories, thoughts, drives and conflicts which cannot be brought into awareness because they are actively repressed (*see below*).

According to Freud, a newborn child possesses a mass of **instinctual drives** or impulses, the aims of which are to derive instant gratification or relief from discomfort, such as cold or hunger. However, these drives rapidly come into conflict with reality, which inevitably dictates that needs cannot be immediately met and a desire for gratification must sometimes wait. Three main elements are involved in developing personality, which becomes clearly differentiated into the **ego** (the 'aware part of the self' whose function is to test reality), the unconscious **id** (containing the instinctual drives) and the **superego**. The latter evolves as the child becomes influenced by the morals, attitudes and judgements of his parents, as well as by the constraints of society. The superego is often likened to the conscience, but in fact represents far more than this. It is not only an incorporation into the self of actual parental and social values, but is also a manifestation of the fantasised standards, qualities and failings that the child attributes to his caregivers.

Character and personality are therefore seen to develop through a perpetual struggle between the ego, the superego and the id, which influence a person's thoughts, emotions and behaviour. For example, a ravenous child may be driven (by the id) to take a bar of chocolate from a shop counter, which (the ego confirms) is a realistic way of satisfying his hunger. His mother or father will need to stop him behaving in this way until such time as parental values become incorporated within the child in the form of the superego, which then controls the ego and the id.

When the gratification of needs is frustrated or conflicts remain unresolved, anxiety results which, because of its unpleasant quality, can only be endured for a limited period of time. Sometimes, anxiety can be consciously dealt with by taking appropriate action, such as earning extra money to overcome financial difficulties. Alternatively, unconscious (sometimes referred to as 'neurotic') **defence mechanisms** may be used which act by distorting reality in some way, thereby protecting the ego. It is important to realise that defence mechanisms are merely hypothetical concepts which help the understanding of certain psychological symptoms or behaviour occurring in response to internal conflicts or external stress. They are employed automatically, without any degree of conscious awareness, and form a part of normal mental activity to help cope with the everyday pressures of life. When they are used inappropriately or excessively, their effect is sometimes harmful and they may then be considered abnormal.

Some of the defence mechanisms which are used include:

1. **Repression**: the exclusion from the conscious mind of unacceptable thoughts or feelings, which if allowed to reach awareness, would create conflict or tension; e.g. a person may repress the memory of a sexual assault in childhood.
2. **Denial**: behaviour which suggests a failure to consciously acknowledge some wish, threat or unpleasant reality, even though the person is acquainted with the necessary facts; e.g. a woman whose husband has recently died may continue to act or converse as if he were still alive.
3. **Reaction formation**: the process of obscuring true feelings or motives from oneself by behaving in an opposite manner. Consequently, a man who adopts an overtly masculine life-style may do so as a reaction against repressed homosexual feelings.
4. **Rationalisation**: unconsciously offering reasonable (but false) explanations for feelings or behaviour which would otherwise be unacceptable; e.g. a candidate short-listed for a job interview, who is unable to cope with the possibility of rejection, may defend against his anxiety by withdrawing his application on the grounds that the job would involve too much travelling.
5. **Projection**: attributing unacceptable aspects of oneself onto some-

one else, so that they become more tolerable. For instance, a man who no longer loves his wife may feel that she is uncaring and disinterested in him, thereby projecting all the blame for their marital difficulties onto her.

6. **Regression:** behaving in a manner which is representative of a younger age. An older child may start to wet the bed again following the birth of a sibling, as a way of dealing with the frustration of having to compete with the new rival.

7. **Sublimation**: an unconscious means of channelling libidinal urges into acceptable behaviour; e.g. aggressive or sadistic impulses may be dealt with by taking up a contact sport, such as boxing or judo.

8. **Displacement**: the transfer of feelings linked with a particular person or situation onto someone or something else. A man who is involved in a car accident may feel angry with his garage for not servicing the brakes properly, rather than being annoyed with himself for driving carelessly.

9. **Introjection** and **identification**: closely related mechanisms in which the subject unconsciously adopts the feelings, attitudes or behaviour of another person in order to deal with the anxiety of separating from them. Thus, a son may become more businesslike following the death of his financially successful father, and start to dress in a manner similar to the deceased.

Freud believed that sexual and other drives (**libido**) exist from birth, and during the first few years of life pass through a number of stages of maturation which influence personality development. At each stage, the developing child derives gratification from activities connected with a particular area of the body on which the pleasure-seeking id focuses.

In the first year, during the **oral phase**, the infant obtains pleasure from sucking, so that in the absence of comfort derived from the breast or bottle, the thumb or other objects are placed in the mouth. At some time during the second year of life, the child enters the **anal phase** and for the first time experiences the influence of imposed control through toilet training. Pleasure is derived from the act of retaining or expelling faeces. In the **phallic phase**, which begins at around the ages of 2–5, the focus of gratification and interest is transferred to the genitalia. At the same time, Freud supposed that libido ceases to be fixated on the self, and instead is eventually directed towards the parent of the opposite sex. In the case of boys, sexual drives focused on the mother are accompanied by feelings of jealousy and resentment towards the father, who is seen as a rival for her affections. This so-called **Oedipus complex** is associated with the child's fear that his desire for his mother will be punished by the father castrating him (**castration anxiety**). The Oedipus complex (and its female equivalent, the Electra complex) becomes devoid of useful meaning if it is interpreted as a literal desire of all children to destroy their mother or father in order to have intercourse with the parent of the opposite sex. Children at this age do not conceptualise intimacy or death in the same way as adults, but certainly they may want a rival for parental affection to be removed in order to achieve greater closeness with their mother or father. The resolution of the conflict is marked by the lessening of anxiety arising from a fear of father's revenge, and the identification with him as a good 'object', rather than as a rival. (In analytical terms, an object is any person who is emotionally significant to the subject.)

Resolution of the phallic phase heralds the onset of a period of **latency**, during which Freud thought interest in the body is replaced by increased attention to the acquisition of environmental skills. Personality development is completed by the **genital phase**, which begins during early adolescence and eventually results in the development of mature sexual relationships.

According to Freud, adult neuroses and certain aspects of character formation result from difficulties encountered at an earlier stage of development, with libido (or life energy) **fixated** at that level. Consequently, he believed that neurotic symptoms and some personality traits involved behaviour originating at the time of the oral, anal or phallic phases which had persisted into adult life. For example, oral fixation is associated with excessive dependence on activities involving the mouth, such as eating, drinking or smoking. By contrast, anal fixation is linked with characteristics which are the adult counterparts of the child's wish to retain his faeces (meanness) or defy parental control over toilet training (stubbornness).

Techniques Used in Dynamic Psychotherapy

Symptoms are thought to result from psychological conflicts, now lost to the conscious mind, which may have arisen many years before. These stem from feelings or desires which were perhaps unacceptable to parental ideals or to the individual's own self-image, but which continue to influence present behaviour and emotions from the unconscious. Access to these basic conflicts is facilitated by encouraging the subject to talk spontaneously about whatever comes to mind, irrespective of its content, a process known as **free association.** The therapist encourages this by saying very little himself and remaining emotionally impassive. His talk will be confined to sometimes **clarifying** what the subject says, **confronting** contradictions and making **interpretations**. At first, the individual may 'filter' his thoughts, only talking about certain topics while clearly avoiding others. This **resistance** may be helpful to the therapist in identifying areas of conflict.

As therapy progresses, the patient begins to develop feelings for the therapist which are evident in both his talk and behaviour. Because the latter reveals little or nothing about himself, many of these feelings and ideas will be distorted, and result from **transference** to the therapist of emotions derived from previous relationships in the subject's life. For example, a patient who consistently feels angry towards the therapist may be reproducing feelings experienced in the past towards a parent. Because the therapist remains detached and does not collude with these notions or expectations, a novel situation is created. An interpretation might then be offered that the subject is behaving as though the therapist were his father, mother or some other important figure from the past. In this way, the patient effectively reproduces within therapy important aspects of his relationships with others, allowing maladaptive and destructive processes to be identified and, in time, changed. Interpretations may at first be rejected, and emotional conflicts will need to be re-experienced many times (**working through**) before insight is gained and changes in patterns of thinking and behaviour can occur. Sometimes, the patient might convey feelings in actions rather than words (such as expressing anger by persistently arriving late for therapy sessions), and such **acting out** will also require interpretation.

Countertransference is concerned with the therapist's feelings towards the patient. In most forms of dynamic therapy, these are not deliberately or overtly revealed, but by acknowledging and exploring the feelings that the patient evokes in him, the therapist can use the countertransference to understand more about the therapeutic relationship.

Other routes to unconscious conflicts include the interpretation of **dreams** and slips of the tongue (**parapraxes**). Freud saw these as expressions of conflicts and wishes buried in the unconscious mind. In the case of dreams, unconscious material often becomes intermixed and incorporated with events and happenings of the previous day. The actual (or **manifest**) dream content was thought to be the result of modified or disguised unconscious material, the latter referred to by Freud as the **latent** dream content. He used free association to reveal the unconscious or real meaning underlying the actual dream.

Other Schools of Dynamic Psychotherapy

Alfred Adler was a colleague of Freud who developed his own school of **individual psychology** in which he saw man's struggle for power and status (rather than the fulfilment of sexual needs) as the main determinant of adult character. Adler viewed existence as a constant striving to overcome inborn feelings of **inferiority**, in which well-adjusted adults had successfully come to terms with the challenges of life. He considered that the development of 'adult neurosis' was a means of obtaining power by a 'retreat into illness', so that superiority was gained by using symptoms to control others or to provide an excuse for not living up to impossible ambitions (**fictive goals**).

Adlerian theory was particularly influential in the USA where several analysts, such as **Fromm**, **Horney** and **Harry Stack Sullivan**, developed concepts which emphasised the importance of external influences (e.g. personal relationships, social pressures and cultural factors) in the formation of the personality.

Carl Jung was a pupil of Freud who developed his own school of **analytical psychology**. Jung considered the mind or 'psyche' as functioning at three levels. The conscious level included the **persona**, the outer layer of the personality, which was the exact opposite of feelings and sensitivities embodied in the underlying level of the personal unconscious. The latter also included the **animus**, the unconscious masculine side of the woman's female persona, and the **anima**, the unconscious feminine side of the man's male persona. Thus Jung saw the manner of the flamboyant, gregarious extrovert as reflecting feelings of shyness, insecurity and introversion within the personal unconscious. The latter was viewed as merely part of the **collective unconscious**, which held the beliefs and experiences of all mankind. Aspects of the collective unconscious can enter the conscious mind in the form of symbols or **archetypes**, which then influence thought and behaviour. Evidence of the collective unconscious is acknowledged through the similarity of myths, symbols and various religious practices throughout the world, as well as in recurring themes of legends, dreams and paintings. Jungian analysts, although concerned with the problems and conflicts of reality, are especially interested in the interpretation of dreams, artistic expression and the inner world of fantasy.

Anna Freud maintained her father's analytical direction, but devoted much of her work to understanding the character development of children from the age of 2 years onwards. She emphasised the importance of ego defence mechanisms on everyday aspects of living, and from her work the concept of **ego psychology** developed. The latter views the ego as a powerful autonomous force which does not merely arise from conflict between the id and the superego. **Melanie Klein** stressed the importance of aggressive drives in determining character from the first few months of life. She also applied Freud's psychoanalytical theories to interpreting the play of young children. Her work was influential in the development of **object relations theory**. This is concerned with the way in which the child's perceptions and fantasies about the relationships between important people or 'objects' in his life (such as between parents, or mother and child) become incorporated into the mind at an early stage of development. These mental constructs of prototypal relationships continue to have a bearing on the capacity of the individual to relate to others throughout life, to sustain emotional ties and to cope with separation.

GROUP THERAPY

Man is a social animal, and since much of life is spent living and working in groups, many of the problems which affect people on a day-to-day basis are appropriately dealt with in a group setting. As with individual work, group therapy may be purely supportive in its aims or more dynamically orientated. **Small groups** usually consist of 6–10 people who meet regularly to pursue a common purpose, and include one or two therapists who act as facilitators or conductors. The group may comprise inpatients on a hospital ward or outpatients who meet at a specified time, usually once a week. **Large groups** (*see later*) consist of 20 or more members.

Groups of any size can be **open,** with a regular turnover of people leaving and being replaced by others, or **closed**, with all members starting and finishing therapy together. Patient selection may be **homogeneous** (such as a group exclusively for obese depressed women) or **heterogeneous**, consisting of people with a variety of different problems. **Time-limited** groups meet for a specified period agreed at the outset (e.g. agoraphobics who meet for eight weekly sessions), while **unlimited groups** continue for an indefinite period.

Dynamic Group Therapy

It is important to realise from the outset that dynamic group therapy is not 'individual therapy' conducted with several people at once. The therapeutic methods are different, and the group setting provides an opportunity to look at interpersonal relationships through the dynamics of the group in terms of its social structure, interactions and the conflicts that develop within it. The most important therapeutic factor is the group itself. By disclosing personal difficulties and concerns, and seeing various aspects of their social, psychological and physical characteristics reflected in others (**mirroring**), its members receive feedback from a number of standpoints. This helps the individual learn about his distorted views of relationships and maladaptive behaviour, and discover ways of modifying them accordingly. Because the group functions as a social microcosm, each member is, in time, likely to act in a manner which reflects his behaviour in the outside environment. For example, a man who has a tendency to be aggressive, or is inclined to manipulate others, is liable to display similar behaviour within the group. The group members utilise this information to help them gain **insight** into their interactions with other people. Understanding alone does not guarantee change, and the group also provides an experiential setting for testing novel ways of behaving and communicating, which will hopefully lead to the diminution of self-destructive activities and the development of more appropriate and satisfying relationships.

Other Therapeutic Factors in Group Therapy

A number of therapeutic factors can be identified which operate in all forms of group therapy. Groups help to **instil hope** in those who are demoralised by allowing them to observe others who have benefited from therapy. **Interpersonal learning** occurs through gaining insight into the positive and detrimental aspects of one's interactions with other people. The idea that one's difficulties are unique is often rapidly dispelled on learning that others share similar concerns, and the ensuing awareness of the **universality** of problems offers considerable relief. The open **expression of emotion** may allow some people to feel better in the short-term, although it is rarely of lasting benefit. More importantly, group members learn how to express their ideas and feelings openly, and see that this does not necessarily have the adverse consequences they often fear.

Imparting of information can help individuals to learn about the meaning of their symptoms. **Imitative behaviour** in groups, in which members model themselves on aspects of the therapist or each other, is an invaluable first step towards discarding rigid, inappropriate or destructive behaviour patterns. Group interactions not only create an opportunity for **developing new socialising techniques**, but the accompanying sense of **altruism** also enhances self-esteem and dispels beliefs of having no useful part to play in society. Subjects may develop a sense of belonging and acceptance (some for the first time in their lives), and for many this feeling of **group cohesiveness** is highly therapeutic. Groups frequently discuss issues of ultimate concern such as death, freedom and the purpose of life. By developing a sense of **existential awareness**, members can learn to come to terms with the limitations of relationships and the problems associated with isolation and loneliness.

Functions of the Group Therapist (Conductor)

The functioning of any group is highly complex, not only because of the multiple interactions which occur between its members, but also as a result of the different levels at which it operates. There is the manifest or observable level (i.e. the overt expression of emotion) and the unconscious level, such as rivalry which occurs between group members in competition for the attention of the parent figure (the conductor). The therapeutic atmosphere which exists within a group can either facilitate expression and communication or inhibit it. For example, if anger or fear predominate, then it will not feel safe for group members to express themselves, and interaction may be minimal. Therefore, it will be necessary at times for the conductor to promote an atmosphere in which self-revelation and frank discussion of intimate matters can take place. In order for the group to function therapeutically, aspects of both individual and group psychopathology need to be recognised and dealt with during sessions. Consequently, the conductor requires the capacity to view the group in terms of its constituent members and as an entity in its own right, paying attention to its structure, processes and dynamics.

Although the conductor sometimes directs the group, he does not lead it. At times, it may be necessary for him to clarify the aims of therapy, make interpretations, encourage communication and deal with disruptive processes. Particularly during the early stages of treatment, group members will often turn to the conductor to cure them. Such attempts need to be resisted in order to prevent the group from **regressing** into a state in which dependency needs are encouraged and adult responsibilities inhibited or denied. **Resistance** within a group is often expressed through anger or silence (so-called 'fight or flight'), superficiality or irrelevance, as well as being acted out in the form of irregular attendance or disruptive behaviour. Sometimes, a group member is repeatedly attacked verbally or rejected by the others. **Scapegoating** of this kind is another manifestation of resistance which prevents the assailants from acknowledging comparable features of their own personalities, or allows some unwanted aspect of the group as a whole to be projected onto the scapegoat. In addition, resistance may be expressed through **pairing**, in which two members of the group form an alliance which separates them from interacting with the others. Irrespective of its mode of presentation, resistance needs to be identified and dealt with appropriately by the group.

The conductor will also be involved in the selection of group members, who will need to be interviewed individually to determine their suitability for therapy. As a general rule, people of similar age, intelligence and cultural background should be chosen, and the group needs to contain an equal number of men and women with a variety of psychological problems. Furthermore, ground rules have to be established to ensure that the group meets regularly at a certain time, and that policy decisions (such as whether or not smoking is allowed) are adhered to. Members are expected not to have contact with one another outside of the sessions (if it is an outpatient group), but if they do, they should report back to the group the details of any meetings.

Large Group Therapy

Many psychiatric wards begin the day with a meeting of all patients and staff members to allow the general problems of living together to be discussed. This also provides the staff with an opportunity to 'keep a finger on the pulse' of the ward by identifying those patients who are distressed, disturbed or withdrawn. Some psychiatric units, particularly those run on the lines of **therapeutic communities** (*see* Chapter 3), hold large groups which operate using a more analytical approach. Staff members can facilitate the ventilation of emotion and conflicts, point out how the group is functioning, and create a forum for social learning. Running large groups involves a different approach to that used in small group therapy, and because the experience can be very stressful for some members, disturbed behaviour is often amplified. Consequently, staff may need to protect vulnerable patients from excessive confrontation by others, and also exclude those who are too ill to attend.

Other Types of Group Therapy

The types of group therapy described so far rely upon talking as the main form of interaction. **Psychodrama** is used by some therapists to allow individuals to re-enact, in a dramatic form, emotionally painful experiences or conflicts from their past. Other group members portray the parts of significant people involved in the situation, and this re-enactment leads the patient to a greater understanding of the problem. **Encounter groups** use either talking or actions to facilitate the expression of emotions in a setting where open communication and self-awareness are encouraged.

FAMILY AND COUPLE THERAPY

Family therapy involves the treatment of the family as a unit, rather than dealing with the problems of its members individually. The purposes of therapy are to relieve symptoms in the member who presents with a problem (often a child), by altering the way in which the family functions. Sometimes, this is facilitated by redefining the complaint from one restricted to the index patient, to another which concerns the whole family. For example, bed-wetting in a young child may be a reflection of tension in the home, resulting from marital conflict between the parents. **Couple therapy** is indicated where conflict arises within a relationship and results in emotional, sexual or behavioural problems in one or both partners. If the survival of the marriage or relationship is under threat, therapy is only indicated where both partners wish it to continue. Several different approaches to treatment are used, some using psychodynamic methods and others behavioural techniques (*see* p. 279).

One style of family therapy commonly used is the **structural approach**, which is based on **systems theory**. This views the family as a 'system' having properties which are greater than the sum of its constituent parts. As a result, it is not directly concerned with the intrapsychic make-up or behaviour of individual family members. Communication and feedback mechanisms are seen as expressions of the power structure within the family and the rules by which it functions. Assessment and treatment involve one or more therapists meeting together with all the family on a regular basis in order to identify, and if necessary help change, the way in which members **interact** and **communicate** with each other. This may include:

1. observing and clarifying verbal and non-verbal patterns of communication which often contradict one another, and viewing the way in which feelings and needs are expressed within the family
2. helping to create boundaries between family members where there is evidence of overinvolvement or enmeshment, and the autonomy of certain individuals is threatened
3. helping inappropriately rigid patterns of interaction between family members to become more flexible
4. defining the manner in which family decisions are made and the responsibility for implementing them is delegated
5. identifying abnormal patterns of interaction used to cope with stress
6. supporting, educating and guiding the family as a whole.

Family therapy should be considered whenever there is evidence of family dysfunction which is related to the problems for which help is being sought. Indications include:

1. marital difficulties and other relationship problems, particularly if the viability of the family unit or the adequate care of children is threatened
2. behavioural problems in children or adolescents, such as eating disorders, enuresis, school refusal and conduct disorder
3. childhood illnesses thought to have a psychological component, such as asthma, psoriasis and eczema
4. family crises: bereavement, divorce, adolescent separation or loss of a job.

GENERAL CONSIDERATIONS IN THE USE OF PSYCHOTHERAPY

The Type of Psychotherapy Offered

Deciding whether to offer individual or group psychotherapy will not only depend on the nature of the problem, but is also, to some extent, a matter of personal choice. Some people feel they cannot work in a group because of shyness or embarrassment about their problem, while others may specifically benefit from such a setting if, for example, their difficulties are concerned with social functioning and interaction. Financial considerations also need to be borne in mind, since the more intensive individual therapies are largely restricted to the private sector, and may therefore be beyond the means of many people.

Supportive psychotherapy is frequently offered to people with emotional difficulties of short duration, or to those who need help in coming to terms with a change in their personal circumstances. Dynamic psychotherapy may be considered for individuals with certain long-standing neurotic disorders, particularly where symptoms of anxiety and depression are prominent. The presenting problem needs to be understandable in psychological terms, and the patient must possess a motivation to change, as well as a readiness to question long-standing attitudes and behaviour. The capacity to tolerate slow and often painful progress and the ability to verbalise emotions are also important.

Dynamic psychotherapy is usually contraindicated in those actively suffering from major mental illnesses, such as schizophrenia and the affective psychoses, although a demonstration of support, sympathy and caring will be beneficial to *all* patients. Psychopathic personality disorders are also largely resistant to a dynamic approach, although some younger patients with other mild forms of personality disorder may benefit.

Because supportive psychotherapy requires less formal training, it is practised by professionals from various disciplines, working in both the hospital and the community setting. Dynamic psychotherapy requires more intensive, long-term training in which the therapist needs to gain a knowledge of analytical and psychodynamic theory, as well as insight into his own personality and psychopathology. This is usually achieved by undergoing a personal analysis and receiving supervised training of a large number of psychotherapy cases.

The Efficacy of Psychotherapy

Not everyone benefits from receiving psychotherapy, and there is a body of opinion which holds that its success rate is no greater than the level of spontaneous recovery observed in people awaiting treatment. Although a considerable amount of research has been conducted to determine the efficacy of psychotherapy, problems with methodology make this a very difficult matter to determine. Nevertheless, a therapist who displays warmth, genuineness and empathy, and is able to convey to the patient that he can and will be helped, will almost certainly produce better results than one who is cold, indifferent or hostile. Explaining to the patient from the outset the aims of treatment and how these are to be achieved is also likely to increase success. Ultimately, it must be left to the individual therapist to decide whether or not his personality and clinical skills can be utilised effectively for psychotherapy.

PSYCHOTHERAPY IN GENERAL PRACTICE

Time is a major constraint when treating patients in the primary care setting, so that psychotherapeutic techniques need to be modified accordingly. Offering advice, support, sympathy and reassurance are important aspects of most consultations, and consequently psychotherapy forms an integral part of the day-to-day work of all general practitioners. In addition, the family doctor may be involved in the specific counselling of patients in times of stress (e.g. following bereavement, divorce or miscarriage), as well as in giving anticipatory guidance (such as to those about to undergo surgery or to parents who have given birth to a handicapped child). Opportunities for conducting analytically-orientated psychotherapy are understandably limited, although general practitioners who are particularly interested in this form of treatment may specifically set aside time for dealing with problems in this way.

The attitude and approach of the doctor towards the patient has a significant influence in determining therapeutic success in almost every clinical setting, but this is especially so in general practice. A pioneer of this approach was **Michael Balint**, who through a number of research seminars involving interested family doctors, revealed that 'the most frequently used drug in general practice was the doctor himself. It was not only the bottle of medicine that mattered, but the whole atmosphere in which the drug was given and taken'. Consequently, it is important for all family doctors to maintain an awareness of the interaction which occurs between themselves and patients during every consultation, and to use it therapeutically.

It is easy for the doctor to become irritated by the apparent triviality of the complaints of certain habitual attenders at his surgery, especially if their symptoms seem resistant to all attempts at treatment, and the patient appears to be ungrateful or hostile. In such cases, the growing frustration of the doctor is likely to be matched only by the patient's increased demands for help, often resulting in a total breakdown of effective communication between the two.

The doctor who 'looks beneath the surface', and is prepared to understand and tolerate his patients' behaviour (and respond accordingly to their needs), is likely to be more effective in the long-term than one who uses the prescription pad inappropriately to bring a swift end to an irksome consultation. A display of aggression or lack of appreciation by the patient might well be camouflaging feelings of anxiety or inferiority, while persistent requests for help may reflect unresolved dependency needs. Allowing the patient an opportunity to express his feelings, and offering reassurance that support will be available in times of genuine need, may be all that is required to prevent the development of a chronic psychological problem.

A patient visiting his general practitioner with a specific problem may also have expectations and fears about the consultation itself. Therefore, in order to create an atmosphere that puts the subject at ease and encourages self-expression, the doctor needs to concern himself with more than just the clinical content of the interview. He should pay attention to the manner in which he greets the patient, the seating arrangements in the consulting room (rather than use his desk as a barrier, he should seat himself to one side of it), the amount of eye contact he makes, as well as his facial expression and tone of voice during the consultation. Most people are aware of the positive effects of a good 'bedside manner', and the opposite impression is likely to evoke feelings of rejection, anxiety and defensiveness in many patients.

A large proportion of the problems seen in general practice have a psychological basis, although this is not always immediately apparent from the nature of the consultation. Sometimes, the presenting complaint is used to determine whether the doctor is likely to be receptive or understanding regarding some other matter, about which the patient feels anxious or embarrassed. It is therefore helpful to adopt an 'open-ended' approach to the interview, allowing the patient some time to talk freely, and avoiding the use of too many direct questions which are only likely to result in direct answers.

A 51-year-old woman attended her general practitioner complaining of vague tightness in the chest. The doctor asked systematic questions regarding the nature of her symptoms, breathing and exercise tolerance, and following a brief physical examination, pronounced that he could find nothing wrong. Rather than reassuring her, this statement caused the woman to burst into tears, at which point the doctor gently enquired if there was anything else worrying her. She admitted that the real reason for her attendance was concern over the discovery of a lump in her breast the day before, but that she had felt too frightened to mention it directly.

This example demonstrates that by limiting questions strictly to the presenting problem, the true reason for the consultation can easily be missed. In other instances, the purpose of the visit may remain undisclosed until the very end of the interview.

A middle-aged woman made an apparently unnecessary appointment to see the doctor in order to collect a prescription for an antacid mixture for her husband. On her way out, she suddenly asked whether someone who felt permanently tired could be suffering from a serious illness. The doctor invited her back into the room and allowed her to elaborate. It emerged that she was concerned about her husband's fatigue, and whether or not this was due to his medication. With further prompting, she tearfully admitted that it was their sex life that was specifically affected, and that otherwise he continued to be his normal energetic self. The doctor offered to see the woman jointly with her husband at a further consultation, to which she readily agreed.

The nature of the relationship between the general practitioner and the patient is such that the doctor has an opportunity to get to know his patients in depth, and to see them in surroundings which are far less formal and threatening than in a hospital consultation. By creating and utilising an environment which promotes the likelihood of self-expression, the family doctor can make full use of his therapeutic skills, both to improve the quality of his patients' lives, and increase his own sense of job satisfaction and fulfilment.

BEHAVIOUR THERAPY

Behaviour therapy is aimed at improving an individual's functioning and well-being by a direct change in behaviour. In contrast to supportive or dynamic psychotherapy, behavioural treatments are not concerned with the underlying causes of symptoms, but are simply directed at modifying or removing them.

Behaviour therapy is useful in the management of many different conditions (*see* Table 13.1). Behaviourists view symptoms as 'maladaptive learned responses' to stress which, by utilising principles derived from learning theory, can be removed completely or replaced with more appropriate coping mechanisms and behaviour.

Behavioural Techniques

Behavioural techniques can be broadly classified into:

1. those for reducing anxiety and inducing relaxation
2. those for minimising unwanted behaviour
3. those for developing new behaviour or increasing wanted behaviour
4. cognitive therapy
5. other behavioural techniques.

1. TECHNIQUES FOR REDUCING ANXIETY AND INDUCING RELAXATION

Relaxation training (*see* p. 57): anxiety and tension usually involve physical and psychological components which are inexorably linked. The subject is encouraged to adopt a comfortable position while lying or sitting, and then starting at the toes and working upwards, is taught to recognise physical tension by contracting and releasing each muscle group of the body in sequence. This technique is used to induce a state of physical relaxation, since the physiological response of muscle is automatically to relax once voluntary contraction ceases. Finally, the subject is taught to control the rate and depth of his breathing, and to concentrate solely on removing tension from his body. Mental relaxation will then follow as a matter of course.

Exposure treatment is the technique of choice for dealing with phobic disorders (agoraphobia, simple and social phobias) and is discussed further on p. 62. It is sometimes used in conjunction with relaxation training. **Graded exposure** involves exposing the subject to the feared stimulus one step at a time. A **hierarchy** of increasingly stressful situations is established, ranging from those which arouse only minimal fear to others which induce feelings of extreme anxiety or panic. Progression to the next stage of the hierarchy does not commence until the subject can confidently cope with the previous level. **Systematic desensitisation** is an elaborate form of graded exposure in fantasy which is now largely obsolete.

Flooding (*see* p. 62) is a variant of exposure in which the subject is exposed to the maximally feared situation straight away without using a hierarchical approach. Provided that contact with the phobic stimulus is maintained for long enough, and avoidance (such as running away) is prevented, the fear will eventually abate. Sometimes, exposure *in vivo* is preceded by maximal exposure in fantasy, which is referred to as **implosion**.

Once the fear has been controlled, it is likely to return unless the subject repeatedly 'rehearses' his exposure to it. **Programmed practice** involves delegating much of the responsibility for treatment to the subject, sometimes enlisting the help of other family members. The individual is encouraged to seek out situations which would formerly have been avoided and to practise ways of controlling anxiety symptoms should these develop during exposure.

Paradoxical intention aims to reduce anxiety by encouraging the subject to carry out the very behaviour he fears. For example, this might involve instructing someone who is afraid of losing control in public to bring on a panic attack, or advising the insomniac who is tense about his inability to fall asleep, to stay awake all night. By encouraging the intentional production of symptoms (which is usually found to be impossible), the subject experiences a change of attitude towards his fear, resulting in a reduction of anxiety.

2. TECHNIQUES FOR MINIMISING UNWANTED BEHAVIOUR

Response prevention (*see* p. 65) is the treatment of choice for dealing with rituals in obsessive compulsive disorders. The subject is instructed to desist from carrying out the unwanted behaviour (such as repeated hand-washing), while simultaneously being exposed to a situation which is likely to increase his need to perform the act, e.g. rummaging through a dustbin. Except in very severe cases, constant supervision does not appear to be necessary, merely telling the subject to refrain being sufficient to control the behaviour.

Aversion therapy aims to reduce maladaptive behaviour by associating it with an unpleasant experience, such as pain or a noxious smell. Techniques of this kind were used in the past for the treatment of sexual deviations, such as cross-dressing, when the subject might be shown a picture of a man wearing women's clothing, following which a small electric shock would be administered. However, the ethical issues surrounding the inflicting of pain as a form of treatment, coupled with the knowledge that behavioural changes which occurred tended to be short-lived, resulted in these methods falling into disuse. Nowadays, aversion therapy is sometimes used in the management of alcohol abuse through the administration of disulfiram (*see* p. 211).

Covert sensitisation is a form of aversion therapy which relies on imagination. The subject is encouraged to think about the undesirable behaviour (such as exposing his genitals) and immediately associate it with a mental picture of something unpleasant, e.g. standing in the dock at the magistrates court. **Thought stopping** (*see* p. 65) is used in the treatment of obsessions. The patient is encouraged to relax and then ruminate, at which point the therapist shouts 'Stop!' By repeating this procedure, the subject finds it increasingly difficult to bring the obsessional thought into his mind, and eventually, he learns to internalise control by shouting 'Stop!' to himself whenever the obsession occurs. The method sometimes employs mildly aversive stimuli as further negative reinforcement, such as pulling and releasing an elastic band placed around the wrist when thought stopping is attempted.

Massed practice involves the subject repeatedly practising the unwanted behaviour until he is fatigued. It has been shown to be of some benefit in the treatment of tics, nail-biting and other habit disorders.

3. TECHNIQUES FOR DEVELOPING NEW BEHAVIOUR OR INCREASING WANTED BEHAVIOUR

Social skills training is used to help those who have difficulty in forming or maintaining relationships with others. Techniques include teaching the importance of non-verbal aspects of communication, such as making eye contact during a conversation, and role-playing commonly encountered social situations, e.g. how to talk to someone at a party. **Assertiveness training** can be of help to those people who lack confidence and have difficulty in expressing themselves in a variety of circumstances, such as when dealing with a store manager who refuses to exchange faulty goods or handling someone who pushes in front in a queue.

Token economies are sometimes used where the development of new behaviour is required among a group of people (particularly those with chronic disabilities) who live together, e.g. in residential accommodation or on a continuing care ward in hospital. In return for performing certain tasks, such as getting out of bed on time or washing and dressing without prompting, the subject receives tokens as a reward, which can then be exchanged for luxuries or privileges such as cigarettes, chocolates or the right to watch television. In this way, a repertoire of personal and social skills can be developed which increase self-sufficiency and minimise disabilities. Critics of the token economy system contend that behavioural changes are often not maintained when the individual moves on to a different environment, and there is also evidence to show that increased involvement of staff may be a sufficiently powerful therapeutic factor on its own, without the use of tokens.

Shaping involves the gradual development of complex pieces of behaviour by reinforcement of the constituent parts. This technique can be used to develop speech and other basic skills (such as eating and dressing) in mentally retarded children or in adults with severe behavioural difficulties resulting from mental disorder. It entails the use of positive reinforcement (e.g. offering a sweet) when behaviour approximates to that which is desired. For instance, while teaching a child to dress himself, a reward may at first be given for merely picking up the clothes, but then further reinforcement is only offered for attempts to put garments on, button them correctly, lace up shoes and so on. The process is often slow and laborious, sometimes requiring several weeks or months before the behaviour is finally 'shaped' to the desired aim.

Contracts may be either verbal or written and can be of use in individual, family or marital work to effect behavioural changes. For example, a husband may commit himself to helping regularly with the household chores in return for his wife agreeing to allow him a night out with his workmates once a week. By 'giving to get', each person can see how they benefit through meeting the needs of others, thereby improving the quality of family relationships and the home atmosphere.

4. COGNITIVE THERAPY (see also Chapter 5)

This form of treatment is based on the principle that maladaptive behaviour and abnormal mood states can be altered by changing thought patterns. It has been mainly used in the management of depression (see p. 100), although its effectiveness in comparison to other forms of treatment has not been satisfactorily evaluated. According to cognitive theory, people who are depressed maintain their low mood by adopting a pattern of thinking which includes:

1. focusing on misfortunes rather than pleasant happenings
2. interpreting events in a negative way without considering alternative explanations ('because my boss appeared angry this morning, he is obviously displeased with my work')
3. attributing excessive importance to trivial mishaps ('forgetting to post that letter proves I am a useless secretary')
4. making unrealistic assumptions ('I can only be happy if I earn a great deal of money').

One aspect of therapy involves the subject noting his assumptions and patterns of thinking throughout each day, and recording them in a diary alongside his interpretation of any significant events which occur. By regularly examining the entries with the patient, the therapist can be of assistance in a number of ways:

1. helping him to adopt a more balanced perspective of his life (by demonstrating that pleasant happenings occur just as frequently as misfortunes)
2. generating alternative explanations to his interpretation of events ('your boss may have looked angry because he'd had a row with his wife')
3. helping him to acknowledge his strengths and attributes, as well as his weaknesses ('despite forgetting to post the letter, you managed to finish typing the chairman's report a day ahead of time')
4. generating alternatives to negative assumptions ('your brother earns very little, and yet you say he's always cheerful').

Over a period of time, maladaptive patterns of thinking are replaced by more creative ones, which in turn should lead to an elevation of mood, increased involvement in pleasurable pursuits and a more optimistic view of the future.

Self-control techniques use a cognitive approach to bring about behavioural changes by requiring subjects to monitor their own progress (e.g. obese women on a slimming programme recording their own loss of weight). When a target is reached or behaviour is acceptably modified, reinforcement is achieved by means of a suitable self-reward, such as the subject buying herself a new outfit.

5. OTHER BEHAVIOURAL TECHNIQUES

Biofeedback is the process of bringing involuntary physiological responses, such as heart rate, muscle tension and blood pressure, under voluntary control. The response being measured is presented to the individual via a signal generator, in the form of a flashing light or audible tone, and changes in rate or intensity are indicated by an alteration in the frequency of the signal. The subject learns how to regulate autonomic responses by identifying which thoughts or feelings bring about certain physiological changes. In this way, biofeedback presents an opportunity to control many of the physical symptoms of anxiety.

Modelling is more simply described as 'learning by imitation', and involves the subject copying behaviour demonstrated by the therapist. In the context of reducing unwanted behaviour, it can be used as an adjunct to other techniques, such as response prevention or graded exposure. For example, the subject may be helped to overcome a fear of spiders by initially watching one crawl harmlessly over the therapist's hand. Modelling can also be helpful in encouraging desirable behaviour, and is widely used by therapists to demonstrate appropriate interpersonal skills in group settings.

Directive sex therapy and the behavioural techniques employed are discussed in detail in Chapter 19.

Advantages and Disadvantages of Behaviour Therapy

Unlike certain forms of psychotherapy, most behavioural techniques are not limited by the patient's intelligence, insight or verbal abilities. Furthermore, treatment can usually be continued by the subject and members of his family outside the therapy session. Although clinical psychologists have particular expertise in designing and implementing behavioural programmes, members of all disciplines can, with adequate instruction and supervision, be effective behavioural therapists.

Certain behavioural techniques are only effective provided the subject's cooperation can be enlisted, as in the case of graded exposure. Furthermore, in those instances where behavioural difficulties are non-specific (free-floating anxiety) or widespread (multiple phobias), constructing a treatment programme can be difficult, because simple and clearly defined goals cannot always be established.

Nevertheless, behaviour therapy remains the treatment of choice for several conditions and a useful adjunctive measure in a number of others, as shown in Table 13.1.

Table 13.1 Indications for the use of behaviour therapy

Condition	Behavioural techniques	Remarks
Disorders in which behaviour therapy is often the treatment of choice		
Agoraphobia	Graded exposure/flooding Programmed practice Relaxation training	Improvement also noted in mood and general adjustment to work and relationships
Simple phobias	Graded exposure/flooding Modelling	Response to treatment usually good
Social phobias	Graded exposure/flooding Social skills training Paradoxical intention	Response to treatment is variable
Obsessive-compulsive disorders	Response prevention Thought stopping	Clomipramine may be useful adjunct where depression is marked
Anxiety states	Relaxation training	Can be used as an alternative or adjunct to drug treatment
Sexual dysfunction	Directive sex therapy	(*See* Chapter 19)
Nocturnal enuresis	Operant conditioning through use of star charts, also bell and pad enuresis alarm	*See* p. 319
Learning problems/ conduct disorders in children	Positive reinforcement, modelling, shaping, negative reinforcement	Often used in children with mental retardation
Disorders in which behaviour therapy may be useful		
Depression	Cognitive therapy	Not suitable for severe cases
Bereavement	Guided mourning	*See* p. 121
Marital and relationship difficulties	Contracts Paradoxical injunction, modelling, communication training, social skills training, assertiveness training, role-play	May be used in conjunction with individual, group or couple therapy
Eating disorders	Self-monitoring and other cognitive approaches	Useful in obesity and bulimia nervosa (*see* Chapter 17)

continued overleaf

Table 13.1 *Continued*

Condition	Behavioural techniques	Remarks
Chronic schizophrenia	Token economy programmes, social skills training	Sometimes used as part of a rehabilitation programme
Habit disorders	Massed practice	May be useful in treating tics
Sexual deviations	Aversion therapy Covert sensitisation	May be ethical problems in their use

OTHER PSYCHOLOGICAL TREATMENTS

Hypnosis

The term hypnosis was coined by James Braid, a nineteenth century physician. Although it suggests sleep (Greek *hypnos*=sleep), it is in fact a heightened state of focal awareness brought about by artificial means. Its use in medicine has had a somewhat chequered history, and the Austrian physician, Anton Mesmer, popularised it under the name of 'animal magnetism'. His opponents vilified him and his treatment, which they dubbed 'Mesmerism'. At the end of the nineteenth century, the celebrated French neurologist, Charcot, held public demonstrations at the Saltpétrière in Paris, showing how hypnosis could bring about dramatic cures in hysterical paralyses and aphonias. The young Sigmund Freud was influenced by Charcot's work, and he used hypnosis in the early development of psychoanalysis, but later discarded it as being unnecessary in this form of treatment. Today, hypnosis is widely accepted as a valid form of medical treatment, and there is a section devoted to it at the Royal Society of Medicine.

Although the hypnotic trance has been extensively studied, uncertainty exists as to its nature. EEG tracings reveal the presence of alpha waves (normally present during wakefulness) and physiologically there is a slowing of the pulse rate, a decrease in blood pressure and generalised muscular relaxation. Psychically, there is a decreased awareness of peripheral stimuli, increased concentration on a central focus, and a distortion of the perception of time. Suggestibility is heightened and the whole state is often referred to as one of dissociation.

A trance state is often quite easily induced by simple methods, and resorting to complicated apparatus, coloured lights and other forms of pseudoscientific 'mumbo-jumbo' is unnecessary. The simplest procedure is to employ eye fixation. The hypnotherapist simultaneously encourages the subject to progressively relax by focusing attention on his eyelids and limbs. Simple tests may be applied to gauge the depth of the hypnotic state, but for most procedures, a light trance is all that is necessary.

Hypnosis has a number of possible clinical applications which include:

1. the reduction of anxiety
2. modifying or eliminating phobic or obsessional states
3. the induction of anaesthesia in minor operations, including dental procedures
4. replacing or supplementing inhalation analgesia in obstetric practice
5. resolving hysterical paralyses or aphonias
6. assisting the abreaction of traumatic emotional events (hypno-analysis).

Hypnosis is a safe procedure, but should not be employed with suspicious or paranoid patients, in psychotic states or in those with abnormal personalities.

Abreaction

Some people who are acutely distressed following a psychologically traumatic event (such as an assault or an accident) are incapable of expressing the strong emotions, such as anger or guilt, which are often associated with these experiences. In some cases, the individual becomes preoccupied with his feelings, and as a consequence, is unable to function or cope with the everyday demands of life. Abreaction is the process of discharging pent up emotions and facilitating their expression. It can be brought about by encouraging the individual to relive the experience within the context of a therapeutic interview, which may be assisted by inducing a hypnotic state or administering a sedative drug. In drug-assisted abreaction, the subject is given a slow intravenous injection of amylobarbitone or a benzodiazepine, in order to lower his level of arousal, and enable him to talk about the experience. Abreaction should only be carried out with the full cooperation of the patient, and should not be performed on psychotic individuals or on those with unstable personalities, in whom the reaction is often unpredictable.

SUMMARY

1. **Psychotherapy** uses talking and listening to relieve specific symptoms, or to help people adjust to and cope with the problems of everyday life. It may be conducted with individuals, couples or groups of people, but in all cases, the relationship which develops between the subject and therapist is important in bringing about change.

2. There are various forms of psychotherapy which differ in their duration and complexity, but they can all be broadly categorised into supportive and dynamic types. Both aim to prevent a breakdown of functioning and bring about symptom relief, as well as increase self-esteem and facilitate the release of emotion. In **supportive psychotherapy**, this is accomplished by allowing the ventilation of feelings, demonstrating empathy and offering advice. Dynamic psychotherapy is also concerned with the development of insight and aims to bring about change by detecting and resolving underlying psychological conflicts.

3. **Dynamic psychotherapy** is based upon analytical theory developed by Freud, in which all aspects of mental life are seen as being influenced by inborn psychological forces which often conflict with each other and the demands of the environment. These forces exist at different levels of awareness: the conscious, preconscious and unconscious. Freud saw character and personality as developing through a perpetual struggle between the ego (that part of the self which tests reality), the id (containing the instinctual drives) and the superego (containing the internalised morals and attitudes of parents and society). Unconscious neurotic defence mechanisms help 'protect' the ego against intolerable anxiety and conflicts by distorting reality in some way. They include repression, denial, reaction formation, rationalisation, projection, re-gression, sublimation, displacement, introjection and identification. Sexual and other drives (libido) present from birth pass through various phases of maturation (oral, anal, phallic, latency and genital) which influence personality development. Adult neuroses are thought to arise from libido becoming fixated at a particular level, behaviour representative of that phase persisting into adult life.

4. **Techniques** used in dynamic psychotherapy aim to give access to the unconscious conflicts which are thought to give rise to symptoms. This is achieved by encouraging free association, identifying areas of resistance, and interpreting dreams and parapraxes. The development of transference (the shifting of the patient's emotions and attitudes from previous experiences onto the therapist) allows maladaptive and destructive relationship processes to be identified and, in time, changed. Counter-transference is concerned with the therapist's feelings towards the patient.

5. Other schools of dynamic psychotherapy have been developed. Adler saw the struggle for power and status as the main determinant of adult character. Jung proposed a model of mental functioning comprising the conscious, personal unconscious and collective unconscious – the latter containing generalised symbols and images (archetypes) common to all mankind. Melanie Klein applied psychoanalytical principles to interpreting the play of young children. Anna Freud further developed her father's theories and stressed the importance of ego defence mechanisms in mental functioning.

6. **Group therapy** (in particular the small outpatient group) provides an

opportunity for members to gradually learn about their distorted views of relationships and maladaptive behaviour, and discover how to modify them accordingly. The group not only provides a therapeutic environment, but is also an experiential setting for testing novel behaviour and ways of communicating. The functioning of any group is highly complex, since it operates at many different levels. The therapist conducts the group but does not lead it. At times, it may be necessary for him to facilitate a therapeutic atmosphere, clarify the aims of therapy, make interpretations, encourage communication and deal with disruptive processes. He is also responsible for selecting group members and establishing ground rules for the functioning of the group.

7. **Family therapy** involves the treatment of the family as a unit, rather than dealing with the problems of its members individually. A structural approach to therapy views the family as a 'system', with treatment aimed at identifying, and if necessary changing, the way in which members interact and communicate with each other. Family therapy should be considered when there is evidence of family dysfunction which is related to the problems presented. Indications include marital difficulties, behavioural problems in children, childhood illnesses which are thought to have a psychological component and family crises.

8. The type of psychotherapy which is offered depends upon the nature of the problem, personal choice and the availability of therapists. Because of methodological problems, it is difficult to evaluate the efficacy of psychotherapy, although the personal characteristics of the therapist are undoubtedly important in producing a favourable outcome to treatment.

9. Time is a major constraint when employing psychotherapeutic techniques in the **general practice** setting. The attitude and approach of the family doctor towards his patients will significantly influence his therapeutic effectiveness. An 'open-ended' manner in conducting consultations is important, since the psychological difficulties underlying many of the problems seen in general practice are not always immediately apparent.

10. **Behaviour therapy** is directed towards improving an individual's functioning and well-being by a change in behaviour. It is the treatment of choice for phobias and obsessive-compulsive disorders, and is also useful in the management of many other conditions. Techniques are broadly classified into:

(a) those for reducing anxiety and inducing relaxation: relaxation training, graded exposure and flooding (used in phobic disorders), paradoxical intention and programmed practice

(b) those for minimising unwanted behaviour: response prevention and thought stopping (in obsessive-compulsive disorders), aversion therapy (for alcohol dependence) and massed practice (for tics and other habit disorders)

(c) those for developing new behaviour or increasing wanted behaviour: social skills and assertiveness training (used for those with relationship difficulties and problems of social interaction), token economies and shaping (used in chronic mental illness and mental retardation) and contracts (as an adjunct to psychotherapy)

(d) cognitive therapy: mainly used in depression to modify negative thought patterns

(e) other behavioural techniques: biofeedback, modelling and directive sex therapy.

11. **Hypnosis** is a heightened state of awareness brought on by artificial means. It has a number of possible clinical applications which include anxiety reduction and the elimination of phobic, obsessional or hysterical symptoms, the induction of anaesthesia in minor operations and as a supplement to analgesia in obstetrics. **Abreaction** is the process of discharging pent up emotions and facilitating their expression, and may be of use in people who are acutely distressed following a psychologically traumatic event. The process can be assisted using hypnosis or intravenous sedation.

REFERENCES AND FURTHER READING

Balint, M. (1964). *The Doctor, his Patient and the Illness*, 2nd edn. London: Pitman.

Brown, J. A. C. (1964). *Freud and the Post-Freudians*. Harmondsworth: Penguin.

Crown, S. (1983). Contraindications and dangers of psychotherapy. *British Journal of Psychiatry*; **145**: 436–41.

Lask, B. (1987). Family therapy. *British Medical Journal*; **294**: 203–4.

Marks, I. M. (1986). *Behavioural Psychotherapy: Maudsley Pocket Book of Clinical Management*. Bristol: Wright.

Maxwell, H., ed (1986). *An Outline of Psychotherapy for Medical Students and Practitioners*. Bristol: Wright.

Roberts, J. P. (1986). In-patient group psychotherapy. *British Journal of Hospital Medicine*; **36**: 367–70.

Shepherd, M. (1984). What price psychotherapy? *British Medical Journal*; **288**: 809–10.

Yalom, I. D. (1976). *The Theory and Practice of Group Psychotherapy*, 2nd edn. New York: Basic Books.

14 COMMUNITY PSYCHIATRY

HISTORICAL BACKGROUND

Until the end of the eighteenth century, 'community care' of the mentally ill in Britain involved their incarceration in prisons, workhouses and madhouses in such appalling conditions, that public indignation eventually led to the creation of the first **mental hospitals**. These **asylums** initially adopted a liberal style of non-restraint, with an emphasis on treating patients in a dignified and humane manner. However, by the late nineteenth century the large influx of mentally ill people into these institutions, combined with a shortage of staff, inevitably led to the development of authoritarian and custodial patterns of care. This frequently created an **institutionalised** culture within mental hospitals, in which patients became apathetic, submissive and showed a marked lack of initiative and drive. The loss of personal identity and self-respect which many of them experienced further added to the handicapping effects of mental illness, making it difficult for them to return to the outside community.

In the 1930s, alternative models of care began to evolve and new legislation allowed asylums to accept psychiatric patients on a voluntary basis. This was followed by the establishment of the first **outpatient** and **after-care** facilities for the mentally ill. Following the Second World War, changes in social attitudes and the inception of the National Health Service hastened the development of psychiatric care facilities outside of hospitals. In the early 1950s, new **drugs** effective in the control of major mental illnesses, such as schizophrenia, became available, and together with the introduction of **open door** policies of treatment, allowed large numbers of patients to be discharged back into the community.

Since the 1960s, there has been a move away from providing inpatient care in large isolated mental hospitals towards a **community-orientated approach**. This has involved the development of psychiatric units that are part of **district general hospitals** situated within the area they serve. In addition, there has been an emphasis towards the provision of community services and facilities which are discussed later on in this chapter.

AIMS OF COMMUNITY CARE

Community psychiatry is based upon the concept that people with psychiatric problems can be most effectively helped when links are maintained with family, friends, work colleagues and society in general. Because many patients and their relatives prefer psychiatric care to be provided in a community setting, services need to be organised in such a way to allow most patients to receive treatment near to their homes. This has the additional advantage of minimising the social and behavioural difficulties, as well as the stigmatisation, which are often associated with living in a large mental hospital.

Elements of community care include the following:

1. Rehabilitation

Rehabilitation programmes should be specifically tailored to meet individual needs and should aim to:

- (a) treat incapacitating symptoms of psychiatric illness, and stabilise mental functioning and behaviour
- (b) prevent or treat the disabilities associated with established mental illness and restore patients to community life as soon as possible
- (c) offer patients who have spent many years in hospital an opportunity to regain their place in the community
- (d) provide support for the chronic mentally ill within the community, so as to reduce their need to stay in hospital.

2. Prevention

To fulfil a preventive role by:

- (a) continuing the provision of treatment for patients living outside hospital
- (b) maintaining regular contact between patients and primary care workers to ensure the early detection of relapsing illness
- (c) providing community care services and facilities (*see later*)
- (d) establishing mental health care centres throughout the community (*see later*).

3. Coordination of Services

It is important that good coordination exists between the various agencies involved in community care, to ensure that services are delivered effectively to the client. This involves adequate liaison between the hospital, social services, primary care workers, probation services, employment officers and voluntary organisations.

4. Education

(a) To increase public awareness of the resources and facilities available for help
(b) To increase public acceptance of mental illness and reduce the stigmatisation associated with psychiatric care.

REHABILITATION

Rehabilitation should begin as soon as possible after admission to hospital, so that all phases of treatment and after-care are seen as an integral part of the process. Where practicable, the aim is to restore the individual to his former degree of functioning prior to the onset of illness, but when this is not feasible, attempts should be made to maintain him at the highest level possible. The process involves the four elements discussed below.

1. Treating Incapacitating Symptoms of Mental Illness

The presence of delusions, hallucinations or altered mood usually affect an individual's ability to function adequately by impairing his judgement, concentration and relationship with others. Stabilising the mental state, through the use of physical treatments and general support from care givers, is therefore a prerequisite to further rehabilitative measures. Other symptoms, especially those associated with the defect state of chronic schizophrenia (i.e. lack of drive and social withdrawal), can be more difficult to deal with, but may be helped by behavioural techniques (*see* Chapter 13).

2. Assessing the Extent of Additional Psychological, Social and Physical Handicaps

Mental illness, whether or not it results in hospitalisation, frequently produces additional psychological handicaps, such as loss of confidence, poor self-image and fear of failure. As a result, difficulties may arise in forming relationships or finding work, thereby increasing the problem of remaining self-sufficient within the community. Social isolation can be further compounded if abnormal movements (such as body-rocking or facial grimacing) have developed during the course of the illness, as people afflicted in this way tend to be avoided or rejected by others because of their 'oddness'. Physical disability, even if present before the onset of psychiatric illness, may subsequently become an intolerable burden for which the patient requires additional help and support. Consequently, assessment must include an appraisal of the patient's level of functioning prior to his illness, his current abilities in terms of personal, domestic and occupational skills, his level of awareness of handicaps and his expectations for the future.

3. Establishing a Rehabilitation Plan

This should include an agreed order of priority for dealing with problems. For example, there is little point in placing a homeless man in a hostel when he currently lacks the ability to wash and dress himself if a prerequisite of living there is self-sufficiency. Rehabilitation must pay attention to the individual's problems regarding:

(a) work
(b) accommodation
(c) level of social functioning
(d) capacity for independent living.

A comprehensive **occupational therapy programme** needs to include the assessment and teaching of a wide range of skills such as:

(a) activities of daily living (self-care, cooking, housekeeping)
(b) community living skills (shopping, budgeting, use of public facilities)
(c) social skills (non-verbal communication, role-playing, etiquette).

As a preliminary towards restarting work, it is helpful to increase confidence in this area by role-playing interviews, offering practice with form filling, and arranging visits to job centres. Practical preparation and new job skills are best provided by a graded approach, using work of varying complexity and responsibility within an occupational or industrial therapy setting (*see later*).

Continuing support and reassurance from care givers is essential in helping people to cope with problems which inevitably arise during any rehabilitation programme. Creative and expressive groups, using suitably trained music, drama or art therapists, may be of benefit to those who lack the necessary verbal skills to express their conflicts or distress. Behavioural training can be helpful in the management of anxiety, and to enhance assertiveness using role-play and video playback. Physical recreation groups emphasise the importance of bodily health in maintaining a sense of well-being through regular exercise and participation in sporting activities.

4. Deciding Which Members of the Multidisciplinary Team Can Best Deal with Identified Problems

The rehabilitative needs of a community cannot be met solely by hospital-based staff, and their contributions should be complemented by primary health care workers such as the general practitioner, field social worker and the community nurse. A team approach to rehabilitation is not only essential for organisational purposes, but also has the advantage of pooling resources and skills, as well as helping to share responsibilities. In many units, it is common practice to appoint a key worker who has overall knowledge of the case, and is best able to decide which services are appropriate for any given patient. This can be *any* team member, and similarly, allocation of responsibility for dealing with problems is not always restricted by conventional roles (e.g. the social worker may undertake to conduct individual psychotherapy with a client). Figure 14.1 shows the members of the multidisciplinary team and the resources available for rehabilitation and after-care.

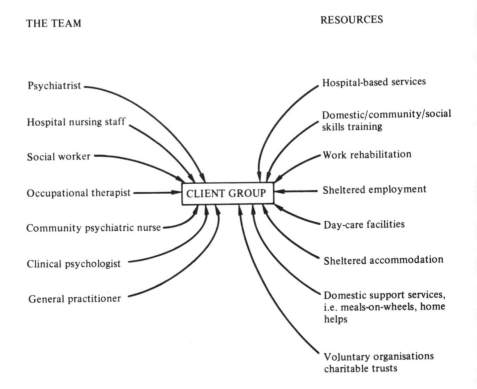

THE TEAM

RESOURCES

Psychiatrist

Hospital nursing staff

Social worker

Occupational therapist

Community psychiatric nurse

Clinical psychologist

General practitioner

CLIENT GROUP

Hospital-based services

Domestic/community/social skills training

Work rehabilitation

Sheltered employment

Day-care facilities

Sheltered accommodation

Domestic support services, i.e. meals-on-wheels, home helps

Voluntary organisations charitable trusts

Fig. 14.1 The multidisciplinary team and resources available for rehabilitation and aftercare

COMMUNITY CARE FACILITIES

In the past, community care generally referred to treatment conducted 'outside the hospital'. However, because the district general hospital is situated in the area that it serves, its facilities must be seen as part of any community care programme, if this is to function smoothly and effectively. Hospital-based services include inpatient and outpatient facilities, domiciliary assessment and day hospital care. Services provided by the local authority include day centres, various forms of sheltered accommodation and domestic services, such as meals-on-wheels and home helps. In addition, within the private sector a number of voluntary organisations and charitable trusts make an important contribution towards the provision of community facilities.

Day Care Facilities

Day hospitals provide an opportunity for observation and assessment, as well as for the treatment of all categories of adult mental illness. A wide range of therapies are within the scope of day hospital care. These include individual and group psychotherapy, behaviour modification, social skills and home management training. The staff also deal with other aspects of treatment, such as the supervision of medication, as well as providing patients with support and offering advice when needed. Day hospitals are intended for those who require more than outpatient supervision (but for whom inpatient care is unwarranted), and for patients needing continuing rehabilitation following discharge from hospital. Although they also fulfil a social function, they are not primarily concerned in dealing with problems of loneliness or isolation, which are more suitably catered for by day centres.

Day centres, unlike day hospitals, are not usually medically staffed. In addition to providing company, they offer leisure activities, meals, and in some cases, a sheltered working environment for those unable to obtain open employment. They are also suitable for people suffering from chronic mental illness who require little medical supervision, but are nevertheless, in need of a supportive and stimulating environment to prevent relapse. A recent survey of day hospitals and day centres showed that in many areas, there is considerable overlap in the type of services each provides. Because of the limited resources currently available, it is likely that the traditional roles of these facilities will be modified to meet the changing needs of community care in the future.

Industrial Rehabilitation

Patients recovering from mental illness may either require help in returning to former employment, or retraining if there has been a change in their level of functioning. A graded approach to industrial rehabilitation needs to be adopted, and the process should commence as soon as it is realistically possible after admission to hospital. This is provided within an occupational or industrial therapy unit, both of which allow for the assessment of capabilities in a variety of work settings. These range from relaxed non-stressful environments, to those in which the discipline and usual restraints of normal working conditions apply. Occupational experience is offered for both skilled and unskilled industrial jobs, as well as for clerical work. In some areas, Employment Rehabilitation Centres exist for the benefit of those who have been off work for some time, and although they do not provide training for skilled employment, they do assess suitability for placement elsewhere. This might be on a training course, a community project, or in sheltered or open employment. Placement may be assisted by the Disablement Resettlement Officer based at the local job centre, who can help in finding suitable employment for those handicapped by, or recovering from, mental or physical illness.

Accommodation

Following discharge from hospital, many people will be able to return to live with their families or to support themselves in the community. Others who have spent a long time in hospital or are permanently impaired may be unable to do so, and therefore require some form of sheltered accommodation in the community. **Hostels** are usually supervised by a warden and/or a team of care-assistants, and offer accommodation mainly to the chronically mentally disordered, whose disabilities are such that they need to live there long-term. They also serve as 'half-way houses' for those continuing to recover from mental illness, but who are not yet ready to live independently. Many hospitals now have **hostel wards** which prepare long-stay patients for life in the community. Medical and nursing supervision are provided to a limited extent, but residents are expected to be totally self-sufficient prior to discharge.

Group homes offer ordinary residential accommodation for four to eight people, who live together on a permanent basis and benefit from mutual support. Group members need to be carefully selected for compatibility, and residents are expected between them to undertake all the domestic responsibilities of a normal household, such as cooking, cleaning, shopping and paying bills. Day-to-day supervision is minimal, although regular contact with psychiatric services is maintained through visits by the community nurse. In some areas, **adult home-finding services** offer patients board and lodgings with families (adult fostering) or 'friendly landladies'. The latter usually have some expertise in dealing with the problems of those handicapped by mental disorder, and are frequently prepared to offer assistance with budgeting, shopping and preparing meals.

Primary Care Workers in the Community

Proper coordination of services is essential in order to identify and provide for the needs of the mentally disordered within the community. Good communication and regular liaison with primary care workers is therefore important. **Community psychiatric nurses** offer an invaluable service in many areas by:

1. supervising treatment (especially with depot neuroleptics) following discharge from hospital
2. providing support and advice to patients (and their families) living in the community, including those in residential accommodation
3. assessing the need for psychiatric intervention in patients referred to them by general practitioners
4. recognising early signs of relapse.

In this way, the community psychiatric nurse provides an important link between hospital services and the general practitioner.

The majority of psychiatric problems within the community are dealt with by the **general practitioner**, and only a small percentage of cases are referred to hospital specialists. The range of psychiatric disorders is wide, but most involve stress-related problems, neurotic symptoms, relationship difficulties and alcohol abuse. By contrast, there is a preponderance of major mental illness among those psychiatric patients who are admitted to acute wards.

In addition to funding residential accommodation and day centres, local authority **social services** also provide community-based social workers, as well as facilities for child care, the elderly, the mentally retarded and the homeless.

THE FUTURE OF COMMUNITY CARE

Developments in community care in the UK have been impeded by a lack of resources and facilities to cover the transition period between running down the large mental hospitals and building up community services. In addition, plans have been further hampered by a growing awareness that not all patients can be supported outside of hospital, and that some will continue to require care within a secure and sheltered environment. This is demonstrated by the growing number of 'new long-stay' patients in

Table 14.1 Comparative advantages and disadvantages of mental hospital and community care

Advantages	Disadvantages
Community care	
Patient lives within a 'natural' environment	High cost of establishing services
Links with community maintained	Stressors of everyday living increase likelihood of relapse in vulnerable individuals
Stigmatisation of being a 'mental patient' reduced	Violent and aggressive patients less easily contained
Reduced risk of institutionalisation	Risk of homelessness and vagrancy increased with inadequate support
Preventive health care possible by early contact with individual	Fragmented resources and expertise
	Problems of coordinating services
Better liaison between hospital and primary health care workers	
Mental hospitals	
Supportive and protected environment	Institutionalisation and stigmatisation
Risk of relapse due to environmental stressors diminished	More 'authoritarian' regime
	Poorer access to community
Disturbed individuals more easily contained	Poorer liaison between hospital and the community
Relatively easy administrative structure	
Concentration of resources and expertise	

mental hospitals who have failed to be reintegrated back into community life. Furthermore, social support has not been as effective as was originally anticipated in dealing with the additional strain placed upon the families of the mentally ill living outside of hospital. The comparative advantages and disadvantages of mental hospital and community-based care are shown in Table 14.1.

Because financial resources are likely to remain limited for the foreseeable future, there is a danger that patient care will suffer due to the underfunding of community services. Although at present there is no simple solution to the problem, alternative concepts in community care have been considered which focus attention on preventive measures.

Other Models of Care

The establishment of community-based **joint assessment clinics**, attended by the psychiatrist, general practitioner and other health care workers, is one means of practising preventive psychiatry by detecting problems at an earlier stage, and helping to minimise relapse in the chronic mentally ill. The potential benefits of this approach are that it reduces the demands on hospital-based services and enhances the skills of the primary health care team. A similar aim can be achieved through consultants conducting clinics in general practice surgeries, although this may not be the most economical use of the psychiatrist's time.

Another approach to preventive psychiatry is through the provision of **counselling services** for those groups who are at high risk of developing mental disorder, such as the bereaved, divorced and unemployed. Counsellors who are specially trained may offer their services at community 'drop-in' centres, or hold groups in hospitals or general practice surgeries.

Because of the logistic and financial difficulties in providing adequate resources to meet the needs of some communities, an alternative method is to identify those areas which have the greatest psychiatric morbidity (such as certain housing estates or high-rise flats) and situate a secondary care unit close by. In the **hive system** (Fig. 14.2), the district general hospital remains the administrative centre of psychiatric care, from which staff travel to a cluster of nearby secondary units, where they provide an appropriate range of treatment facilities (in a manner analogous to worker bees in a hive).

Crisis intervention services have been established in certain parts of the UK, whereby a team (usually consisting of a doctor, psychiatric nurse and a social worker) provide either 24 hour or daytime cover to deal with crises experienced by individuals or families living within a designated

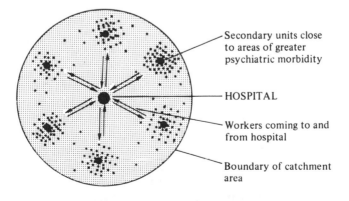

Fig. 14.2 The hive system

(Reproduced by kind permission of the British Journal of Psychiatry)

catchment area. The service is based on the principle that when faced with a crisis (e.g. marital breakdown or loss of a job), the individual may either deal with it effectively and emerge with increased coping skills and an enhanced sense of identity, or be damaged by the experience. The latter can lead to the development of mental disorder, or result in further maladaptive responses in the face of subsequent adversity. Crisis theory proposes that people are most susceptible to change at a time when levels of stress are high, and internal and external coping resources are being mobilised. If an approach is sought which temporarily alleviates distress without solving the problem (e.g. admission to hospital or prescribing sedatives), the individual is more likely to break down when dealing with future crises.

In response to a request for assistance, a domiciliary visit is made by the team (sometimes on more than one occasion) in order to assess the nature of the crisis and where possible, bring about an effective solution. This may involve identifying precipitants and exploring new ways of dealing with the crisis, encouraging problem-solving behaviour, promoting communication between family members and facilitating the expression of emotion. Sometimes, it is necessary to refer the individual or family to an appropriate agency for further help, or remove responsibility temporarily by allowing the person to adopt the sick role and accept hospital admission. The overall benefit of this approach to treatment, in comparison to more traditional methods, has yet to be clearly evaluated.

SUMMARY

1. In recent years, there has been a move away from providing psychiatric care in large, isolated mental hospitals towards a community-orientated approach. This is based upon the concept that psychiatric patients can be most effectively helped when links with the community in which they live are maintained. **Community care** is concerned with preventive aspects of mental health, the rehabilitation of patients with acute and chronic psychiatric disorders, as well as with public education regarding mental illness.

2. The process of **rehabilitation** should begin as soon as possible after admission to hospital, and aims to restore the individual to his previous standard of functioning or the highest level possible. Incapacitating symptoms of mental illness need to be treated before establishing and implementing a rehabilitation programme, which should be based upon the assessment of psychological, social and physical handicaps. Treatment is concerned with helping the individual learn or relearn skills associated with domestic and community living, work and recreation.

3. **Community care facilities** encompass those provided by the hospital, local authority and charitable organisations. They include domestic and

work rehabilitation, day care, domestic support services and sheltered accommodation. Additional facilities are also provided by local authorities for child care, the elderly, the mentally retarded and the homeless. The delivery of effective care is contingent upon close liaison between all agencies and professionals concerned with the individual's rehabilitation.

4. The progress of community care in the UK has been impeded by a lack of resources and facilities, as well as by a growing awareness that not all patients can be supported outside of the hospital environment. Although there are no simple solutions to these problems, alternative concepts in community care are being considered which place an emphasis on preventive rather than curative measures.

REFERENCES AND FURTHER READING

Caplan, G. (1961). *An Approach to Community Mental Health.* London: Tavistock.

Department of Health and Social Security (1975). *Better Services for the Mentally Ill.* Cmnd 6233, London: HMSO.

Edwards, C., Carter, J. (1979). Day services and the mentally ill. In *Community Care for the Mentally Disabled* (Wing, J. K., Olsen, R., eds). Oxford: Oxford University Press.

Hume, C., Pullen, I. (1986). *Rehabilitation in Psychiatry.* Edinburgh: Churchill Livingstone.

Levene, L. S., Donaldson, L. J., Brandon, S. (1985). How likely is it that a district health authority can close its large mental hospitals? *British Journal of Psychiatry*; **147**: 150–55.

Tyrer, P. (1985). The hive system: a model for a psychiatric service. *British Journal of Psychiatry*; **146**: 571–75.

Vaughan, P. J. (1985). Developments in psychiatric day care. *British Journal of Psychiatry*; **147**: 1–4.

Waldron, G. (1984). Crisis intervention: is it effective? *British Journal of Hospital Medicine*; **31**: 283–87.

Wallace, M. (1987). A caring community? The plight of Britain's mentally ill. *The Sunday Times Magazine*; 3 May: 25–38.

15

The link between 'mind and body' is interesting not only from a theoretical viewpoint, but also because it has important implications in everyday clinical practice. The significance of this interrelationship will become apparent to most students by virtue of the large number of patients they will see on medical and surgical wards with psychological complaints, as well as those under psychiatric care who report physical symptoms.

THE CONCEPT OF PSYCHOSOMATIC MEDICINE

The idea that psychological factors were influential in the development of physical illness has existed since the time of Ancient Greece, although a resurgence of interest in this association occurred towards the end of the nineteenth century. In the 1920s and 1930s, a number of medical reformists in the USA developed the concept further, and established the foundations of **psychosomatic medicine**. This approach embraced the theory that emotional conflicts had an important role in the development of a number of physical disorders*, and that psychological factors were also responsible or the perpetuation and exacerbation of these conditions. It was further suggested that a direct relationship might exist between particular personality types and the development of specific illnesses or pathological processes. Although the theories attracted a great deal of interest, research findings have failed to produce any clear evidence to substantiate them. Nevertheless, the term 'psychosomatic' is still regarded by many as meaning the psychological causation of bodily disorders.

The psychosomatic movement expressed its disenchantment with contemporary medical research, particularly concerning its tendency to concentrate on the biological causation of disease, to the exclusion of

---

* The 'psychosomatic' conditions identified were ulcerative colitis, asthma, eczema, rheumatoid arthritis, essential hypertension, peptic ulceration and thyrotoxicosis.

psychological and social influences. It opposed the artificial division between mind and body, since it saw the two as inexorably linked, and proposed a 'whole-person' approach to the causation and treatment of illness. It is this latter concept which gives rise to the modern meaning of psychosomatic medicine as:

1. the study of the interrelationship between biological, psychological and social variables in health and disease (the latter assumed to be multifactorial in origin)
2. the holistic approach to the practice of medicine, in which the mind and body are seen as a single unit
3. clinical activities at the interface of medicine and psychiatry, termed **liaison psychiatry** (*see later*).

Current research in psychosomatic medicine is concerned with the role of psychosocial factors (such as stressful life events) in the development of physical illness in general, rather than limiting investigations to specific conditions. Other studies have concentrated on attempting to establish the endocrine, autonomic and immunological mechanisms which mediate between emotional experiences and the physical changes which are associated with them.

Because there is no clear evidence to support the concept that psychological factors are a *direct* cause of physical illness, the complex association between disorders of psyche and soma is best considered in terms of:

1. physical and psychiatric disorders which coexist
2. physical illness and its psychological effects
3. psychiatric disorders which present with physical symptoms
4. psychological factors which predispose to physical illness.

PHYSICAL AND PSYCHIATRIC DISORDERS WHICH COEXIST

Several studies conducted in a variety of settings (general practice, psychiatric and general hospitals) have demonstrated that physical and psychiatric disorders frequently coexist. Where the symptoms of one illness predominate, the other can easily be overlooked, and research findings have confirmed that a substantial number of psychiatric disorders occurring in patients admitted to medical wards go unrecognised. Apart from the protracted suffering this is likely to cause, the persistence of untreated psychiatric symptoms can also prolong the course of a physical illness and, in some cases (such as with depression), may increase the risk of suicide.

PHYSICAL ILLNESS AND ITS PSYCHOLOGICAL EFFECTS

Organic brain disease or systemic dysfunction can produce psychological symptoms which are characterised by features of acute or chronic **organic reactions** (*see* Chapter 9). Where treatment of the underlying pathology is possible, resolution of the psychological symptoms is likely.

Psychological reactions to physical illness, especially anxiety and depression, are common. **Anxiety** is often prominent in the early stages of an illness (particularly if the outcome is uncertain), and if persistent, has been shown to affect prognosis adversely in a number of conditions, notably peptic ulceration and myocardial infarction. **Depression** is a recognised feature of several organic conditions (*see* p. 92), and is also likely if illness results in some form of loss, which may be anatomical (such as amputation), functional (e.g. paralysis following a stroke) or symbolic (the loss of child-bearing ability after hysterectomy). Depression during convalescence may delay recovery, and prevent a return to work and the resumption of normal responsibilities. Elderly people who become physically ill, and as a consequence suffer intractable pain or social isolation, are particularly at risk of becoming depressed and committing suicide.

Some people cope with illness by an unconscious rejection of any associated unpleasant facts or emotions (*see* p. 263). In the early stages of illness, such **denial** may be of benefit in protecting the individual from otherwise overwhelming anxiety. For example, patients who seem to use mechanisms of denial in the first few days following a heart attack, appear to have a lower mortality rate than those who straightforwardly accept the implications of their condition. Alternatively, denial can result in delay in seeking help for conditions which are serious or potentially life-threatening (such as following the discovery of a breast lump), as well as lead to a failure to comply with treatment.

In contrast to those who deny illness, some people develop an excessive **preoccupation** with their physical condition. This may result in the patient spending a great deal of time reading and enquiring about his illness, while constantly challenging the degree of knowledge shown by his care givers. An increasing involvement with the details of treatment sometimes results in instructions or therapeutic procedures being followed to extremes, often to the exclusion of other activities and interests.

Psychological responses to physical illness are influenced not only by the subject's personality and the significance he attributes to his condition, but also by the reaction of his family and friends. The duration and severity of the illness, as well as social and cultural influences, will have some additional bearing on the response.

The Influence of Personality

People with obsessional personalities characteristically find difficulty in coping with uncertainty, so that they may experience severe stress where there is doubt about the diagnosis and outcome of the illness. Those with narcissistic tendencies, who are preoccupied with their appearance, are particularly vulnerable when illness results in disfiguration or loss of bodily function. On the other hand, dependent personalities may readily accept their disabilities, especially if the increased attention of others satisfies their need to be cared for. Patients with paranoid personalities might blame someone else, such as a relative or doctor, for their plight. Irrespective of the premorbid personality, illness is more difficult to contend with when coping resources for dealing with sickness are underdeveloped, due to lack of past experience. In this respect, the young are particularly vulnerable.

Personal Significance of the Illness

The personal meaning which the patient attaches to his condition can significantly affect its course and outcome. This will in part be influenced by how much a person knows about his illness, and whether this is based upon accurate information or is elaborated from popular myth or 'old wives' tales'. In the latter case, undue significance may be attached to relatively minor symptoms, resulting in the development of anxiety or depression, either of which can delay recovery. Similarly, the prognosis may be adversely affected in those who regard their illness as an unfair punishment, and as a consequence become bitter and resentful. In contrast, patients who adopt an attitude of stoicism and determination towards overcoming their condition often fare better than those who capitulate and resign themselves to their fate. Psychological responses are also influenced by the significance and value that the patient attributes to the part of the body which is affected and any ensuing dysfunction. For example, the implications of a broken finger for a concert pianist are understandably greater than a similar injury occurring in someone whose livelihood does not depend to the same extent on the use of his hands.

Family, Social and Cultural Influences

Appropriate emotional support from the family is an important factor in aiding recovery from ill health. However, families that readily condone the sick role, or an illness which arises in the setting of a relationship difficulty, can result in the prolongation of physical symptoms. For example, an unhappily married woman with severe epilepsy, who repeatedly fails to take her anticonvulsant medication, is perhaps using her seizures as a way of simultaneously expressing her wish to be cared for and her anger towards an indifferent husband. Similarly, a man with chronic back pain may readily accept his symptoms as a means of avoiding intimacy within an unhappy marriage.

Domestic and financial responsibilities can have an important bearing on illness behaviour. The impact of illness is likely to be far greater for a self-employed man with dependents, than for someone who is financially cushioned by the benefits of working for a large organisation, with only himself to support. Cultural factors also have an influence on illness response. For example, several studies have indicated that people from Mediterranean countries tend to seek medical help earlier, and respond to pain in a more emotional fashion, than those of Anglo-Saxon origin.

The Duration and Severity of the Illness

Psychological problems are often encountered in those suffering from severe, life-threatening illness, especially if hospital treatment is provided in an environment which is perceived as highly technological and perilous, such as a coronary care or intensive therapy unit. The duration and course of the illness may also be significant, in that the prospect of long-term disability which arises with some chronic physical disorders (such as rheumatoid arthritis) may lead to persistent psychological symptoms.

PSYCHIATRIC DISORDERS WHICH PRESENT WITH PHYSICAL SYMPTOMS

Psychiatrists are frequently called upon to see patients who report physical symptoms for which no underlying organic cause can be established. Mostly, these are demonstrated to be somatic manifestations of anxiety or depression (*see* Table 15.1), but symptoms of this type are also encountered in association with certain personality disorders, neuroses and psychotic illnesses. In the latter case, for example, the patient may describe somatic delusions, in which the structure or function of parts of the body are believed to have changed.

Under normal circumstances, recovery from illness results in the patient relinquishing the **sick role** and resuming former activities and responsibilities. However, if this role is maintained beyond the time when physical recovery has taken place, then the individual may be obtaining some advantage by remaining a patient. **Abnormal illness behaviour** may therefore be perpetuated by **gain**, which can take the form of abrogation of responsibilities by not returning to work, increased attention from members of the family or possible financial compensation. Where the gain is conscious, the behaviour is described as malingering; if the gain is unconscious, then **hysterical mechanisms** may be operating (*see* Chapter 4). Furthermore, patients who have difficulty in expressing their feelings verbally may unconsciously use physical symptoms as a way of communicating their distress to relatives or doctors, a mechanism referred to as **alexithymia**. **Hypochondriacal** individuals who demonstrate a preoccupation with illness or bodily function, and never seem completely well, may be utilising a similar process (*see* Chapter 4). Alternatively, they might have become entrenched within the sick role due to reinforcement of their illness behaviour (*see above*).

Subjecting the patient to repeated and extensive physical investigations which yield negative results may only serve to intensify symptoms and increase his anxiety that something is amiss. The need for considering a psychological cause, and explaining its relevance to the patient during the early stages of assessment, is therefore vital. If such a possibility is ignored and only considered after failure to demonstrate an organic cause, the patient's attitude towards his condition may well have become fixed, by which time he is unlikely to be receptive to the idea that his problem has a psychological basis.

Anxiety states in which symptoms of autonomic overactivity predominate are sometimes mistaken for primary physical conditions, such as thyrotoxicosis, cardiac disease or gastrointestinal disorder (*see* Table 15.1).

Somatic complaints and physical changes that are prominent features of a **depressive illness**, such as alterations in sleep, appetite or weight, may overshadow any mood disturbance and thereby disguise the true nature of

Table 15.1 Some of the somatic symptoms of anxiety and depression

Somatic symptoms of anxiety	Somatic symptoms of depression
Headache	Weight loss
Breathlessness	Loss of appetite
Frequency of micturition	Constipation
Palpitations	Lethargy
Chest or abdominal pain	Loss of libido
Tremulousness	Sleep disturbance
Paraesthesiae	Pain — head, face, back, abdomen, limbs
Tiredness	or genitalia
Dry mouth	Difficulty in swallowing
Difficulty in swallowing	
Sweating	
Flushing	
Sleep disturbance	
Dizziness	
Bowel upset	
Nausea and retching	
Sexual dysfunction	
Generalised muscle aching	

the diagnosis. This becomes a particular problem when a physical complaint occurs in isolation and not as part of a recognisable constellation of depressive symptoms. A lowering of the pain threshold may also occur in depression, resulting in increased sensitivity to visceral sensations and minor aches or pains. Consequently, depression should always be considered in patients who repeatedly seek medical help for apparently trivial complaints.

When evaluating somatic symptoms that are suspected to have a psychological basis, care must be taken to establish when the subject was last completely well, the time of onset of symptoms and their temporal relationship to any significant life events. This information may help to explain their cause, as well as encourage the doctor to review potential problem areas in the patient's life. It is also important to determine if symptoms, other than those which are reported spontaneously or focused on during the interview, are present. For example, a man who complains of severe headaches may disregard and fail to report his dry mouth, palpitations and urinary frequency. Even though the subject might insist that he has no worries, evidence of psychological conflict or emotional difficulties can emerge after information has been gathered from other sources, such as family, friends or work colleagues. More than one interview may be required before the patient feels sufficiently confident to reveal his anxieties and concerns. Increased or reduced levels of stress which act as exacerbating or relieving factors are further indications that the symptoms might have a psychological basis (e.g. headaches that occur before going to work, but not at weekends).

A 51-year-old woman was referred for a psychiatric opinion by the otolaryngology department of her local hospital. She gave a 6-month history of intermittent hoarseness and difficulty with articulation ('My tongue keeps sticking to the roof of my mouth'). Examination of her vocal cords had been unremarkable, and there was no neurological abnormality to account for her symptoms. The history revealed that her problem had developed shortly after the death of her common-law husband. They had been a devoted couple with no children and few friends. She denied feeling depressed and said that his passing had been a relief, because of the terrible pain he had suffered prior to his death. At interview, she was cooperative and spoke intermittently in a hoarse whisper, whilst at other times her voice was normal. The mucous membranes of her mouth and lips were noticeably dry (which appeared to account for her difficulties with articulation), she was breathing rapidly and had a prominent tremor. Having excluded other causes of autonomic overactivity, her symptoms were diagnosed as secondary to somatic manifestations of anxiety (dry mouth and hyperventilation).

The patient's past medical history, or that of other family members, can occasionally be helpful in explaining the pattern of current symptoms, which may be modelled upon a previous illness. Further enquiries might reveal that the subject has had a lifelong history of hypochondriacal complaints, with no clear organic basis ever having been established. The description of symptoms can be confusing or misleading when dealing with people from different cultures, and this must be taken into account when trying to establish the nature of their problems (*see* Chapter 22).

PSYCHOLOGICAL FACTORS WHICH PREDISPOSE TO PHYSICAL ILLNESS

Although there is no evidence that psychological factors are a direct cause of physical disorders, it is widely accepted that stress may contribute to the evolution of physical illness, alongside biological and social determinants.

The role of stressful **life events** in the development of physical illness is perhaps most strikingly illustrated in the case of bereavement (*see* Chapter 7). One study demonstrated a 40% increase in the mortality of widowers during the first 6 months following the loss of their wives, when compared with an age-matched group of married men. Many of the deaths were reported as due to myocardial infarction, and one explanation offered was that the physiological changes accompanying the stress of bereavement may have placed an intolerable burden on cardiovascular systems with pre-existing disease, thereby lending some credence to the popular concept of dying from a 'broken heart'. Other studies have indicated that the relationship between life events and the onset of physical illness is more complex. It has been suggested that only individuals who first experience a psychological reaction to the life event are then predisposed to the subsequent development of a somatic disorder.

The adverse effects of stress on physical health have also been investigated with respect to certain personality types and the **lifestyle** that such people lead. For example, studies have demonstrated that coronary heart disease appears to be twice as common in so-called 'type A personalities' as opposed to 'type B personalities'. Type A individuals are characterised by men who are competitive, aggressive and strive for achievement with a sense of 'time urgency'. In contrast, type B individuals are more placid, tend to take life as it comes and are not motivated by a drive to succeed.

LIAISON PSYCHIATRY

This area of work is concerned with the role of the psychiatrist in the general hospital and other clinical areas where psychological problems occur in association with physical disorders. The liaison psychiatrist can provide a service in a number of ways. He may adopt a traditional consultative role, offering help or advice to non-psychiatric colleagues with regard to the diagnosis and treatment of psychological problems which arise in their patients. In addition, he might also focus on the doctor-patient relationship and its bearing on clinical management and overall progress. For example, a poor interaction between physician and patient may adversely affect treatment compliance or result in the development of inappropriate illness behaviour.

In some hospitals, liaison psychiatrists regularly attend ward rounds or clinical conferences on general medical, surgical and obstetric units. These occasions not only offer a chance to advise on psychological problems which are presented, but also allow an opportunity for teaching. Students and other staff members can learn the advantages of adopting an holistic approach to patient care, which emphasises the importance of social and interpersonal aspects of treatment. This might include advice on psychologically preparing people prior to surgery, the necessity of adequately explaining treatment procedures, the significance of finding time to listen and talk to patients, and the value of offering support to relatives. Sometimes, the liaison psychiatrist may need to suggest ways of improving the general ward atmosphere, especially if conflict among staff or patients affects management.

Another important role is that of advising on the psychological care of the dying, as well as dealing with problems experienced by their care givers. This is discussed further in chapter 7.

SUMMARY

1. **Psychosomatic medicine** is the study of the interrelationship between biological, psychological and social variables in health and disease. It also describes an approach to the study of medicine in which the functions of mind and body are viewed as an integral unit.

2. The association between disorders of psyche and soma is complex. Physical and psychiatric disorders frequently coexist, and where one group of symptoms predominates, the other can easily go unrecognised, often leading to protracted suffering and delayed recovery. Psychological reactions to physical illness, particularly anxiety and depression, are common and may adversely affect the prognosis. Denial can sometimes be of benefit in the early stages of illness, but may also lead to delay in seeking help or a failure to comply with treatment. The individual who continues to exhibit 'illness behaviour' beyond a time when physical recovery has taken place, may be deriving some form of gain (either conscious or unconscious) by maintaining the sick role. Factors which have a bearing on the psychological response to physical illness include the subject's personality, the reaction of family and friends, the duration

and severity of the illness, as well as social and cultural influences.

3. Physical symptoms, for which no underlying organic cause can be established, are frequently demonstrated to be somatic manifestations of anxiety or depression. In such cases, it is important to consider a psychological cause early in the assessment process. This avoids unnecessary investigations being repeatedly performed, which only serve to increase the patient's anxiety and diminish the likelihood of him accepting an alternative cause for his symptoms. Where it is difficult to determine the true nature of a somatic complaint, a careful and detailed history taken from both the patient and other informants will often help to establish the correct diagnosis. Although there is no evidence that psychological factors are a direct cause of physical disorders, it is widely accepted that stress may contribute to the evolution of physical illness alongside biological and social determinants.

4. **Liaison psychiatry** is concerned with the role of the psychiatrist in the general hospital and other clinical areas where psychological problems occur in association with physical disorders. The liaison psychiatrist can provide a conventional consultation service to non-psychiatric colleagues, or adopt a wider approach. In the latter case, he may attend ward rounds or clinical conferences, and focus on aspects of care which have an important (but less obvious) bearing on management and prognosis, such as the doctor-patient relationship or the ward atmosphere.

REFERENCES AND FURTHER READING

Creed, F. H., Pfeffer, J. M., eds (1982). *Medicine and Psychiatry: a Practical Approach*. London: Pitman.

Lipowski, Z. J. (1974). Consultation-liaison psychiatry: an overview. *American Journal of Psychiatry*; **131**: 623–30.

Lloyd, G. G. (1977). Psychological reactions to physical illness. *British Journal of Hospital Medicine*; **18**: 352–58.

Maguire, G. P., Granville-Grossman, K. L. (1968). Physical illness in psychiatric patients. *British Journal of Psychiatry*; **114**: 1365-69.

Parkes, C. M., Benjamin, B., Fitzgerald, R. G. (1969). Broken heart: a statistical study of increased mortality among widowers. *British Medical Journal*; **i**: 740–43.

16

CHILD PSYCHIATRY

Children are occasionally brought to the attention of psychiatrists because their parents or teachers are concerned about some aspect of their behaviour, emotional state or rate of development. Judging whether the presenting problem constitutes a psychiatric disorder, and therefore requires treatment, will depend on several factors. First, because childhood is a time of rapid physical and psychological changes, it is important to have an understanding of the limits of normality at any stage of development (Table 16.1). Only then is it possible to decide whether the parents' anxiety that 'something is wrong' is justified, or perhaps reflects over-concern on their part. For example, occasional temper tantrums are quite common in a 2-year-old, whereas persistent behaviour of a similar nature in a child of 10 is almost certainly abnormal.

Second, the child's reliance on adults for meeting most of his important needs is such that emotional or behavioural problems in a care giver might well result in the development of some form of disturbance in the child. Treatment under these circumstances may need to be directed towards a change in the behaviour or attitudes of parents or teachers. Finally, the child's problems might be a reflection of some difficulty or tension between close relatives, so that to complete the assessment, an evaluation of the whole family and the interactions between its members is required.

As a corollary of the above, childhood psychiatric disorder may be considered as a **deviation** from normal conduct, emotions or rate of development, which results in **suffering** to the child or care givers, or produces **impairment of functioning**.

CLASSIFICATION

A **multiaxial system** is sometimes used to classify disorders, in which recognition is given not only to the diagnostic category, but also to associated aetiological factors, developmental delay, intellectual capacity and the child's level of functioning over the previous year. Childhood psychiatric disorders can also be considered in terms of the categories shown in Table 16.2.

Table 16.1 Important developmental milestones from infancy to adolescence

Period	Sensorimotor, speech	Social/emotional
4 weeks		Begins to smile
3 months	Starts to hold head erect, sits up with help	
6 months	Begins to sit up unaided, reaches out for toys, places things in mouth	Begins to distinguish between self and other objects, smiles selectively at mother
7–10 months	Starts to crawl, sits unsupported for a few minutes, tuneful babbling	Attachment behaviour, separation anxiety (parting child from mother results in distress), fear of strangers
12–18 months	Walks unaided, speaks first words, understands simple commands	Temper tantrums common as a sign of resistance to social learning, begins to make choices, waves goodbye
18–24 months	Vocabulary expands — able to make simple sentences; can build a tower of four cubes, able to use a cup and spoon	Becomes a 'member' of the family, begins toilet training, develops clear gender identity
2–3 years	Complex speech develops, able to use a fork	Asks for potty, dry by day, actively follows parent figure to avoid separation, begins to test behavioural boundaries
3–4 years	Dresses with help, able to copy a circle and a square	Dry by night, begins symbolic play, likes listening to stories, experiences rivalry and jealousy, develops egocentricity
4–5 years	Fluent speech, dresses and washes unaided	Develops conscience, enjoys telling stories
5–12 years	Learns to read and write and deal with figures	Starts school and extends social horizons beyond the family; personality becomes clearly established, develops concept of achievement, ability and personal limitations; understands gender identity and position in family; standards of social behaviour refined

continued overleaf

Table 16.1 *Continued*

Period	Sensorimotor, speech	Social/emotional
Adolescence	Accelerated growth, development of secondary sexual characteristics	Capability for abstract thought, increased awareness of personal identity and sexuality Early adolescence — separation from parental ethos Middle adolescence — development of peer group identity Late adolescence — finding a sexual partner, establishing a work role

EPIDEMIOLOGY

A number of population studies conducted in the 1970s attempted to determine the extent of childhood psychiatric disorder in both urban and rural settings, and to identify the demographic factors which may influence its development.

The **Isle of Wight study** (Rutter *et al.*, 1976) screened all 10- and 11-year-old children living on the island using standardised questionnaires. The overall prevalence of psychiatric disorder was found to be approximately 7%, with twice as many boys affected as girls. Its development was found to be associated with epilepsy, brain damage, specific reading retardation (*see later*), low intelligence and physical illness, although no simple link was established between social class and psychiatric disorder.

The **Camberwell study** (Rutter *et al.*, 1975) found the prevalence of psychiatric disorder among a similar age group in an urban environment to be 13%, almost twice that in the Isle of Wight. An increased rate of family problems, combined with the additional burden of a number of social disadvantages (poor housing, overcrowding, poor schooling), were thought to account for the difference.

The **Waltham Forest study** (Richman *et al.*, 1975) found that over 20% of 3-year-olds had some form of psychiatric disorder, but with only one-third (a comparable figure to the Isle of Wight study) demonstrating serious, persistent problems. The sexes were affected equally, and the development of psychiatric disorder was found to be associated with language delay, social disadvantage, parental discord and maternal depression.

Table 16.2 A classification of childhood psychiatric disorders

Conduct disorders	
Emotional disorders	Neuroses, school refusal
Symptomatic disorders	Elimination disorders (enuresis, encopresis), habit disorders (tics, stammering etc.), eating disorders (*see* Chapter 17), sleep disorders (*see* Chapter 21)
Specific delays in development	E.g. specific reading retardation
Childhood psychoses	Infantile autism, disintegrative psychosis
Hyperkinetic syndrome	

In ICD 10, it is likely that infantile autism and disintegrative psychosis will be classified as 'pervasive developmental disorders', and no longer regarded as childhood psychoses.

ASSESSMENT OF THE CHILD

Nowadays, many clinics offer an appointment to the whole family, and the assessment may take several sessions to complete. Depending on the nature of the problem, the child may or may not be seen separately. However, when assessing any problem in child psychiatry, it is essential to view the child both in relation to the family and in the context of the community. In addition, it is necessary to consider **why** the problem is being presented now, **what** are the precipitating and perpetuating factors, and **who** is asking for help (e.g. parents or professionals). Early on in the assessment process, it is important to establish the type of help which will be of greatest use to the child and his family.

A multidisciplinary approach is commonly used, and there is often considerable variation in the roles and responsibilities undertaken by the different professional groups that work with children. Although history-taking and examination of the mental state are important aspects of assessing disturbance in childhood, the manner in which they are undertaken differs in several ways from that practised in adult psychiatry.

The **history** is normally obtained from the parents or care givers, except in the case of older children, who may be able to provide some of the information themselves. It is often helpful to begin by asking questions about non-emotive topics (such as hobbies or what the child enjoys) before moving on to problem areas. The history should include details of any current problems, information about the family background, structure and relationships, as well as a systematic enquiry into the child's recent health, emotional state and behaviour. Information is also obtained regarding the child's development and schooling, since these are comparable to the personal history and work record of the adult. The degree of social adjustment needs to be considered, and will be reflected by the way he occupies his day, his role within the family, as well as his friendships and interests.

The **mental state examination** includes a record of the child's appearance, general behaviour, speech and mood. The thought content can be determined by noting any fears and anxieties, preoccupations or fantasies, as well as the child's attitude towards others. Unobtrusively observing the child at play may yield much of this information, as well as providing an indication of his developmental level, attention span, intellectual capabilities, inventiveness and socialisation. The interviewer should also note the family relationships and interactions, since these may contribute towards an understanding of any abnormal dynamics which might adversely influence the child's mental health or perpetuate symptomatic behaviour.

In order to create a profile of how the child functions at school and at home, parental permission is usually sought for additional reports from teachers and social workers. Formal tests of intelligence may also be conducted by the educational psychologist to assess performance levels in a number of skills involving reading, spelling, arithmetical ability and problem solving. In this way, a comprehensive picture is built up of the child's level of functioning in a variety of settings, allowing the identification of problem areas which need specific attention.

GENERAL ASPECTS OF TREATMENT

Children needing psychiatric assessment and treatment are sometimes seen in a hospital setting, but most are referred to their local **child guidance clinic**. Referrals are received from various sources such as general practitioners, health visitors, social workers and parents. The clinic is based in the community and is staffed by a multidisciplinary team which may include a child psychiatrist, educational psychologist, child psychotherapist and social worker. Close links are maintained with other professionals, such as paediatricians and teachers, who might need to be involved in management decisions.

Social case work may highlight difficulties within the family which can be helped by simple measures, such as lending emotional support or offering practical advice to parents about their child. **Psychotherapeutic approaches** to treatment are often employed, and involve the use of both individual and family-orientated methods. Psychotherapy with young children is conducted through the medium of play, while in older children a conversational approach is usually more appropriate. **Behavioural** and **cognitive techniques** are sometimes used in the management of those conditions where a change in behaviour is the primary aim of therapy, or in helping parents to manage their children more effectively. Many of the techniques applied in adult psychiatry, such as positive reinforcement, modelling and shaping, are also effective in children (*see* Chapter 13).

Drug treatments have a limited use in child psychiatry, but may be helpful in certain conditions such as the hyperkinetic syndrome and enuresis.

In cases where learning is compromised as a result of psychiatric or behavioural problems, special **educational measures** may be necessary to overcome specific learning disabilities and improve socialisation. In order to maximise the child's potential, remedial teaching can be provided, and since the passage of the 1981 Education Act, it is now official policy to integrate children with 'special needs' into ordinary schools. Sometimes, transfer to a specialised unit is considered necessary, and schools exist specifically for children with behavioural problems, physical dysfunctions or learning disorders. These usually offer a well-structured and intensive teaching programme, combined with the advantages of a high staff/pupil ratio.

Therapeutic separation of the child from the family is occasionally necessary where he is at risk from neglect, emotional deprivation and physical or sexual abuse. Options include fostering, placement in a local authority group home or in a boarding school.

CONDUCT DISORDERS

Occasional acts of antisocial behaviour in childhood are common, but where they become persistent and extreme, or result in suffering to the child or his care givers, a conduct disorder is said to be present. Conduct disorders differ from **juvenile delinquency**, which simply describes law-breaking behaviour, although there is inevitably a degree of overlap between the two entities. Antisocial behaviour can present in various ways including repeated stealing, lying, truancy, fighting, disobedience or fire-setting. Conduct disorders are most commonly seen in boys and are more prevalent among children from the lower social classes.

Aetiology

Factors associated with the development of conduct disorder include poor parenting, large discordant families, a difficult temperament from an early age, brain damage and epilepsy. The influence of the child's peer group may also contribute significantly to the development of antisocial behaviour. The Isle of Wight study demonstrated a strong association between **specific reading retardation** (*see later*) and conduct disorder, although the reasons for this are not clearly established.

Management

Advising parents to provide a consistent and firm approach to the handling of their child may be the only treatment necessary in mild cases.

Where the conduct disorder is more severe, family therapy or behavioural modification might be indicated. Remedial teaching should be considered if reading difficulties are evident. When all other forms of intervention fail, separation of the child from the family is sometimes necessary. The long-term prognosis is generally poor, with more than half of all conduct-disordered children continuing to display antisocial behaviour in adult life.

SCHOOL REFUSAL

Children who fail to attend school may do so as a result of:

1. truancy: wilful avoidance of school without parental knowledge of the child's whereabouts
2. genuine physical illness
3. parental influence/encouragement to stay at home, such as an agoraphobic mother who keeps her child away from school in order to cope with her own feelings of anxiety
4. school refusal: a persistent reluctance or inability to attend school because of fear (hence the former term 'school phobia').

Unlike children who truant, school refusers tend to come from overprotective middle-class families and are often high academic achievers. Truancy has a clear male predominance and is usually confined to adolescents, whereas school refusal affects the sexes equally and also occurs in younger children. Two main groups can be identified: the first category (5–7-year-olds) display transient anxiety about separating from their parents, or have specific fears regarding the school environment. Older children in the second category (aged 11–14) often present with chronic symptoms and are likely to become socially withdrawn. In addition, they tend to demonstrate poor adaptation to change, low self-esteem, depressive symptoms and specific concerns about changing schools.

Generally, school refusers display signs of anxiety at the time they should normally leave home for school, which may manifest as physical problems (such as abdominal pain or vomiting) restricted to weekday mornings. These are sometimes accompanied by tantrums or aggressive behaviour, and if actually made to leave the house, the child often returns home shortly afterwards in a state of panic. In either age group, the problem may follow a significant life event such as moving house, experiencing a death in the family, changing teachers, suffering a physical illness or starting menstruation.

Management

The recognition of school refusal is dependent upon differentiating the condition from other causes of non-attendance at school, together with an appraisal of any adverse factors which might have precipitated or perpetuated the disorder, such as bullying or fear of exams. Management requires close liaison with both the parents and teachers, as well as the involvement of the school's educational psychologist and welfare officer.

Where school refusal has only persisted for a short time, the problem can often be resolved by adopting a firm and consistent attitude, and **returning the child to school** as soon as possible on a date agreed by all concerned (*see* flooding. p. 277). However, when there is a longer history, it may be necessary to adopt a behavioural approach which aims for a graded return to school (*see* graded exposure, p. 277) under parental responsibility. For example, this might initially involve doing school work at home, followed by the child making trips to the school locality, then sitting in on selected lessons, and eventually building up to full attendance. In extreme cases, a programme of this type may need to be preceded by hospital admission, in order to treat any associated psychiatric symptoms and ensure that the child continues to receive a proper education. Parents sometimes fail to accept that help is needed, or openly collude with the child. If family therapy is agreed to under such circumstances, it may be more effective if the education authority, rather than the clinician, deals with its legal responsibilities for ensuring the child's attendance at school.

The response to treatment is generally good, particularly in younger children and those with a secure and supportive family environment. A minority of cases, usually adolescents, go on to develop neurotic disorders in adult life.

NEUROSES

Neurotic symptoms occurring in childhood are similar to those seen in adults, although they tend to be of shorter duration and more variable in nature. In the majority of cases, spontaneous resolution occurs without treatment.

Anxiety states are prevalent throughout childhood and adolescence, particularly among children who are timid and have difficulty in separating from their parents. They may present with a variety of symptoms such as nightmares, headaches, abdominal pain, diarrhoea, vomiting or nausea.

Fears and **phobias** concerning certain objects or situations (such as the dark, animals and insects) are common, but seldom produce significant handicap.

Obsessive-compulsive neurosis is rare, although transient childhood rituals are frequent (e.g. avoiding stepping on cracks in the pavement). **Hysterical phenomena** are more likely to occur among adolescents than in younger age groups, but their overall prevalence in childhood remains low.

Depressive symptoms are common in children, especially in response to unhappy circumstances or events, although adult-type depressive illnesses are infrequent and tend to be confined to adolescents. **Suicide** is extremely rare and virtually unknown below the age of 10.

ENURESIS

Enuresis is defined as repeated involuntary urination beyond an age at which continence is expected. It may occur during sleep (**nocturnal enuresis**) and/or during waking hours (**diurnal enuresis**). Primary enuresis describes those cases in which urinary continence has never been achieved, while the secondary form applies to children who become enuretic after dryness has been attained. Daytime bladder control is normally achieved first, and most children can be expected to be fully continent between the ages of 3 and 4. Consequently, nocturnal enuresis is generally considered 'a problem' if bed-wetting occurs after the age of 5. Estimates of prevalence vary, but it is thought that approximately 10–15% of 5-year-olds are bed-wetters, this figure falling to 5% by the age of 10 and less than 1% in adolescence. Boys are affected two to three times more frequently than girls, and there is an increased prevalence among the lower social classes.

Aetiology

The causation of enuresis is considered to be multifactorial. In over two-thirds of cases, there is a history of bed-wetting among first-degree relatives, suggesting an inherited component. Other factors implicated as being aetiologically significant include delayed maturation of bladder control, urinary tract infections, a small bladder capacity, low intelligence and associated psychiatric disorder. Environmental influences, such as large families, institutional upbringing, social deprivation and stressful life events, may exert their effect by modifying normal continence training.

Management

Assessment of the enuretic child begins by taking a **history** to determine:

1. if the problem is nocturnal or diurnal (the latter is more likely to be due to a physical cause, such as urinary tract infection)

2. whether the enuresis is primary (possible anatomical defect or delayed maturation) or secondary (environmental stress or acquired physical disorder)
3. the duration and frequency of symptoms
4. if there has been any recent life event (such as moving house, birth of a sibling, family bereavement, domestic conflict or changes in sleeping arrangements)
5. the parental attitudes to the problem and the types of treatment attempted so far.

Physical examination should aim to exclude anatomical or neurological abnormalities such as hypospadias, ectopic bladder or spina bifida. **Investigations** routinely include urine microscopy and culture, as well as urinalysis for protein or glucose.

Once any underlying physical or psychiatric disorder has been excluded, attention should be turned towards exploring and dissipating family tensions. For example, simple measures such as offering **support** and **reassurance**, as well as discouraging parents from punishing the child for wet beds, might in themselves be sufficient to resolve the problem. Encouraging the child to empty his bladder before sleep may also be of benefit.

A **star chart** is a useful means of determining the frequency of enuresis, and also helps to establish a reward system for dry nights (wet nights being ignored). This method is often successful in effecting a cure, but resistant cases may respond to the additional use of a **bell and pad enuresis alarm**. This device consists of two mesh or foil pads separated by a sheet, each of which is connected to a buzzer. When urine starts to be voided the circuit is completed and a bell sounds, waking the child and his parents. The child is then required to get up, switch off the alarm and complete urination in the toilet. Before returning to sleep, he should strip and remake the bed under parental supervision, and also reset the alarm. Provided this procedure is carefully followed, the success rate is high, and continence is usually achieved in 3–4 weeks. **Tricyclic antidepressants** in small doses are often rapidly effective in overcoming nocturnal enuresis (their efficacy being unrelated to any antidepressant action), but relapse is common on discontinuing medication and the side-effects can be troublesome.

ENCOPRESIS

Encopresis or **faecal soiling** is defined as defaecation in inappropriate places (notably clothing or receptacles) beyond an age at which bowel control is expected — about 4 years old. The problem is much less common than enuresis, affecting approximately 1% of children aged 5–11, with boys outnumbering girls by 4:1. It is more frequent among children from socially deprived backgrounds and where there is evidence of family discord.

Aetiology

Faecal soiling may be retentive or non-retentive.

RETENTIVE TYPE

The child develops retention of faeces with subsequent overflow due to either:

1. physical conditions such as anal fissure or Hirschsprung's disease
2. emotional stress: overzealous parental toilet training causes the child to become anxious and unable to 'defaecate to command'; the resultant constipation eventually leads to retention with overflow. This is the most common form of encopresis.

NON-RETENTIVE TYPE

Faeces escape freely and the condition is either primary (constantly present since birth) or secondary (develops after a period of faecal continence).

1. The primary form is most commonly due to inadequate toilet training or developmental delay (often associated with enuresis), which may be related to low intelligence.
2. Secondary encopresis may be regressive (the child reverts to an earlier stage of development in response to stress) or aggressive (a defiant response to attempts at parental control, resulting in deliberately inappropriate defaecation). Rarely, secondary encopresis arises from inflammatory bowel disease.

Management

A carefully taken **history** should attempt to establish the duration, severity and likely cause of the problem, as well as identifying any family stresses which often centre around parental disapproval of the soiling. **Abdominal palpation** and sometimes rectal examination is necessary to determine whether or not there is retention or any underlying physical disorder. Occasionally, plain abdominal x-rays or barium studies are needed to establish the diagnosis.

Once any underlying organic cause has been excluded, treatment begins with **reassurance** and **explanation** to the family as to how the soiling has developed, and the measures necessary to correct the problem. It is important to decrease tensions and anxieties which exist regarding cleanliness and bowel habit, and to make the parents aware that, in most cases, the behaviour is not wilful.

When retention is present, **the rectum must be emptied**, and oral laxatives or bulking agents are helpful under these circumstances. Faecal lubricants, enemata or bowel washouts may also be necessary if impaction is severe. **Behavioural techniques** can be employed to encourage appropriate defaecation through the implementation of star charts, and by rewarding correct use of the toilet. Most children respond well to this approach, but difficult cases may require hospital admission in order to carry out treatment.

TICS

Tics are sudden, rapid, repetitive, non-goal directed movements, which although involuntary, can be suppressed with effort at the expense of mounting anxiety. They most commonly occur in the face and neck (as well as involving the vocal cords), and tend to be coordinated. Tics are accentuated by periods of tension or excitement, but disappear during sleep. Approximately 10% of children develop movements of this kind at some stage in their lives, with the average age of onset at about 7 years, boys being affected three times more frequently than girls.

In up to one-third of cases there is a family history of tics, and onset occasionally follows an emotional upset, although causation often remains unknown. The majority of tics are simple rather than multiple in nature, and they usually resolve spontaneously. More severe cases may respond to the administration of neuroleptic drugs, such as haloperidol, or be helped by behavioural techniques involving relaxation training or massed practice (*see* Chapter 13). Gilles de la Tourette syndrome is a rare disorder involving multiple facial and vocal tics (*see* Chapter 23).

OTHER HABIT DISORDERS

Stammering is usually a transient phenomenon of uncertain causation and is more commonly found in boys. Where treatment is necessary, speech therapy is sometimes helpful, although psychotherapy may be indicated if there is associated emotional stress.

Temper tantrums and **breath-holding attacks** are common in both toddlers and young children, but generally cease by school age. Parents should be encouraged to adopt a calm and consistent approach, in order to avoid perpetuating the behaviour. **Thumb-sucking** and **nail-biting** are common childhood habits and only require treatment if they become severe or compulsive. **Head-banging** and **body-rocking** occur in normal toddlers, but may also be a feature in autistic and other mentally retarded children.

SPECIFIC READING RETARDATION

Some children demonstrate a specific impairment of reading ability, despite having normal intelligence and receiving adequate teaching. When the reading age is 28 months or more below that expected, the problem is termed one of specific reading retardation. The condition was found in 4% of children in the Isle of Wight study, with the prevalence increasing to 10% among those living in an inner city environment. In both studies, boys outnumbered girls, and the disorder appeared more frequently in children from the lower social classes.

The **aetiology** is uncertain, but in many cases there is a family history of reading difficulties. One-third of affected children have a coexisting **conduct disorder** (*see* p. 315), and there may be other features of developmental delay such as general clumsiness, bed-wetting and delayed speech. Other associated factors include poor concentration, large family size, cerebral palsy and epilepsy. Having excluded general educational backwardness, **treatment** consists of remedial teaching and encouraging parental involvement in helping the child to read. Despite these measures, the **prognosis** is usually poor, and problems with reading may persist into adult life.

CHILDHOOD PSYCHOSES

Adult-type mental illnesses, such as schizophrenia and affective psychoses, are extremely rare before adolescence. However, two disorders specific to children result in serious disturbances of behaviour, emotion and social interaction, and are therefore classified as childhood psychoses.

Infantile Autism

First described by Kanner in 1943, this syndrome has a recognised onset before the age of 30 months and affects 2–4 children in every 10 000. The male:female sex ratio is 4:1, and although some studies have indicated an increased prevalence among the upper socioeconomic classes, the validity of this association is doubtful.

CLINICAL FEATURES

Three central features are recognised, all of which must be represented in order to make the diagnosis.

1. **Autistic aloneness**: children with the disorder are often described as unresponsive to cuddling and other close contact during infancy. As they get older, autistic children have a tendency to treat individuals as objects rather than people, and their limited capacity to form social relationships sometimes leads parents to suspect that they may be deaf or mentally retarded. Eye contact is poor, and their preference for solitude is also reflected in a lack of shared play.

2. **Impaired communication**: speech is nearly always delayed and sometimes there is a complete failure to talk. Abnormalities of speech are often conspicuous, with a tendency to repeat phrases and 'echo' the words of others, or to display pronominal reversal (e.g. referring to themselves as 'you'). Comprehension is poor, and some children do not respond at all when spoken to. Those who learn to read appear to do so mechanically, demonstrating little understanding of the written word . Non-verbal communication is also affected, with a paucity or inappropriateness of gesture, as well as a lack of creativity and symbolic play.

3. **A desire for sameness** : difficulty in coping with change is reflected by a propensity for routines and rituals. The child may insist on eating the same type of meal or wearing the same outfit every day, and even minor alterations in routine are met with emotional outbursts and signs of distress. Play is often repetitive and aimless, with a preoccupation for unusual objects (such as switches or wheels) which have a mechanical function, but little use for imaginative or creative activity. Toys or household items are sometimes arranged in patterns or systematically lined up in a particular way, with any attempt to move them being strenuously resisted.

Abnormal body movements are often evident, and these may become pronounced if the child is upset. Pirouetting, body-rocking and a curious tendency to flap the hands or examine the fingers closely are sometimes seen. In addition, there may be unexpected bouts of overactivity accompanied by emotional outbursts. Self-mutilation is occasionally a problem.

Most autistic children are **intellectually impaired**, with an IQ below 70. However, disabilities vary from severe forms of the condition, where the child is totally inaccessible and mute, to mild cases, where functional ability is only slightly impaired. Isolated areas of excellence, such as musical ability, drawing or feats of memory, are sometimes seen in individuals who are otherwise severely handicapped (**idiot savant**). Autistic traits (in the absence of the full syndrome) are occasionally evident in otherwise normal children.

AETIOLOGY

Although the causation of autism remains unclear, the findings from twin and family studies (*see* p. 7) suggest that the disorder may have a genetic component. An organic cause is likely in most cases (as suggested by the development of epileptic seizures in about one in four sufferers by the time they reach adolescence), even though clear evidence of brain damage or neurological abnormalities is not always demonstrable.

MANAGEMENT

Living with an autistic child is often demanding and distressing for other members of the family. Consequently, both parents and siblings require considerable support and advice in order to help cope with the behavioural problems, learning and communication difficulties which can arise. The **National Society for Autistic Children** may be able to offer help in some of these areas, as well as providing information, advice and contact with other affected families.

Behavioural techniques can be useful in some cases to promote linguistic skills, increase social interaction and diminish unwanted behaviour. Many autistic children require placement in a **special school**, where intensive methods are employed to minimise cognitive and social handicaps. The use of **medication**, such as haloperidol or other major tranquillisers, is occasionally indicated to control aggressive or overactive behaviour. When all therapeutic measures have failed, and the child cannot be managed at home, **residential care** will need to be considered.

PROGNOSIS

The outcome is generally poor, with most autistic children remaining severely handicapped as adults. One-half never learn to talk, and only one in six attain the necessary skills which enable them to receive normal schooling or to work in open employment. Consequently, considerable support is needed in later life, especially with difficulties that may arise regarding relationships. These can be particularly troublesome at the time of adolescence, with the emergence of adult sexuality, and later at work, when interaction with other employees may be a problem.

Disintegrative Psychosis

This disorder is distinguished from infantile autism in that the onset of symptoms is after the age of 30 months and follows a period of 2–3 years of normal development. The clinical picture is one of rapid and progressive social withdrawal and intellectual deterioration, associated with loss of speech. Some children exhibit disturbed and overactive behaviour, together with mannerisms and stereotypies.

Several uncommon organic brain disorders, including encephalitis, Wilson's disease, the lipidoses and tuberous sclerosis, are associated with the development of this syndrome. As with autism, treatment is entirely symptomatic and the prognosis is generally poor, with many cases resulting in severe mental retardation or death at an early age.

THE HYPERKINETIC SYNDROME

Episodes of overactivity in children are a relatively common reason for seeking expert help, but most cases are simply variants of normal behaviour. In the USA, **hyperactivity** is a term used to describe a disorder in which children are overactive in specific situations (typically at school) and show evidence of distractability, together with impulsive and excitable behaviour. More than one-third of American children are described as 'overactive' by parents or teachers, and even when they fulfil all of the above criteria, the prevalence is still high (about 5%). Consequently, some authorities believe that hyperactivity disorder is overdiagnosed in the USA, and many cases may in fact be either conduct disorders or variants of normal behaviour.

The term **hyperkinetic syndrome** is more strictly applied in the UK to those children who demonstrate:

1. severe, pervasive overactivity (in two or more situations, e.g. both at home and at school) that is excessive for the child's age and IQ, and is a handicap to development
2. evidence of marked inattentiveness and restlessness from direct observation by the diagnostician
3. absence of childhood autism or affective disorder.

It is a rare disorder affecting approximately one in 1000 children, the majority showing evidence of neurological dysfunction or mental retardation, although some are of normal intelligence. Boys are affected more commonly than girls, and the age of onset is characteristically before 6 years. The **cause** is unknown, but may be associated with an underlying neurophysiological abnormality. Typically, the child is relentlessly over-active, and unable to concentrate or apply himself to tasks for anything other than a short period of time. Consequently, learning difficulties are common and persistently disruptive behaviour often evokes punitive responses from exhausted teachers and parents.

Initial **management** of the hyperkinetic syndrome involves the provision of adequate support for both the family and teachers, as well as helping all concerned to adopt a consistent approach in handling the child. This can be augmented with **behavioural techniques** or (paradoxically) **stimulant drugs** such as dexamphetamine, both of which have proved to be effective in reducing overactivity. The latter should be administered with caution, because of its tendency to cause growth retardation. **Remedial teaching** may be required and should be implemented in a structured classroom environment, in order to provide firm boundaries to the child's behaviour. Restricting certain **food additives** from the diet is thought by some to be helpful in controlling symptoms, although this remains controversial.

In most cases, overactivity diminishes by the time the child reaches adolescence, although associated disabilities are more likely to continue into adulthood.

ELECTIVE MUTISM

This rare disorder constitutes a persistent refusal to talk in certain situations, particularly at school, while speaking freely in others (such as the home). The condition occurs equally in boys and girls, and the onset in most cases is at the age of starting school. The aetiology is usually unknown, but the behaviour may be attention-seeking or a response to extreme stress, such as an assault. Some children become electively mute as a phobic response to the supposed consequences of speaking. Spon-taneous remission is frequent in the younger child, although older children have a less favourable prognosis and may require behavioural or psychotherapeutic intervention.

CHILD ABUSE

Each year in the UK, an increasing number of cases are detected where children have been subjected to physical violence, sexual abuse or neglect. It is estimated that annually between 5 and 10 children in every 1000 under the age of 18 are victims of some form of abuse, although the actual figure may be much higher due to considerable under-reporting.

Recognition of Child Abuse

Early detection of the problem, and prompt action following its discovery, is vital to minimise the risk of further harm. Any injury occurring in a baby under the age of 12 months should always raise the question of child abuse. As children become ambulant, the likelihood of an accident being genuine increases. Nevertheless, suspicions should be aroused where there is delay or avoidance in reporting the incident, the parents' account of what happened does not tally with the injuries sustained, or there are other obvious inconsistencies in the stories given. Child abuse needs to be considered when the following injuries are present:

1. multiple bruises of different ages, especially if suspected strapmarks or fingermarks are present
2. black eyes
3. unusual or unexplained burns or lacerations
4. human bite marks
5. petechial haemorrhages on the face
6. any fracture, especially in babies or toddlers
7. subdural haematoma or visceral rupture.

Children who are victims of abuse or neglect sometimes appear dishevelled and unkempt. Young babies may fail to thrive or show other evidence of inadequate care, such as chronic nappy rash. Toddlers tend to be perpetually miserable and cry constantly, while older children often have a cowered appearance or seem excessively vigilant and apprehensive of adults ('frozen watchfulness'). Sometimes, the problem comes to light due to poor attendance at school.

Aetiological Factors

Most acts of violence towards children are not premeditated and often occur in response to a sudden release of frustration or anger after a period of mounting tension. Less commonly, the abuse is calculated and inflicted with sadistic intent. Child abuse is more likely to occur when one or both parents were themselves mistreated in childhood, or where either of them have a history of violence or criminal behaviour. Young unmarried mothers, especially those isolated from their families, are particularly prone to harm their children. Tensions which lead to aggressive outbursts may be increased if the child is particularly demanding or the family are forced to live in cramped or otherwise unsuitable living accommodation. Most parents who maltreat their children are not mentally ill, although abuse of alcohol or drugs increases the likelihood of violent or irresponsible behaviour. Unwanted or complicated pregnancies, poor maternal bonding or lengthy separations from parents are additional factors which increase the risk of subsequent child abuse.

The Management of Child Abuse

If the injuries are severe, the child should be immediately admitted to hospital under the provisions of a **Place of Safety Order**. In less extreme cases, a careful physical examination for further evidence of abuse needs to be performed, and an explanation obtained from the responsible adult as to how the injury occurred. In many areas, a district policy of the procedure for handling cases has been set out, and **child abuse teams** have been established (comprising a senior doctor, nurse and social worker), who should be informed when non-accidental injury is suspected. Attention must then be given as to whether or not it is safe for the child to return home. If removal from parental care is under consideration, it is preferable that no action be taken until a **case conference** has been held. This provides an opportunity for all professionals involved to share information that is known about a family, to assess the significance of the available facts and to draw up a plan of action.

Under certain circumstances, it may be preferable for the child to remain at home, provided appropriate **support** and **help** are available to the parents. When it is too dangerous to consider this option, it is possible to offer the parents relief by receiving the child into care on their own voluntary application. If they refuse, then it is necessary to obtain a magistrate's warrant for a Place of Safety Order to remove the child into care for a period not exceeding 28 days. During this time, further assessment and investigations can be carried out, following which it may be decided to extend the order for a further period, return the child home or consider permanent separation.

It is vital that the details of all children who are designated as being **at risk** are maintained on a social services register, following which the local authority has a statutory obligation to follow them up at regular intervals. The family will need to be supervised by medical and social services to ensure that any further abuse is quickly detected. Parents should also be offered help and support in dealing with problems they have in caring for their children. The **family doctor** fulfils an important role in this capacity, and is able to liaise with other supportive agencies who may need to be involved.

ADOLESCENT PSYCHIATRY

Adolescence is a time of rapid physical and psychosocial changes. Presenting problems can be a perpetuation of childhood disorders, or herald the onset of adult psychiatric conditions. However, certain disturbances may be specifically attributable to the stresses of adolescence. Concerns about sexual orientation and attractiveness, peer relationships, 'the meaning of life', dependency needs and religious convictions can give rise to a sense of inner turmoil, in which feelings of uncertainty, misery and low self-esteem are sometimes expressed. Ideas of reference and rebellious behaviour are commonly seen, and may be viewed as a response to the search for personal identity and independence.

When reactions of this kind are transient, they can be considered a normal part of the transition to adulthood. However, in some instances they may result in a decline in academic performance or social functioning, so that some form of therapeutic intervention is necessary. Experimentation with alcohol or drugs (especially solvent abuse, *see* p. 224) is fairly common, although only in a minority of cases does this lead to significant psychiatric or social disturbance. Eating disorders frequently have an onset during adolescence (*see* Chapter 17) and major functional illnesses, such as schizophrenia (*see* Chapter 8), can also occur at this time.

The assessment and management of the adolescent can often prove difficult, and therefore require particular skills. Therapeutic approaches vary according to the degree of maturity of the individual, although younger adolescents may be managed using treatment methods outlined earlier in this chapter. In contrast, older subjects will require a more adult-orientated approach, in which their autonomy is respected. Psychotherapy is sometimes helpful in providing a forum for the ventilation of feelings and the exploration of doubts and fears. Anxiety can be reduced by offering support and reassurance, and psychotherapy also allows the development of a trusting relationship with an adult. Occasionally, where psychological disturbance is severe, admission to a specialist adolescent unit may be necessary. Suicide rates are rising in this age group, so that the estimation of suicidal risk is an increasingly important aspect of assessment (*see* Chapter 6).

SUMMARY

1. **Childhood psychiatric disorder** may be considered as a deviation from normal conduct, emotions or rate of development, which results in suffering to the child or caregivers, or produces impairment of functioning. Disorders are sometimes classified using a multiaxial system in which aetiology, developmental delay, intellectual capacity and level of functioning are recorded in addition to the diagnostic category. The interplay of genetic, physical, psychological and environmental factors is involved in the development of many childhood psychiatric disorders, which are generally more common in boys.

2. **Assessment** often involves the whole family, and the child should be

viewed both in relation to the family unit and in a wider social context. Attention should be paid as to why the problem is presenting at this time, the precipitating or perpetuating factors, and who is asking for help. Most children are assessed at a Child Guidance Clinic staffed by members of a multidisciplinary team. History-taking usually relies on information provided by parents or care givers, and it is important to observe the child at play and when interacting with others. Further information may be needed from teachers, social workers and educational psychologists to complete the assessment.

3. **Conduct disorders** are more common in boys and in children from socially deprived backgrounds or disturbed families. There is a strong association with specific reading retardation and organic brain disorder. Mild cases may respond to a firm and consistent parental approach, while family therapy, behavioural modification, remedial teaching or separation from the family might need to be considered in more severe cases. The prognosis is generally poor. **School refusal** is a persistent reluctance or inability to attend school due to fear, and needs to be distinguished from other causes of non-attendance, in particular truancy. The condition sometimes develops following a significant event in the child's life. In young children the problem is often acute, and management involves firm and consistent handling, together with a prompt return of the child to school. When there is a longer history, a phased return to school is often required.

4. **Nocturnal enuresis** occurs in 10–15% of 5-year-olds, particularly those from deprived backgrounds, with boys outnumbering girls by 3:1. Causation is considered to be multifactorial. Treatment should aim to reduce family tensions, and offer reassurance and support to child and parents. Specific measures involve encouraging the child to keep a star chart, the use of the bell and pad enuresis alarm, and the occasional administration of tricyclic antidepressants. **Encopresis** or faecal soiling is much less common than enuresis, and is more prevalent in children from socially deprived backgrounds and discordant families. Boys outnumber girls by 4:1. Retentive and non-retentive types occur. Treatment involves reassurance and explanation to the family as to how the soiling has developed, followed in retentive cases by emptying of the rectum, and the use of behavioural measures to ensure appropriate defaecation in the toilet.

5. **Tics** affect about 10% of children at some time in their lives. In most cases they resolve spontaneously, but when severe, behavioural treatment or the administration of neuroleptic drugs may be necessary. **Specific reading retardation** is more common in boys than girls, and in one-third of cases there is a coexisting conduct disorder. Remedial teaching may help, but problems with reading often persist into adult life.

6. **Infantile autism** is a condition of unknown aetiology, affecting 2–4 children/10 000. It is four times more common in boys than girls, and has

an onset before the age of 30 months. The diagnosis is made in the presence of three central features: autistic aloneness, impaired communication and a desire for sameness, the latter manifesting as routines and rituals. Most autistic children are intellectually impaired and 50% never learn to talk. Many exhibit abnormal body movements. Treatment includes the provision of advice and support for other family members, behavioural methods to promote linguistic skills and social interaction, medication to control overactivity and aggressive behaviour, and special schooling to minimise cognitive and social handicaps. The prognosis is generally poor.

7. The **hyperkinetic syndrome** is a rare disorder of unknown causation. Affected children demonstrate severe hyperactivity in several situations, associated with marked inattentiveness and restlessness. Consequently, learning difficulties are common and remedial teaching may be necessary. Behavioural techniques can help to control overactivity, and the paradoxical use of stimulant drugs is also sometimes effective. Overactivity usually diminishes by the time the child reaches adolescence.

8. An increasing number of children each year are victims of **child abuse**. Early detection of the problem, and prompt action following its discovery, is vital to minimise the risk of further harm. If the injuries are severe, immediate separation from the parents should be undertaken, if necessary under the provisions of a Place of Safety Order. In every instance, long-term decisions about the child's future should only be considered after a case conference has been held. Children 'at risk' who remain under parental care need to be maintained on a social services register, and must be regularly followed-up by the medical and social services. Ongoing help and support should be made available to the whole family.

9. **Adolescence** is a time of rapid change, so that some degree of psychological distress during this period is inevitable. In most cases, such reactions are transient, but occasionally they can lead to a decline in academic performance or social functioning. Eating disorders and major functional illnesses, such as schizophrenia, may begin during adolescence, and experimentation with alcohol and drugs is fairly common. The assessment and management of adolescent problems requires special skills, and depending on the age and maturity of the subject, the therapist may draw on techniques used in either child or adult psychiatric practice.

REFERENCES AND FURTHER READING

Barker, P. (1983). *Basic Child Psychiatry*, 4th edn. London: Granada.
Berg, I. (1984). School refusal. *British Journal of Hospital Medicine*; **31**: 59–62.
Hill, P. (1986). Child psychiatry. In *Essentials of Postgraduate Psychiatry* (Hill, P., Murray, R., Thorley, A., eds) pp. 81–137. London: Grune and Stratton.
Richman, N., Stevenson, J., Graham, P. (1975). Prevalence of behaviour

problems in 3 year old children: an epidemiological study in a London borough. *Journal of Child Psychology and Psychiatry*; **16**: 277–87.

Rutter, M., Tizzard, J., Yule, W., Graham, P., Whitmore, K. (1976). Isle of Wight studies, 1964–1974. *Psychological Medicine*; **6**: 313–32.

Rutter, M., Yule, B., Quinton, D., Rowlands, O., Yule, W., Berger, M. (1975). Attainment and adjustment in two geographical areas: III. Some factors accounting for area differences. *British Journal of Psychiatry*; **126**: 520–33.

17 EATING DISORDERS

General interest in eating disorders has increased considerably in recent years, particularly with regard to anorexia nervosa and bulimia nervosa. In both conditions, abnormal eating habits are associated with a fear of fatness, and an undue sensitivity to change in weight is often accompanied by a distortion in the perception of body image. In many cases, a familial tendency towards obesity or a personal history of being overweight is noted. The symptomatic interrelationship between anorexia nervosa, bulimia nervosa and obesity is shown in Fig. 17.1.

Although the management of obesity is not usually the province of the psychiatrist, the psychological effects of being overweight or of a failure to lose weight can sometimes precipitate emotional disturbance or mental disorder.

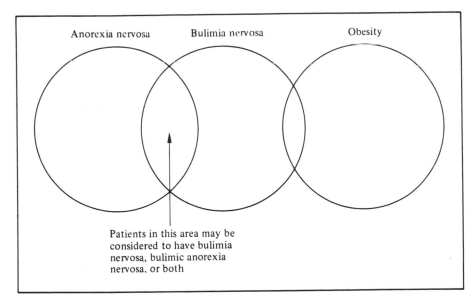

Fig. 17.1 The symptomatic interrelationship between anorexia nervosa, bulimia nervosa and obesity

Reproduced by kind permission of the British Journal of Hospital Medicine

OBESITY

Obesity refers to an **abnormally high percentage of body fat** which, in most cases, is related to an increase in body weight of 20% above standard weight. There are notable exceptions to this rule, such as athletes and weightlifters, whose extra weight is likely to be due to an increase in muscle bulk rather than fat. It is estimated that approximately one-third of adults in the UK are above the weight range appropriate for their sex and height, obesity being especially prevalent among women in lower socioeconomic classes.

Aetiology

Rarely, obesity is attributable to an underlying hypothalamic disorder, but in most instances this is not so. **Genetic factors** have been implicated as a result of family and twin studies (*see* p. 7), although psychological and social influences are also important in both its cause and perpetuation. **Psychoanalytical theory** considers obesity to be a manifestation of an 'oral personality', whereby eating is seen as a substitute for deriving comfort from the mother's breast (*see* p. 264). However, this view is at dissonance with several studies which have shown that the personality and temperament of obese people are not markedly different from those encountered in the general population.

Somewhat surprisingly, most obese people have been found to have similar caloric intakes to the non-obese, and their extra fat deposition is perhaps due to **deficient utilisation of energy**. In some cases, **abnormal eating patterns** are identified, such as consuming food when unhappy or stressed, getting up at night to have a meal or indulging in bouts of excessive and uncontrolled eating (binges). **Psychotropic drugs**, particularly neuroleptics, antidepressants and lithium, can induce weight gain, and overeating may also occur as a result of an affective or schizophrenic illness.

Management

Cases of mild obesity may respond to simple **dietary advice**, whereas other people sometimes derive help from slimming clubs or 'calorie counting'. Referral to a general practitioner or psychiatrist is indicated when an obese person fails to lose weight, and as a result becomes depressed or suicidal. Management begins by taking a **weight history** and assessing current **eating habits**. The personal and social implications of being overweight should be determined, as these sometimes offer a clue as to the factors which have precipitated or are perpetuating the problem. Finally, a physical examination needs to be performed to exclude possible organic causes or serious complications, such as hypertension or ischaemic heart disease.

Much of the treatment of obesity utilises **behavioural techniques**, in which positive rewards (such as peer approval) are given for weight loss. Attempts can be made to modify eating habits by encouraging the consumption of controlled amounts of food only at meal times. An alteration in eating style (e.g. consuming food more slowly), and identifying and avoiding the cues which are likely to induce eating (such as watching television), may also be helpful.

Results using such measures are generally disappointing, in that short-term weight losses are not often maintained. **Appetite suppressant drugs** are similarly limited in their effect, and carry the added risk of addiction. Individual or group **psychotherapy** is sometimes helpful if overeating is associated with poor self-esteem or relationship difficulties. Microdiets that provide a very low intake of energy (such as the Cambridge diet) are only suitable for the moderately obese, and any benefit derived from them is likely to be temporary. In severe cases, especially where massive obesity is potentially life-threatening, **surgical intervention** (in the form of jaw-wiring, gastric reduction or jejuno-ileal bypass) is occasionally warranted.

ANOREXIA NERVOSA

Descriptions of clinical states resembling anorexia nervosa appeared in medical books as long ago as the seventeenth century, but the condition was first clearly outlined by Gull in 1874. It is a disorder primarily affecting adolescent females, with only 5–10% of cases occurring in males. Because secrecy and denial are common, its prevalence is difficult to determine accurately, although there are thought to be approximately 10 000 severely affected individuals in the UK at any one time. It is more common among the middle and upper social classes, and tends to be limited to developed societies throughout the world.

Clinical Features

The central psychopathology of anorexia nervosa is a **morbid fear of fatness.** As a consequence, high-calorie foods (especially carbohydrates) are avoided, which in turn leads to **substantial weight loss**, resulting in a body weight more than 25% below normal. Associated endocrine changes also occur, producing **amenorrhoea** in females and loss of libido and impotence in males.

Symptoms characteristically begin within a few years of the onset of puberty, and sometimes develop from **dieting** in response to adolescent plumpness. In the early stages of anorexia nervosa, appetite is not diminished. At this time, the individual's thoughts and behaviour appear to be governed by an internal conflict between on the one hand, hunger and a desire to eat, and on the other a fear of losing control and gaining weight. A **preoccupation with food** is common, so that the subject will happily absorb herself in cooking for others, often displaying a detailed knowledge of the caloric content of every item involved, while eating nothing of the meal herself. Many hours may be spent shopping for food and then hoarding purchases, and some anorectics resort to shoplifting in order to satisfy their fixation.

Food-related **rituals** are often conducted secretively, and the extent of weight loss may be concealed by wearing bulky clothing. Relatives sometimes collude with such behaviour, but even if the subject is directly confronted about her actions, such challenges are frequently met with abject **denial** of anything being wrong. Consequently, medical help is usually sought by parents, by which time the patient will have already lost a considerable amount of weight. She may be reluctant to give details of the duration or extent of her problem, while vociferously objecting to any suggestion that she is underweight or needs to eat more. **Distortion of body image** is frequent, resulting in the subject grossly overestimating the size of various parts of her body. In certain individuals, the hunger drive intermittently overcomes their fear of fatness and results in occasional bouts of uncontrolled excessive eating (**bingeing**), which may be followed by self-induced vomiting, laxative or diuretic abuse as a means of weight control (*see later*).

Many anorectics remain remarkably **energetic** despite evidence of gross emaciation, and some use strenuous exercise as a way of further controlling their weight. **Early morning wakening** is a common symptom but, in contrast to the type seen in depressive illnesses, feelings of dysphoria are not marked at this time. However, some anorectics do become clinically **depressed** and may even be suicidal, while others display obsessional features or multiple phobic symptoms.

At referral, weight is often less than 35 kg and, in addition to a history of amenorrhoea, **physical examination** may reveal evidence of gross muscle wasting, dehydration, anaemia and other signs of starvation, although breast atrophy does not usually occur. The extremities are sometimes cold and blue (acrocyanosis) and ankle oedema may be present (occasionally associated with a low serum albumin). Pubic and axillary hair are retained, and a fine down (lanugo hair) also appears on the trunk and limbs. Bradycardia, hypotension and hypothermia can occur and constipation may be severe. Vomiting and laxative abuse sometimes cause a hypokalaemic alkalosis, which can result in the development of renal problems, cardiac arrhythmias and seizures. Growth hormone and plasma cortisol levels are raised, while those of gonadotrophin are reduced.

A 15-year-old schoolgirl started dieting in response to constant teasing by her friends for being overweight. At that time, she weighed 65 kg (10 st 3 lb), and being only 1.6 m (5 ft 3 in) tall, she felt 'very fat'. She followed a low-carbohydrate, high-protein diet, and within 6 months her weight had dropped to 49 kg (7 st 9 lb), by which time she had stopped menstruating. Although at first pleased with their daughter's weight loss, her parents' concern grew when she began to miss meals. When they pressured her to eat, she began to take food up to her room while doing her homework, secretly disposing of it later down the toilet.

After considerable coercion by her parents, she was eventually persuaded to visit the family doctor. She told him that she felt extremely well, and resented the fuss her parents were making. She did not accept that she had lost an excessive amount of weight, and was concerned that her hips and thighs were still too fat. Over the next 3 months, her weight dropped to 38 kg (5 st 13 lb). She rejected all efforts to help her, and it was only when her weight reached 29 kg (4 st 8 lb), with compulsory admission to hospital being considered, that she agreed to inpatient treatment, by which time she was grossly cachectic and physically weak.

Aetiology

The interplay of several factors is probably involved in the development of this condition. A **genetic predisposition** is suggested by an increased concordance rate among monozygotic compared with dizygotic twins (*see* p. 7). The mothers of anorectic children often have a history of psychiatric disorder, and in some cases, may have suffered from the condition themselves.

A common theme of the numerous **psychological theories** that have been advanced to explain the disorder proposes that avoidance of fattening foods is due to a fear of mature body weight, and results in a regression to a more primitive (oral) level of functioning (*see* p. 264). By retaining the 'body of a child', problems of adulthood, sexuality and separating from parents need not be faced.

Abnormal family processes are seen by some as paramount in the causation of anorexia nervosa. The development of symptoms in the 'patient' is viewed as a means of avoiding conflict between family members, thereby allowing them to continue functioning as a unit. The pattern of interaction is such that members are frequently inflexible in their roles (rigidity), problems and disagreements are seldom resolved (lack of conflict resolution), individual identities are poorly defined (enmeshment), and there is evidence of overprotectiveness. The subject is often described as being a 'model child' — shy and introverted in nature, and conscientious and compliant to the wishes of others.

The reduction in sex hormone levels and lowered basal metabolic rate which occur in anorexia nervosa have led to the proposal that the condition might result from a primary **hypothalamic disorder**. Although there have been a few case reports of the condition developing in association with a hypothalamic tumour, post-mortem findings usually show no such abnormality. Since nearly all the physical changes are reversed when body weight is restored, they are most probably the effects of starvation.

The **pursuit of thinness** is to some extent encouraged by media pressure for women to conform to a 'sexual stereotype', in which femininity and attractiveness are equated with slenderness. A further emphasis is placed on the desirability of remaining slim and healthy, and the dangers of being overweight. This may explain why the condition is more common in females from middle- and upper-class backgrounds, who are perhaps most susceptible to **social pressures** of this type. Certain groups, such as models and ballet students, seem to be at particular risk, since weight control is an integral part of their working lives.

The disorder sometimes follows a **life event** which, if perceived as a threat to the individual's self-esteem, can lead to feelings of ineffectiveness. Under these circumstances, dieting behaviour may represent a means of regaining control, and is reinforced by feelings of attractiveness, the attention of others and a sense of achievement due to weight loss.

Management

Before commencing treatment, a careful **assessment** should be made of both the patient and her family. This not only serves to establish the diagnosis and explore the family dynamics, but also helps to gain the individual's trust and confidence, and to achieve agreement upon a management plan. Additional information is usually obtained from another source, such as a relative, since the patient is frequently a reluctant recipient of psychiatric help. Details of personal and family **background** should be supplemented by a dietary, weight and menstrual **history**, together with information regarding self-induced vomiting or the abuse of purgatives. It is also important to determine the subject's concept of her ideal weight and body image.

The **mental state examination** should aim to identify any evidence of depression or suicidal ideation, and to exclude other psychiatric disorders (such as schizophrenia) where abnormal ideas about food and eating may exist. A **physical examination** and **investigations** are performed to assess the extent of malnutrition, emaciation and other somatic complications, in particular electrolyte disturbance. Rarely, it may be necessary to consider alternative causes of weight loss or endocrine dysfunction, such as pituitary failure, thyrotoxicosis, malignancy, diabetes, occult tuberculosis or malabsorption.

Treatment should at first concentrate on **restoring normal body weight**. This is best achieved by setting a target weight and obtaining the individual's agreement to remain in treatment until it has been reached. A programme of organised refeeding is then established over a period of 2–3 months. When weight loss is severe, **hospital admission** is usually required, although milder cases are occasionally treated on an outpatient basis. Token resistance is often encountered, but in response to a firm and caring approach, most patients capitulate and accept the need for treatment. In some cases, especially where the condition is life-threatening, compulsory admission to hospital will need to be considered.

Various therapeutic regimens have been described, but most advocate an initial period of **bed-rest** following admission to hospital, combined with a programme of **controlled refeeding**, ensuring that at least 3000 calories are being eaten daily. Successful treatment is dependent upon the nursing staff's ability to establish a trusting relationship with the patient, and yet remain firmly in control when necessary (e.g. in determining the amount and type of food eaten). Such an approach requires patience and perseverence, since many anorectics are intent on deceiving their care givers by hiding food, swallowing excess water before being weighed or vomiting after meals. Even so, staff must maintain a supportive and caring role, and try to deal with problems as they arise.

With effective treatment, a weight gain of about 1–2 kg a week can be expected, and sustained increases are rewarded by allowing the patient more time out of bed. Further positive reinforcement can be achieved by granting additional privileges, such as permission to watch television, listen to records or receive visits from friends, while demonstrating the gain in weight on a clearly visible wall chart.

As weight increases, many patients who have been depressed begin to acknowledge an improvement in their mood and a reduction in their preoccupation with food. Individual or group **psychotherapy** is an important aspect of treatment, which creates an opportunity to encourage maturity and independence by dealing with issues such as the responsibilities of adulthood and fears about sexuality, as well as promoting normal attitudes towards food and weight. Some form of **family therapy** is usually indicated, particularly in younger girls where the family dynamics are clearly disturbed. Ongoing support and treatment are important aspects of after-care, and therapy will often need to be continued for a considerable time following discharge home. With this aim in mind, a number of self-help organisations have been established, such as 'Anorexic Aid' and 'Overeaters Anon'. There is no evidence that appetite stimulants, such as chlorpromazine, are of any additional benefit in management, although antidepressants are sometimes prescribed if depressive symptoms are severe.

Prognosis

Although the short-term prognosis is generally good, the course of the illness is variable, and periods of remission are often interspersed with recurrent cycles of weight loss followed by re-admission to hospital. Factors associated with a poor outcome include a later age of onset, male sex, severe weight loss, bulimic symptoms, vomiting and purgative abuse, and a protracted illness.

Results of long-term studies indicate that approximately two-thirds of patients have maintained a normal weight for several years following treatment, while the remainder are moderately or severely underweight. However, more than half of all anorectics continue to display abnormal eating habits, and suffer from persistent psychiatric symptoms and relationship difficulties.

Adequate follow-up and continuing support are important in order to deal with adverse events and personal crises when they arise, as well as to minimise the frequency and severity of relapse. Despite this, 5% of cases end in death from starvation or suicide.

BULIMIA NERVOSA

Bulimia or **binge-eating** refers to episodes of excessive and uncontrolled food intake. Although bulimic symptoms can occur in both obesity and anorexia nervosa, they are also the central feature of the disorder known as bulimia nervosa. In this condition, otherwise referred to as the 'dietary chaos syndrome', individuals report frequent bingeing, for which they compensate by **self-induced vomiting**, **diuretic** or **laxative abuse** and **dieting**. In contrast to anorexia nervosa, body weight is frequently normal or above normal, and many women continue to menstruate. Bulimics are highly sensitive to changes in their weight or shape and, as with anorectics, usually express a **fear of fatness** or of losing control over eating.

The syndrome of bulimia nervosa is confined almost exclusively to women, the age of onset tending to be later than for anorexia nervosa, usually in late adolescence or early adulthood. The prevalence is not known, although the rate of case referral appears to be increasing, possibly because of media exposure and a growing awareness among the medical profession that abnormal eating behaviour can exist in those of normal body weight.

Clinical Features

Characteristically, **eating habits are grossly disturbed**, and attempts at dietary restraint are disrupted by frequent binges, which are usually conducted in secret. Bingeing sometimes occurs in response to specific 'cues', such as an unpleasant event or a life crisis, or can be provoked by feelings of depression, loneliness or boredom.

Initially, binge-eating may relieve tension and be experienced as enjoyable, but as the amount of food consumed increases, it is rapidly followed by feelings of guilt, despair and loss of control. Carbohydrate-rich foods such as cakes, bread and biscuits are commonly chosen, and are frequently of a consistency which makes swallowing easy. Bulimics often binge at least two or three times a day (although it can be considerably more), and unless interrupted, each episode may continue until all the available food has been eaten or physical exhaustion occurs. It is usually followed by self-induced vomiting in order to regurgitate food before it is absorbed, and some purge themselves with laxatives. Diuretic abuse, excessive exercise and dieting are additional methods employed to control weight.

Dichotomous thinking is a common feature of bulimia nervosa, the subject tending to view certain aspects of herself or her behaviour in uncompromisingly positive or negative terms. Consequently, she may see herself as either 'fat or thin', or her eating behaviour as 'in or out of control', which is often reflected by **fluctuations in mood**. Because bulimics are aware that their eating habits are abnormal, feelings of disgust and regret frequently occur during or after an episode of bingeing. Preoccupations about food and eating often conflict with fears of obesity and a wish to be thin, or with a desire to reach and maintain an 'ideal weight'. This commonly results in feelings of anxiety and tension, and a sense of depression or despair may ensue, sometimes leading to suicidal thoughts or acts. Other aspects of the bulimic's life, in terms of relationships, sexual behaviour and drinking habits, may be equally chaotic. Some repeatedly indulge in antisocial or attention-seeking activities such as shoplifting, sexual promiscuity or self-mutilation, which may be related to alcohol or drug abuse.

Although weight usually remains within the normal range, **physical complications** can result from self-induced vomiting, diuretic or purgative abuse. Hypokalaemia may cause cardiac arrhythmias, tetany, paraesthesiae, seizures, muscle weakness and renal damage. Vomiting and the resultant acid regurgitation can produce erosion of dental enamel (perimolysis), painless enlargement of the salivary glands, hoarseness, and oesophageal stricture, while purgative abuse may lead to the development of steatorrhoea. Finger clubbing is sometimes evident, as well as calluses on the knuckles due to repeated abrasion against the teeth when inducing vomiting. Rarely, overeating can produce acute dilatation of the stomach.

Aetiology

A past history of anorexia nervosa is found in nearly half of all bulimic patients. Many have a familial tendency towards obesity, so that their diet needs to be constantly controlled in order to attain the degree of desired slimness. However, it has also been demonstrated that such individuals rapidly abandon all restraint over their food intake once they believe they have eaten something with a high caloric content. Some of the factors

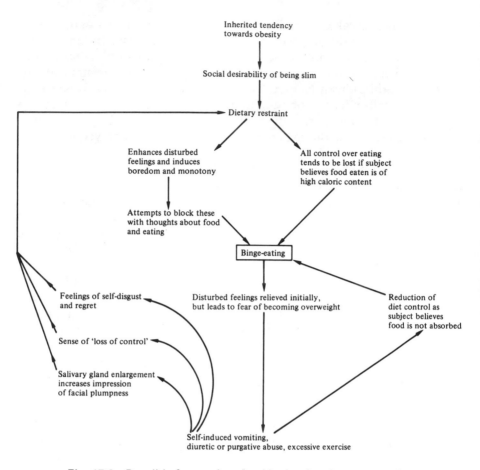

Fig. 17.2 Possible factors involved in the development and perpetuation of symptoms in bulimia nervosa

which are thought to be involved in the establishment of abnormal eating behaviour in bulimia nervosa are shown in Fig. 17.2.

Management

Assessment should follow a similar pattern to that described on p. 338. There seems to be little advantage in providing inpatient care along the lines used in anorexia nervosa, except where symptoms of that condition coexist, or where there is a high risk of suicide.

In addition to providing support, **psychotherapy** helps to focus on events and feelings which act as stimuli to binge-eating. This can be assisted by encouraging the subject to keep a daily diary of eating behaviour, and of the cues which lead to bingeing. Group work adopting a **cognitive–behavioural approach** to treatment has also been advocated, in

25% less than body mass index *(handwritten)*

Table 17.1 Comparison of the main features of the eating disorders

♀ 1% ♂ 0.01% *(handwritten)*

Features	Obesity	Anorexia nervosa	Bulimia nervosa
Body weight	Increased	Decreased	Within normal range
Age of onset	Any age	Early adolescence	Late adolescence or early adulthood
Sex distribution	Females>males	Females≫males	Females≫males
Social class	Mainly lower	Mainly upper and middle	Mainly upper and middle *(lower)*
Prevalence	Common	Uncommon	Unknown
Psychopathology	No distinctive features, may become depressed	Morbid fear of fatness Denial of illness Distorted perception of body image Affective changes common	Fear of fatness Preoccupation with 'ideal weight', dichotomous thinking Anxiety and tension common, may be depressed Insight retained
Eating behaviour	Often normal, may intermittently diet and binge	Restricted food intake Avoid carbohydrates Bingeing and vomiting sometimes a feature	Chaotic eating behaviour Dietary restriction followed by frequent and recurrent bingeing, vomiting or purging
Menstruation	Variable	Absent	Variable
Other physical complications	Yes	Yes	Yes
Response to treatment	Initial weight loss, but relapse common	Initially good, but variable long-term outcome	Not clearly established, although probably poor

Endocrine
↓ FSH, LH
& TRH
↑ cortisol *(handwritten)*

Not seen *(handwritten)*

which information is given about the dangers of self-induced vomiting, purgation and excessive dietary restraint, and a regimen is established whereby food is only eaten at specified times. The subject is helped to anticipate future problems and deal with them appropriately and effectively.

Prognosis

The outcome is uncertain, but those with a preceding history of anorexia nervosa probably have a worse prognosis. This group often demonstrates a fluctuating life-long tendency towards abnormal eating behaviour.

SUMMARY

1. **Obesity** refers to an abnormally high percentage of body fat, and is associated with excessive body weight. Genetic, psychological and social influences are probably involved in its development and, in many cases, extra fat deposition is attributable to inefficient utilisation of energy. Occasionally, weight gain is due to psychotropic drugs or mental illness. Mild cases may respond to simple dietary advice, peer pressure or modification of eating habits. Surgical intervention is sometimes indicated in severe obesity.

2. **Anorexia nervosa** primarily affects adolescent females, the central psychopathology being a morbid fear of fatness associated with avoidance of high-calorie foods. This results in substantial weight loss and amenorrhoea. A preoccupation with food is common and denial of the illness may be maintained, even in the presence of gross emaciation. Bulimic episodes sometimes occur and distortion of body image is frequent. Anorectics often describe a sense of happiness and contentment, although some become profoundly depressed. The endocrine and other physical changes which occur are nearly all reversible when normal weight is restored. Genetic, physical, psychological and social mechanisms have all been implicated in the aetiology of the condition. The initial aim of treatment is to restore normal body weight through a programme of controlled refeeding, usually in hospital. Psychotherapy should help to promote maturity and independence, as well as develop appropriate attitudes to food and weight. Family therapy aims to deal with disturbed interpersonal dynamics. Although the short-term prognosis is generally good, the course of the illness is variable and relapse is common. Around 5% of cases have a fatal outcome due to starvation or suicide.

3. **Bulimia nervosa** is a condition characterised by grossly disturbed eating habits and mainly affects women in late adolescence or early adulthood. Attempts at dietary restraint, due to fears of fatness and losing control over eating, are disrupted by recurrent bingeing, which is followed by self-

induced vomiting, purging or diuretic abuse. The body weight usually remains within normal limits and menstruation may continue. Mood disturbance and dichotomous thinking are common, often reflecting the degree of control the subject experiences over her weight and eating habits. Other aspects of the bulimic's life, in terms of relationships, sexual behaviour and drinking habits, may be equally chaotic. Physical complications can result from self-induced vomiting or diuretic or purgative abuse. The aetiology of the disorder seems uncertain and complex, and treatment using psychotherapeutic and behavioural methods appears to produce only modest results.

REFERENCES AND FURTHER READING

Crisp, A. H. (1983). Anorexia nervosa. *British Medical Journal*; **287**: 855–57.

Fairburn, C. G. (1982). Binge-eating and its management. *British Journal of Psychiatry*; **141**: 631–33.

Fairburn, C. G., Cooper, P. J. (1984). The clinical features of bulimia nervosa. *British Journal of Psychiatry*; **144**: 238-46.

Gull, W. (1874) Anorexia nervosa (apepsia hysterica, anorexia hysterica). *Transactions of the Clinical Society of London*; **7**: 22–24.

Hsu, L. K. G. (1980). Outcome of anorexia nervosa: a review of the literature (1954–1978). *Archives of General Psychiatry*; **37**: 1041–46.

Russell, G. F. N. (1979). Bulimia nervosa: an ominous variant of anorexia nervosa. *Psychological Medicine*; **9**: 429–48.

Treasure, J. (1987). The biochemical and hormonal sequelae of the eating disorders. *British Journal of Hospital Medicine*; **37**: 301-3.

18 MENTAL RETARDATION

Mental retardation (also referred to as mental handicap, mental impairment, amentia and subnormality) is defined by the International Classification of Diseases as 'a condition of incomplete development of mind which is especially characterised by subnormality of intelligence'. It therefore includes individuals in whom intellectual development is predictably impaired from conception by **genetic influences**, as well as those in whom it would otherwise have proceeded normally, but has become arrested at some stage due to **environmental factors**.

Intelligence refers to an individual's powers of reasoning and understanding, the level of which will have some bearing on his ability to maintain an independent existence in society and to protect himself from danger or exploitation by others. Consequently, those who are intellectually impaired often have difficulty in dealing with the demands of everyday life and in establishing some direction and overall purpose to their behaviour. Services for the mentally retarded are therefore concerned with the general care and protection of such people, as well as with their specific social, educational, medical and psychiatric needs.

INTELLIGENCE TESTS

The level of intelligence is usually determined by means of a standardised test, the **Wechsler intelligence scale** being one of the most commonly used. Different formats are available for both adults and children, and scores are commonly expressed in terms of an **intelligence quotient** (or **IQ**) which was originally derived from the equation:

$$\frac{\text{Mental age}}{\text{Chronological age}} \times 100 = IQ$$

However, in adulthood the difference between the mental and chronological ages has little meaning, so that IQ scores (no longer a quotient) are instead calculated from tables in which a standard score of

346

100 (average intelligence) is assigned for each age group.

The Wechsler adult intelligence scale (**WAIS**) and intelligence scale for children (**WISC**) measure both verbal and performance skills. The WAIS consists of six verbal subtests which deal with words or numbers, and five subtests of performance which include the arrangement of spatial patterns, object assembly and picture arrangement. The full IQ score is derived from the combined scores of all the subtests. Other intelligence tests which are sometimes used include **Raven's progressive matrices** (a diagram completion test which assesses performance skills) and the **Mill Hill vocabulary test** (a two-part exercise of verbal ability involving recall and recognition of words). Both give results in terms of centile rankings, which indicate the percentage of the population scoring lower than the subject under test.

There are a number of limitations associated with the use of intelligence tests. Certain abilities, such as general creativity or artistic and musical skills, are not measured by standard testing. Furthermore, the scores obtained may be subject to errors resulting from variations in the way the tests are applied or the responses are interpreted. They can also be inaccurate if the subject is anxious, uncooperative or poorly motivated.

Intelligence in the general population has a normal distribution, centred around a modal IQ score of 100 (Fig. 18.1). Thus 95% of the population have an IQ between 70 and 130 (representing two standard deviations above and below the population mean), although more people have an IQ below the normal range than above. This excess is attributed to various genetic and environmental factors which are discussed later.

Although intelligence tests provide a reasonable indication of a person's current level of functioning, the results on their own cannot be used to diagnose mental retardation. The child's or adult's capabilities need to be assessed over a period of time in various settings before the presence of any intellectual handicap can be confirmed. It is generally accepted that mental retardation encompasses people who have an IQ below 70, but this is not defined in law. Educationalists refer to the **educationally subnormal** or ESN (for those with an IQ of 50–70) and the **severely educationally subnormal** or ESN (S) (for those with an IQ below 50). Under certain circumstances, people who are mentally retarded can be compulsorily detained in hospital. The 1983 Mental Health Act refers to mental impairment and severe mental impairment (rather than retardation), the distinction between the two being simply a matter of degree, without specifying IQ scores or the extent of social dysfunction (*see* Chapter 24 for definitions).

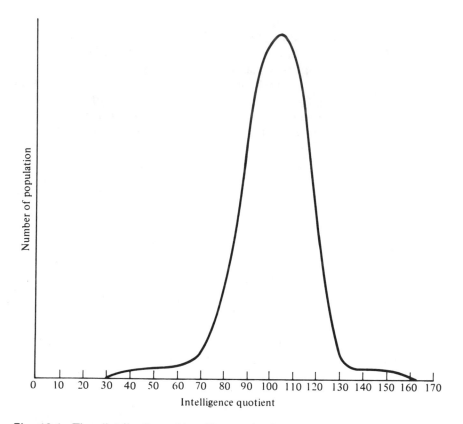

Fig. 18.1 The distribution of intelligence in the general population

EPIDEMIOLOGY

The prevalence of mental retardation in the general population is approximately 3%, with a slight excess of males. The majority (about 85%) are mildly retarded with an IQ of 50–70, the remainder being more severely impaired with an IQ below 50. An identifiable cause can now be established in two out of every three cases.

AETIOLOGY

The causes of mental retardation can be considered in terms of factors which operate before (**prenatal**), during (**perinatal**) or after birth (**postnatal**), as shown in Table 18.1. Mild cases do not usually have a single identifiable cause and probably result from an interplay of several factors. However, specific disorders are more likely to be established in those who are severely retarded.

Table 18.1 Some causes of mental retardation

Prenatal causes	
Chromosomal abnormalities	Down's syndrome, Patau's syndrome, Edward's syndrome, 'cri du chat' syndrome, Klinefelter's syndrome, XYY syndrome, Turner's syndrome, fragile X syndrome
Genetic defects	Tuberous sclerosis, neurofibromatosis, Wilson's disease, cretinism, phenylketonuria and other inborn errors of metabolism, Lesch-Nyhan syndrome, 'true' microcephaly, congenital hydrocephalus
Intrauterine infections	Rubella, cytomegalovirus, syphilis, toxoplasmosis
Physical hazards in pregnancy	Irradiation, drugs, alcohol, smoking, physical trauma, starvation
Complications of pregnancy	Diabetes, hypothyroidism, antepartum haemorrhage, toxaemia, placental insufficiency, Rhesus incompatibility, severe anaemia and other serious maternal illnesses
Perinatal causes	Complicated labour, birth trauma, premature and 'small for dates' infants, neonatal hypoxia, hypoglycaemia, hypothermia
Postnatal causes	
Infections	Encephalitis, meningitis
Toxins	Hyperbilirubinaemia, lead poisoning
Trauma	Non-accidental injury, domestic and road accidents
Subcultural factors	Poor diet, social deprivation (poor schooling, poverty, overcrowding, poor housing), low parental intelligence

1. Chromosomal Abnormalities

DOWN'S SYNDROME

This disorder is responsible for approximately one-third of all severe cases of mental retardation and occurs once in every 600 live births. It most commonly results from the presence of three (rather than two) chromosomes at position 21 (**trisomy**), so that those affected have a total complement of 47. However, in approximately 5% of cases the extra chromosome becomes attached (**translocated**) to one of another pair at positions 13, 15, or 22. The condition can be detected antenatally by

Table 18.2 The clinical features of Down's syndrome

Birth	Often premature and low birth weight
Skull and face	Small round head with brachycephaly (anteroposterior shortening with skull increased in height), slanting ('mongoloid') palpebral fissures, epicanthic folds, 'Brushfield spots' (white speckling of the iris), cataracts and squint commonly present, small nose and ears, high arched palate, protruding and fissured tongue, abnormal dentition
Musculoskeletal	Generalised hypotonia and joint laxity, stunted growth, shortened limbs and neck, square-shaped palms with a single transverse (simian) crease, shortened fingers and toes (sometimes webbed), fifth finger often incurved
Other abnormalities	Congenital cardiac defects, peripheral cyanosis, bowel atresia, Hirschsprung's disease, increased susceptibility to infection (respiratory, blepharitis), leukaemia and thyroiditis, umbilical hernia, scanty beard and axillary hair growth, decreased libido

examining the chromosomes of cells drawn off from the amniotic fluid. Because the incidence of Down's syndrome increases with **maternal age**, amniocentesis should ideally be offered to all pregnant women over the age of 35 and to any woman who previously has had a child with the condition. The main clinical features of Down's syndrome are shown in Table 18.2.

The degree of retardation is variable, although usually severe, so that very few people with Down's syndrome are able to lead an independent existence. Most are placid in nature, with affectionate and cheerful personalities. Life expectancy on average is lower than that of the general population, due to a tendency to age prematurely, although some people with Down's syndrome are now living up to 70 or 80 years. **Patau's** and **Edward's syndromes** are other examples of autosomal trisomy, but those affected usually die in infancy.

OTHER CHROMOSOMAL ABNORMALITIES

Cri du chat syndrome results from the deletion of the short arm of chromosome 5 and is so named because of the characteristic cat-like cry made by these children at birth. The condition gives rise to severe retardation, spasticity, microcephaly, stunted growth and facial abnormalities. Survival beyond infancy is rare.

Sex chromosome abnormalities are sometimes associated with mild mental retardation, although the degree of physical and mental impairment tends to increase with the presence of each additional X chromosome.

Klinefelter's syndrome (XXY karyotype) is the commonest of this group of disorders, occurring in approximately one in 500 males. Those affected are infertile as a consequence of hypogonadism, and the absence of male secondary sex characteristics is associated with the development of female bodily proportions, although they are often tall. Klinefelter males tend to be timid and withdrawn, and although mental retardation is usually mild, other psychiatric disorders (particularly neuroses and personality disorders) are common. **XXX** ('superfemales'), **XYY** and **Turner's** (XO karyotype) **syndromes** are only rarely associated with intellectual impairment (*see* Glossary for details).

Fragile X syndrome is thought to account for about 10% of mental retardation in males (although it is less common in females), and results from fragmentation or detachment of the terminal portion of the long arm of the X chromosome. Some of those affected are noted to have large floppy ears, macro-orchidism and prognathism, although the fragile X anomaly has also been demonstrated in otherwise normal individuals.

2. Single Gene Abnormalities

Disorders arising from single gene abnormalities may be autosomal dominant, autosomal recessive or sex-linked recessive in their mode of transmission. Most are extremely rare, but a few of the more commonly encountered conditions are discussed below.

AUTOSOMAL DOMINANT DISORDERS

Tuberous sclerosis (epiloia) is a condition in which hard nodules of neuroglial cells are distributed throughout the substance of the brain, often resulting in the development of mental retardation and epilepsy. However, the clinical presentation is variable due to poor gene penetrance. An overgrowth of sebaceous glands produces a characteristic facial rash after the age of 4 years. Fibromata, thickened skin patches and areas of depigmentation (café-au-lait spots) are found on the trunk and limbs, while grey-white patches (phakomata) are observed on the retina. Smooth muscle, vascular and fatty tumours also develop and may be found in the heart, lungs and kidneys.

Neurofibromatosis (von Recklinghausen's disease) is a condition characterised by pigmented skin patches associated with multiple neurofibromata (tumours arising from cells of the nerve sheaths). Intracranial tumours can also develop, and in one-third of cases some degree of mental retardation is present.

AUTOSOMAL AND SEX-LINKED RECESSIVE DISORDERS

These disorders include many inborn errors of metabolism, of which phenylketonuria and homocystinuria are the most common. Other conditions of this type are listed in Table 18.3.

Phenylketonuria (PKU) occurs once in every 12 000 live births, although as many as 1 in 50 of the general population are heterozygous carriers. Due to a deficiency of the enzyme **phenylalanine hydroxylase**, affected infants are unable to adequately convert the amino acid phenylalanine to tyrosine. Unless the defect is detected shortly after birth, excessive phenylalanine accumulates in the bloodstream, resulting in irreversible brain damage and mental retardation.

Associated features include low birth weight, reduced pigmentation of the skin and hair, blue eyes, eczema and epilepsy. Routine screening for phenylketonuria is now carried out between 6 and 14 days after birth using the **Guthrie test.** A small sample of blood taken from the baby's heel is introduced into a culture of *Bacillus subtilis*, to which an inhibitory substance has previously been added. The degree of culture growth is proportional to the level of phenylalanine present in the blood, which in homozygous individuals is high. In such cases, a low phenylalanine diet is implemented and maintained throughout early childhood in order to prevent intellectual retardation.

Homocystinuria occurs once in every 50 000 live births. A deficiency of the enzyme **cystathionine synthetase** results in raised blood levels of the amino acids homocystine and methionine. In addition to mental retardation, affected children suffer a number of physical disabilities, including dislocation of the lens of the eye (ectopia lentis), osteoporosis and other skeletal abnormalities, thromboembolism and epilepsy. Children with homocystinuria characteristically have fair skin and hair, as well as a prominent malar flush. Mental retardation may be prevented by early treatment with a low-methionine diet.

3. Infections

Several maternal infections acquired during pregnancy can cross the placenta and harm the developing fetus, sometimes resulting in mental retardation and physical abnormalities (Table 18.4). Teratogenicity is most likely to occur during the first 3 months of pregnancy, when organogenesis is at its most critical stage.

Encephalitis or **meningitis** in childhood may affect the developing brain and, in addition to mental retardation, can produce neurological abnormalities, personality change and (in the case of meningitis) hydrocephalus.

Table 18.3 Some inborn errors of metabolism associated with mental retardation

Disorder	Metabolic error	Main clinical features
Disorders of protein metabolism		
Phenylketonuria	Deficiency of phenylalanine hydroxylase	*See text*
Homocystinuria	Deficiency of cystathionine synthetase	*See text*
Argininosuccinic aciduria	Deficiency of argininosuccinase	Short brittle hair, epilepsy, chorea
Maple syrup disease	Deficiency of ketoacid decarboxylase	Epilepsy, spastic paresis
Hartnup disease	Defective renal transport of amino acids, especially tryptophan	Photosensitive skin, weight loss, pellagra, ataxia
Disorders of carbohydrate metabolism		
Galactosaemia	Deficiency of phosphogalactose uridyl transferase	Accumulation of galactose producing liver and renal damage, cataracts
Glycogen storage disorders: Pompe's disease (glycogenosis)	Deficiency of phosphorylase kinase	Failure to thrive, fits, liver and brain damage
Von Gierke's disease	Deficiency of amylo-1,6-glucosidase	
Disorders of lipid metabolism		
Tay-Sachs disease	Deficiency of hexosaminidase-A	Blindness, cherry-red spot on macula, fits, spasticity, ataxia; commoner in Jews
Niemann-Pick disease	Deficiency of sphingomyelinase	Similar to Tay-Sachs, plus hepatosplenomegaly, skin pigmentation and anaemia
Gaucher's disease	Deficiency of cerebroside beta-glucosidase	Splenomegaly, nerve palsies, pathological fractures, skin pigmentation
Refsum's disease	Deficiency of phytanic acid oxidase	Blindness, deafness, ichthyosis, cerebellar signs

continued overleaf

Table 18.3 *Continued*

Disorder	Metabolic error	Main clinical features
Disorders of connective tissue (Mucopolysaccharidoses)		
Hurler's syndrome	Defect of alpha-L-iduronidase	Large head, gross facial appearance (gargoylism), short stature, kyphosis, corneal opacities, hepatosplenomegaly, cardiac defects
Hunter's syndrome (X-linked recessive)	Defect of L-iduronosulphate sulphatase	As in Hurler's syndrome, except for deafness and lack of corneal opacities
Sanfilippo syndrome	Defect of heparan sulphate sulphamidase	Milder physical features, but mental retardation often more severe
Other metabolic disorders		
Congenital hypothyroidism (cretinism)	Defect in thyroxine synthesis	Apathy, protruding tongue, umbilical hernia, failure to thrive, yellowish puffy skin, low body temperature, characteristic deep cry
Lesch-Nyhan syndrome (infantile hyperuricaemia) (X-linked recessive)	Deficiency of hypoxanthine-guanine phosphoribosyl transferase leading to accumulation of uric acid	Spasticity, cerebral palsy, choreoathetosis, anorexia, excessive thirst, self-mutilation
Nephrogenic diabetes insipidus (X-linked recessive)	Not known, but there is failure of renal tubules to respond to ADH	Polyuria, dehydration, epilepsy, excessive thirst

NB Mode of inheritance is autosomal recessive unless otherwise stated.

4. Other Causes

Sturge-Weber syndrome is a rare disorder characterised by the presence of a naevus (port-wine stain) distributed variably over one half of the face, neck and upper trunk. There is an associated underlying angiomatous growth involving the meninges on the same side as the external lesion, which may result in contralateral hemiparesis, convulsions and severe mental retardation. The mode of causation is unknown, although the

Table 18.4 Mental retardation due to maternal infection

Type of infection	Degree of retardation	Main clinical features
Rubella	Severe if acquired during the first few weeks of pregnancy	Microcephaly, cataracts, glaucoma, deafness, congenital heart defects, stunted growth, hepatitis, thrombocytopenic purpura
Cytomegalovirus	Variable, but may be marked even if infection is acquired late in pregnancy	Premature birth, microcephaly, jaundice, hepatosplenomegaly, thrombocytopenic purpura, cerebral palsy, epilepsy, intracerebral calcification
Syphilis	Variable	Stunted growth, 'saddle-back' nose, deafness, Hutchinson's teeth, epilepsy, corneal opacities, squint, anaemia
Toxoplasmosis	Variable	Microcephaly or mild hydrocephalus, spasticity, epilepsy, hepatosplenomegaly, intracranial calcification, choroidoretinitis

condition may be genetically determined.

Lead poisoning can occur in infants and children who suck or chew paint containing lead, or who inhale lead dust. In severe cases, a confusional state can result which, if untreated, may progress to the development of convulsions, blindness, deafness and mental retardation.

PROBLEMS ASSOCIATED WITH MENTAL RETARDATION

Physical Disorders

Physical disabilities are common in the mentally retarded, particularly where intellectual impairment is severe. **Sensory dysfunction**, involving defects in sight or hearing, may accentuate intellectual impairment and cause behavioural problems due to communication difficulties. In addition to limiting functional capacity, **motor disorders** (such as spasticity and abnormal movements) and **poor sphincter control** can result in social rejection and stigmatisation.

Epilepsy frequently occurs among the mentally retarded, especially where there is evidence of underlying brain damage. It is estimated that almost one in three of those with severe intellectual impairment experience a fit at some time in their lives. Anticonvulsant medication is often required, although care should be taken to minimise unwanted side-effects by regularly reviewing the drug regimen, and if necessary, changing to an alternative preparation.

Psychiatric Disorders

All forms of mental illness are recognised in the mentally retarded, and some studies have suggested that the prevalence of psychiatric disorder among this group is at least three times that in the general population. Diagnosis becomes increasingly complex in those with very low intelligence because language problems (both of comprehension and expression) make assessment of the mental state very difficult. As a result, changes in **observed behaviour** may be of greater diagnostic significance than described experiences.

The features of **schizophrenia** can be similar to those found in people of normal intelligence, although poverty of thought, disturbed behaviour and motor disorders (such as mannerisms and stereotypies) are often more prominent. When described, delusions and hallucinations tend to be of a simple nature. The diagnosis should be considered where there is a significant worsening in behaviour, or a deterioration in social or intellectual functioning. Where doubt exists, it may be necessary to administer a trial of an antipsychotic drug, although these compounds need to be used with caution because of their epileptogenic tendency.

The development of a **depressive illness** does not always result in the expression of feelings of sadness or despair, and the mentally retarded patient often presents with somatic complaints or behavioural changes such as agitation, withdrawal or apathy. **Mania** is frequently associated with overactivity or unusually aggressive behaviour. The treatment of affective disorders is discussed in Chapter 5.

Behavioural problems are very common and are sometimes dangerous, as with those who resort to head-banging, self-mutilation or pica (eating non-edible objects). Aggressiveness, temper tantrums, body-rocking, hair-pulling, masturbating in public and other types of socially unacceptable behaviour are also commonly encountered. The sudden onset of behavioural difficulties should always raise the possibility of the development of a psychiatric disorder, although they can also result from feelings of frustration or boredom.

Functional and Social Disabilities

Impaired intellectual functioning often results in problems with learning and the ability to perform practical skills, as well as diminished powers of reasoning. In cases of mild mental retardation, disabilities may be insignificant, whereas those with more severe impairment will frequently be seriously limited in terms of their work capability, the capacity to lead an independent existence and to communicate adequately. The implications for the individual and his family are discussed later in this chapter.

A lack of social awareness sometimes leads to promiscuous or disinhibited sexual behaviour, and women may be at risk of exploitation, occasionally resulting in unwanted pregnancy. Nevertheless, it is important to acknowledge and respect the sexual needs of men and women who are mentally retarded, and to provide contraceptive and other advice where necessary.

THE ASSESSMENT OF A CASE OF SUSPECTED MENTAL RETARDATION

Mental retardation may be suspected for a variety of reasons. The **physical characteristics** of a disorder, such as Down's syndrome, which is known to be a cause of mental retardation might alert the doctor or the parents shortly after birth. **Developmental delay**, **poor performance at school** or **behaviour disorders** in childhood are other reasons for querying intellectual deficit.

In a case of suspected mental retardation, assessment is normally conducted by members of a **multidisciplinary team** (Table 18.5). Where possible, the child should be assessed at home, but if this is not feasible, an outpatient setting is usually adequate. Irrespective of the location, several assessment interviews will usually be necessary, and close liaison with the parents is important. As the child grows, assessment will need to be under constant review.

THE CARE OF THE MENTALLY RETARDED

The needs of the mentally retarded are often complex and require input by the health and education authorities, as well as by social services. The coordination of resources is the responsibility of the **care planning team**, comprising members from the various disciplines involved in hospital and community care of the mentally retarded.

The Provision of Community Care and Hospital Services

During the past few decades there has been an increasing trend away from **institutionalised care** towards the mentally retarded living at **home** or in small **residential units**. By encouraging independence and allowing even

Table 18.5 The assessment of mental retardation

Type of assessment	Suggested responsible team members	Investigations	Aims
Medical	Paediatrician/physician	Comprehensive family history, history of pregnancy, birth and subsequent development; full physical examination to include height, weight, skull circumference; auditory, visual, speech and other physical defects	To identify and, where possible, treat specific causes of retardation and any associated physical handicap
		Laboratory investigations including FBC, thyroid function tests, serum Ca and bilirubin, blood glucose, chromosomal analysis, serum lead levels, amino acid chromatography, serology for syphilis, skull X-ray	
Psychological	Clinical psychologist, speech therapist, physiotherapist	Tests of intelligence, language and motor skills	To assess intellectual and developmental levels of ability
Social	Occupational therapist, general practitioner, community nurse, social worker	Rating of self-care activities, degree of socialisation and communication skills; family attitudes, home circumstances, degree of community support	To determine social needs and the most appropriate placement for the child
Educational	Remedial teacher, educational psychologist	Assessment of current and future educational needs	To determine where and how the child should be educated — in a special school or remedial teaching in an ordinary school
Psychiatric	Psychiatrist with a special interest in mental retardation	Full psychiatric history and mental state examination; evaluation of family dynamics; identification of behavioural problems	To identify and treat any psychiatric disorder or behavioural difficulties

those with severe handicaps to lead as normal a life as possible, social and functional abilities are likely to be maintained at an optimal level. Two-thirds of severely mentally retarded children under the age of 16 live at home with their families, although the proportion of similarly affected adults who live in the community is considerably smaller. It is possible that half of those currently residing in long-stay hospital wards could live and work in the community with adequate support.

Those with mild mental retardation may be suitably placed in a **hostel** or **group home**, the latter involving a small number of people living together under some degree of supervision and support from professional carers. Short-stay and holiday homes largely exist within the private sector, and are usually run by landladies with expertise in dealing with the needs and problems of the mentally retarded. Privately funded organis-ations, such as **MENCAP**, offer help and information to parents and relatives regarding accommodation facilities, and may also provide financial support for home care.

Hospitals provide **long-term care** for those who cannot be supported in the community, as well as **holiday beds** for short-term admissions to give relatives a break once or twice a year from their responsibilities. They also offer an **assessment service** and provisions for the mentally retarded when they become physically sick. The needs of the severely handicapped in hospital are met primarily by the nursing staff and occupational therapists.

Home support is a hospital-based service which offers care and assistance to mentally retarded people living in the community through the provision of:

1. appliances and aids to assist with activities of daily living
2. behaviour modification programmes to improve social functioning (*see* Chapter 13)
3. financial support and advice to ensure that disability benefits and allowances are received and put to maximum use.

Educational and Employment Services

Education should be provided for **all** mentally retarded children from as early an age as possible, however disabled they may be, and will often need to continue well beyond the normal school-leaving age. In some cases, placement in a special school is considered necessary, but many believe that **remedial teaching** in an ordinary school reduces stigmatis-ation and provides a more normal environment for the developing child. Continuing education is offered through **adult training centres** which, in addition to teaching recreational activities and work skills, also provide sheltered employment. Many mildly retarded people will subsequently be able to work in open employment, but some may benefit from assessment at an **industrial rehabilitation unit** (*see* Chapter 14).

Advice and Support for Families with a Mentally Retarded Member

The discovery that a child is mentally retarded can have a profound impact on all members of the family, and skilled counselling is often necessary to help them cope with their reactions. In some cases, the handicap is evident at or shortly after birth, and it is important to inform the parents as soon as possible, so that they can come to terms with the implications of both the diagnosis and prognosis. Understandably, many questions will follow and parents should be given ample opportunity to have these answered sympathetically by the staff. In addition, they should be informed as to what support is available, and what they can do to enable their child to function at an optimal level.

Reactions are variable, in that some parents may initially express feelings of revulsion, anger or outright rejection, while others become overprotective towards their child. A sense of loss for the 'perfect child' is common, although this may be preceded by denial and shock before the more familiar signs of bereavement emerge. Most parents eventually adjust to their situation, but in some cases, continuing feelings of stigmatisation sometimes lead to social withdrawal and isolation.

With adequate support, the family and child can be helped to deal successfully with the various problems, both foreseeable and unexpected, which need to be overcome during the formative years and later life. Anticipation is the key to success, and crises can often be prevented by additional input from caregivers when the family is liable to be under increased stress. The times at which additional help is most likely to be needed are when the child is due to start school (as parental feelings of protectiveness can sometimes lead to separation difficulties), and at the age of school-leaving, when the issues of independent living, work and adult relationships need to be considered. As parents grow older, they will need increasing reassurance that their offspring will be adequately cared for when they are no longer in a position to do so themselves.

The Role of the Psychiatrist in Managing the Mentally Retarded

In addition to the diagnosis and management of mental illness, the psychiatrist fulfils an important role in providing effective leadership for the multidisciplinary team and coordinating the efforts of its members. Caring for the mentally retarded is often demanding for family members and professional workers alike. One area in which the psychiatrist is able to use his skills is by offering support and advice to other care givers to help them cope with their responsibilities. Administratively, the consultant psychiatrist has a part to play in securing and deploying resources, as well as in planning the future needs of the service. Many also undertake a commitment to teach general practitioners and hospital doctors about the care of the mentally retarded.

THE PREVENTION OF MENTAL RETARDATION

Although a great deal can be done to help the intellectually impaired attain an optimal level of functioning, a significant reduction in the incidence of mental retardation might also be achieved by appropriate preventive measures (Table 18.6).

Subcultural Handicap

In order for normal intellectual development to occur, children must receive adequate stimulation. In particular, **subcultural handicap** is recognised as being not only due to inherited factors, but also to social, cultural and educational deprivation. It has been demonstrated that the use of intensive educational programmes has some beneficial effect in improving the level of intellectual functioning in this group of children. Consequently, efforts should be made to identify those at risk and to offer appropriate educative and social intervention where necessary.

SUMMARY

1. **Mental retardation** is defined as 'a condition of incomplete development of mind which is especially characterised by subnormality of intelligence'. The intellectual impairment which results often interferes with the individual's ability to maintain an independent existence and to protect himself from danger or exploitation by others. Services for the mentally retarded are concerned with the general care and protection of such people, as well as with their specific social, educational, medical and psychiatric needs.
2. **Intelligence** is usually measured by means of standardised tests, results being expressed in terms of an IQ score. The normal range of IQ in the general population is between 70 and 130, mental retardation encompassing those who have an IQ below 70 (3% of the general population). The majority are mildly retarded (85% have an IQ between 50 and 70), while the remainder are more severely impaired with an IQ below 50. An identifiable cause can be established in about two-thirds of all cases.
3. The **aetiology** of mental retardation can be considered in terms of:

   (a) prenatal causes: chromosomal abnormalities, genetic defects, intrauterine infections, physical hazards and other complications of pregnancy
   (b) perinatal causes: complications of labour and childbirth, premature and 'small for dates' infants
   (c) postnatal causes: infections, toxins, trauma, 'subcultural factors'.

Table 18.6 The prevention of mental retardation

Genetic counselling	Offered to those couples planning a pregnancy who already have a mentally retarded child, or where there is a family history of retardation which may be inherited. In some cases, the couple can be informed of the risks involved, and in the light of this knowledge are better equipped to make a decision about the planning of their family
Antenatal measures	Good quality **obstetric care** is an important preventive measure to ensure the well-being of both mother and fetus. Particular aspects include maintaining an adequate maternal diet during pregnancy, and minimising fetal exposure to adverse physical agents such as x-rays, alcohol, tobacco and other drugs
	The increased availability of **amniocentesis**, **fetoscopy** and **ultrasound scanning** in pregnancy has led to the early detection of several conditions which are associated with mental retardation, such as Down's syndrome, neural tube defects, Rhesus incompatibility and some inborn errors of metabolism. **Maternal screening** for alpha-fetoprotein levels, Rhesus blood grouping and syphilis antibodies are other useful investigative measures. In cases where severe mental and/or physical abnormalities are likely, **termination of pregnancy** can be offered to those women who request it
Perinatal measures	These include the detection of inhibited fetal growth, the adequate care of premature infants, and the early identification and proper management of difficult deliveries (i.e. twins, breech, transverse lie), so as to minimise birth trauma, hypoxia, hypothermia, hypoglycaemia and hypocalcaemia
Postnatal measures	**Infant and childhood health care programmes** should include: (1) neonatal screening for metabolic disorders e.g. phenylketonuria and congenital hypothyroidism; (2) early diagnosis and treatment of neonatal and infant infections, such as meningitis; (3) regular checks to detect developmental delay and sensory impairment; (4) identification of those at risk of non-accidental injury; (5) accident prevention measures in the home, on the roads and in the school
	Immunisation programmes involve vaccinating infants against pertussis and measles, immunising schoolgirls against rubella, and giving anti-D antibodies to Rhesus-negative women shortly after childbirth. (Allergic reactions to pertussis vaccination resulting in encephalitis have been reported)

4. Associated **physical disabilities**, especially sensory dysfunction, may accentuate intellectual impairment and cause behavioural problems and communication difficulties. Epilepsy is a common accompaniment of severe mental retardation, especially where there is underlying brain damage. All forms of **psychiatric disorder** occur in the mentally retarded, and overall it is three times more common than in the general population. Diagnosis becomes increasingly complex in those with very low intelligence, and consequently changes in observed behaviour may be of greater diagnostic significance than described experiences. Behavioural problems, **functional and social disabilities** are common, and often result in limited work capability, a diminished capacity for independent living and problems in forming relationships.

5. Mental retardation may be suspected as a result of the physical characteristics of certain disorders, developmental delay, poor performance at school and behaviour disorders. **Assessment** is usually performed by members of a multidisciplinary team, and subsequent management will encompass the patient's medical, psychological, social, educational and psychiatric needs.

6. **Provision of care** for the mentally retarded requires a coordination of efforts by the health and education authorities and social services under the auspices of a care planning team. Most mentally retarded people now live at home or in small community residential units, rather than in large institutions. Hospitals provide long-term care for those who cannot be supported in the community, as well as holiday beds and short-term admission for assessment or for the treatment of physical illness. Education should be provided for all mentally retarded children from as early an age as possible, and often needs to continue well beyond the normal school-leaving age. Those with mild or moderate handicaps are usually capable of going on to work in sheltered, or occasionally open, employment. Offering advice to the parents and supporting the families of the mentally retarded are other important aspects of care.

7. A reduction in the incidence of mental retardation might be achieved by a number of **preventive measures**. These include genetic counselling, improved obstetric and neonatal care, infant and childhood health care services, immunisation programmes and the identification of those at risk of developing subcultural handicap.

REFERENCES AND FURTHER READING

Brimblecombe, F. S. W. (1985). The needs of young intellectually retarded adults. *British Journal of Psychiatry*; **146**: 5–10.

Dupont, A. (1986). Socio-psychiatric aspects of the young severely mentally retarded and the family. *British Journal of Psychiatry*; **148**: 227–34.

Kinnell, H. G. (1987). Fragile X syndrome: an important preventable cause of mental handicap. *British Medical Journal*; **295**: 564–65.

Kirman, B. (1983). A current appraisal of Down's syndrome. *British Journal of Hospital Medicine*; **29**: 293–96.

Reid, A. H. (1982). *The Psychiatry of Mental Handicap*. Oxford: Blackwell Scientific Publications.

Taylor, E., Bicknell, J. (1986). The psychiatry of mental handicap. In *Essentials of Postgraduate Psychiatry* (Hill, P., Murray, R., Thorley, A., eds) pp. 165–94. London: Grune and Stratton.

19

SEXUAL DISORDERS

The term 'sexual disorder' is difficult to define because wide variations are encountered in human sexual behaviour, and the concept of 'sexual normality' is equally diverse among different cultures. In broad terms, it may be described as 'sexual behaviour which causes suffering in the form of psychological or physical discomfort to the person or partner, or is outside the range of what is generally accepted as normal by the society concerned'. On this basis, disorders may be considered in terms of either sexual dysfunctions (which form the majority of cases seen by therapists) or the much rarer sexual deviations.

SEXUAL DYSFUNCTIONS

Few sexual relationships are consistently 'perfect', and many problems which arise are either transient or resolve when the adverse circumstances causing them change. Sexual dysfunction may be defined as the *repeated* failure either to achieve or to enjoy 'normal' sexual intercourse. The sexual response in both the male and female passes through a number of recognised phases: **desire**, **arousal**, **orgasm** and **resolution**. Dysfunction can occur during any of the first three stages, resulting in some difficulties which are common to both men and women, and others which are gender specific. In addition, the perception of a problem will to some extent be contingent upon individual expectations. For example, one partner may be satisfied with intercourse once a week, while the other finds this insufficient. Sexual dysfunction appears to be a common condition among both sexes, with men usually complaining of performance difficulties and women more likely to present with lack of desire or enjoyment.

Sexual Dysfunctions Specific to the Male

1. ERECTILE IMPOTENCE

Erectile impotence is defined as the inability to achieve or sustain an erection despite adequate desire and stimulation. It is a disorder of arousal and is increasingly common with advancing age; it is estimated that approximately 7% of males are impotent at the age of 50, this figure increasing to 55% by 75 years. In younger men, the most frequent reasons for erectile dysfunction are anxiety and intoxication with alcohol, while in middle and old age, a mixture of organic and psychosocial causes is more likely.

Organic causes include diabetes mellitus, multiple sclerosis, spinal injuries, drugs (*see* Table 19.1), testicular atrophy and arterial obstruction due to trauma or vascular disease. Peyronie's disease is a rare idiopathic condition in which the development of fibrous tissue in the corpora of the penis prevents engorgement and erection.

2. PREMATURE EJACULATION

Premature ejaculation is the inability to control the ejaculatory reflex to the satisfaction of both partners. It is the commonest orgasmic disorder in young men, and is nearly always due to anxiety.

3. DELAY OR ABSENCE OF EJACULATION

This sometimes occurs despite adequate stimulation and a sustained erection. It may result from psychological difficulties, such as sexual inhibition and a fear of 'losing control', or have an organic basis. The latter can be caused by an autonomic neuropathy (most commonly due to diabetes or multiple sclerosis), or following the administration of certain hypotensive drugs such as methyldopa, guanethidine and bethanidine.

Sexual Dysfunctions Specific to the Female

1. VAGINISMUS

Vaginismus is the involuntary spasm of the vaginal (and often adductor thigh) muscles in response to attempts at penetration. The cause is usually psychological, and often relates to guilt or anxiety about sex. Less frequently, vaginismus can develop as a consequence of disease or injury to the genital region, such as atrophic vaginitis or scarring caused by a difficult childbirth.

2. DYSPAREUNIA

Dyspareunia is pain on sexual intercourse, which may be superficial or deep. Superficial pain can result from psychological causes, inadequate lubrication, scarring, inflammation and other lesions of the vulva or vagina. Deep dyspareunia is more likely to be associated with pelvic disease such as infection, endometriosis, cysts or tumours.

3. ANORGASMIA

Anorgasmia is the persistent inability to achieve orgasm despite adequate desire and arousal. Approximately 10% of women never achieve orgasm, and of the remainder, few do so consistently. Poor sexual technique accounts for some cases, while inhibition, relationship difficulties and a fear of 'losing control' are other causative factors.

4. GENERAL UNRESPONSIVENESS (FRIGIDITY)

This is a disorder of arousal characterised by a failure of vaginal lubrication despite adequate stimulation. Although it may be due to a lack of sexual desire (*see below*), it can also result from poor technique, anxiety or postmenopausal changes in the vagina.

Sexual Dysfunctions Common to Both Sexes

1. LOSS OF DESIRE

Diminished libido is more frequently complained of by women than by men. A loss of sexual desire towards a specific person is often due to relationship difficulties, whereas a generalised reduction in sex drive may result from advancing age, mental illness (especially depression) or stress. Other factors include loss of confidence (following disfiguring surgery), the use of certain drugs such as oral contraceptives, hormonal imbalance (i.e. testosterone deficiency or hyperprolactinaemia in men) and chronic physical illnesses such as renal, cardiac or respiratory disease.

2. SEX PHOBIA

This is an uncommon disorder predominantly of females, and takes the form of a fear of sexual intercourse, or of the genitalia of the opposite sex.

Table 19.1   Some causes of sexual dysfunction

Physical causes

Congenital/physiological conditions	Ageing, mental retardation, chromosomal abnormalities
Drugs	Neuroleptics, antidepressants, antiparkinsonian drugs, alcohol, opiates, disulfiram, benzodiazepines, oral contraceptives, cimetidine, spironolactone, antilibidinal drugs, hypotensive agents
Systemic illness	Cardiorespiratory disorders, renal disease, hepatic disease, malignancy, tuberculosis, arthritis, autoimmune disorders, acromegaly, Addison's disease, hypogonadism, diabetes, thyroid disorder
Neurological disorders	Brain damage, spinal lesions, multiple sclerosis, autonomic neuropathy
Physical conditions causing loss of confidence	Colostomy or ileostomy, mastectomy, amputation, skin disease, scarring
Local conditions	Genitourinary infections, pelvic disease, atrophic vaginitis, trauma and scarring, vascular obstruction, anatomical abnormalities, Peyronie's disease

Psychosocial causes

Psychiatric disorders and sexual deviations	Depression, dementia, eating disorders, anxiety, obsessional and phobic neuroses, fetishism, homosexuality, transsexualism
Other psychological factors	Ignorance, disgust, inhibition, fear, guilt, anger, poor self-image
Social and environmental stresses	Relationship difficulties, lack of privacy, lack of time or comfort, fatigue, change in family dynamics, e.g. childbirth, cultural taboos and myths

Aetiology

The physical and psychosocial causes of sexual dysfunction are summarised in Table 19.1. Aetiology may be multifactorial, especially from middle age onwards, although psychological causes predominate in younger age groups.

Assessment of Sexual Dysfunction

The treatment of sexual dysfunction should be preceded by a full assessment, involving a detailed sexual, medical and psychiatric **history** from both partners, followed by a **physical** and **mental state examination** supplemented by any necessary **special investigations**. In cases of erectile impotence, these might include blood glucose, serum testosterone, prolactin and gonadotrophin levels. Nocturnal tumescence studies using penile strain-gauges may be of help in distinguishing between organic and psychological causes of impotence, since erections during REM sleep should still be recordable in the latter case. The assessment should determine the **nature** and **cause** of the problem (*see* Table 19.1), and whether the dysfunction is:

1. **primary** or **secondary**: has there always been a problem or has the condition arisen after a period of normal sexual relations?
2. **functional** or **organic**: is there an underlying physical cause (i.e. metabolic, endocrine or anatomical disease), or evidence of psychiatric disorder, stress or other psychosocial problems?
3. **situational** or **global**: does the dysfunction only occur with a specific partner or in a certain setting, or is it present irrespective of circumstances?

Joint interviewing is the most valuable means of assessing how the couple communicate with each other. In addition, the interview should be used to determine the extent of any mistaken ideas they may have about sexual functioning or technique, the level of their **knowledge**, their general **attitudes** towards sex and their **capacity and motivation for change**. Time should also be allowed to see each partner separately, as there may be sensitive issues which demand confidentiality, such as extramarital liaisons, secretive cross-dressing or bisexual behaviour.

Management of Sexual Dysfunction

Management should initially be directed towards treating any organic or psychiatric disorders that have been identified as possible aetiological factors. Following this, therapy is considered in terms of general measures and specific behavioural techniques.

GENERAL MEASURES

Education is an important aspect of therapy when dealing with matters of poor technique, or with fears and other difficulties which arise from a lack of knowledge about sexual functioning or anatomy. Essential information can be imparted by the use of simple diagrams, models and self-examination. The couple should be made aware of the need for choosing an environment which is conducive to love-making, and ensuring that they have adequate privacy, time, warmth and comfort. Teaching and creating an awareness of sexual technique can be helpful in overcoming problems brought about by insufficient foreplay, poor attention to personal hygiene or lack of sensitivity to the other's needs.

Specific worries, such as fears about pregnancy or sexually transmitted diseases, can be resolved by giving appropriate advice (e.g. regarding contraception). Many of the fears and fantasies that people have about sex may be quite irrational, but until they are openly discussed, there is little that can be done to dispel them.

Facilitating better **communication** within a relationship, by encouraging a fuller understanding of each partner's needs and emotions, may bring about spontaneous resolution of sexual dysfunction. More specifically, partners need to tell each other about their sexual likes and dislikes, and sometimes verbalise these during love-making.

SPECIFIC TECHNIQUES

Sexual dysfunction often responds rapidly to behavioural techniques (known as **directive sex therapy**) which aim to reduce anxiety and inhibitions, as well as increase confidence and pleasure. They are often used in combination with each other, as well as with psychotherapeutic and (occasionally) physical measures. Behavioural methods used include 'sensate focusing', graded exposure and a form of biofeedback known as the 'squeeze' technique.

Sensate focusing concentrates on the pleasurable aspects of sex (touching, cuddling and caressing), and aims to dispel fears about sexual performance or failure by initially forbidding intercourse. Couples are usually seen once a week, at which time precise goals for treatment are agreed upon, and they are set tasks or 'homework' to carry out before the next session. 'Giving pleasure to get pleasure' is axiomatic of sensate focusing, and graded exercises are prescribed which progress from non-erotic contact, through erotic and genital stimulation, to mutual masturbation and finally, full sexual intercourse. The couple do not move on from one stage to the next until both feel comfortable about doing so. Erectile impotence, delayed or absent ejaculation and female anorgasmia/ frigidity may all respond to this method of treatment.

Graded exposure is the treatment of choice for vaginismus. The involuntary spasm of vaginal and adductor thigh muscles can be overcome by gradually 'acclimatising' the woman to the idea and sensation of something within her vagina. Initially, she is encouraged to attempt insertion of her fingers, which may be followed by the use of vaginal dilators of increasing size, until these can be accommodated without any reflex spasm occurring. A similar gradual introduction of her partner's penis is then attempted, until full intercourse is eventually possible.

The management of premature ejaculation by the **squeeze technique** is a form of **biofeedback** which allows the development of control over an autonomic body function. This method involves the woman stimulating her partner to the point of orgasm, and then squeezing the glans of his penis firmly between thumb and fingers until the pre-ejaculatory sensations are lost. Stimulation or intercourse then recommences until orgasm is once again nearly reached, and the squeeze is repeated. Ejaculatory control is eventually gained after a number of sessions.

Dynamic psychotherapy, conducted individually or with the couple, is sometimes used as the mainstay of treatment or as an adjunct to behavioural methods, particularly when sexual problems are closely related to inter- or intrapsychic difficulties.

In about 1–2% of cases, lack of desire and erectile dysfunction in males is found to be associated with an identifiable endocrine cause, such as reduced serum levels of testosterone. Under these circumstances, administration of **exogenous hormone** by injection or orally may improve sexual interest and performance. More recently, erectile impotence has been effectively treated by self-injection of an alpha-receptor blocking agent, such as **phenoxybenzamine**, directly into the corpus cavernosum of the penis. This causes penile engorgement, which may be sufficient for sexual intercourse to take place. **Surgical treatment** is occasionally offered for intractable cases of erectile dysfunction, in which semi-rigid implants inserted into the penis allow a degree of vaginal penetration.

A general practitioner referred a couple for sex therapy because they had been unable to consummate their relationship after 2 months of marriage. The doctor had tried to treat the wife's vaginismus using a behavioural approach, but had been unable to make any progress.

The therapist began his investigations by taking a detailed history from both partners, and discovered that although the husband had several sexual partners prior to marriage, his wife had been a virgin. The woman admitted to difficulties in discussing sexual matters, but with support and encouragement she began to talk more freely. She admitted that she had never examined herself internally as she thought her vagina was filled with long slender tendrils, which she feared would be easily damaged during intercourse. With the aid of diagrams and a model, the therapist was able to demonstrate the anatomy of the vagina and reassure her of its durability. During that session, the woman succeeded in inserting a finger into her vagina, and by using a graded approach to treat her vaginismus, the couple progressed to having intercourse within 6 weeks.

SEXUAL DEVIATIONS

Sexual deviation is said to exist when a person displays or engages in recurrent sexual behaviour which departs from that generally considered to be normal. Some practices may also be harmful and cause suffering to either the self or others. However, in certain societies, some activities (such as homosexuality) are viewed as acceptable variations of normality, rather than as deviant behaviour.

Homosexuality

Homosexuality is defined as sexual attraction towards a person of the same sex. In most societies, sexual orientation extends along a continuum, ranging from people who are exclusively heterosexual at one extreme, to those who are totally homosexual at the other. Male and female homosexual practices include kissing and caressing, mutual masturbation, orogenital contact and, between men, anal intercourse. A minority of homosexuals adopt the mannerisms, habits and style of dress of the opposite sex.

The **aetiology** of homosexuality remains unknown, and although some studies have proposed a genetic or hormonal basis, there is no clear evidence to support either of these hypotheses. Other research suggests that homosexual men or women were likely to have had a poor relationship with the parent of the same sex during childhood, who may have been either weak and ineffectual, or cold and indifferent. These abnormal family influences are said to impede the development of heterosexual behaviour.

In England and Wales, homosexual behaviour in private is legal between consenting males over the age of 21, although there are no specific laws regarding similar acts between females. Epidemiological studies indicate that about **4%** of males and **2%** of females are exclusively homosexual throughout their lives.

The majority of homosexuals neither need nor seek psychiatric help. However, there are some who find it difficult to come to terms with their sexual orientation, and consequently feel guilty and uncertain about their feelings or behaviour. **Crises** can arise when young people, on realising that they are predominantly homosexual, are faced with a dilemma of whether or not to inform their family and friends.

Many homosexuals form enduring, lifelong relationships, while a minority are highly promiscuous and indiscriminate in their choice of partners. The latter group are particularly vulnerable as they grow older, since their unstable lifestyle makes them more prone to loneliness and depression as their attractiveness wanes. **Psychiatric disorder** occurring in homosexuals is not necessarily related to problems of sexual orientation, but nevertheless, it is important to establish if such an association exists.

Modifying homosexual behaviour (in those who request it) is extremely difficult, and behavioural approaches have little to offer other than to reduce anxiety. Intrapersonal conflicts and relationship problems may be helped by individual, joint or group psychotherapy.

Paedophilia

Paedophilia is the condition of being sexually attracted to children, and sometimes indulging in sexual activity with them. Most offenders are men who may be **homosexual**, **heterosexual** or **bisexual** in their inclinations. Paedophilic activity usually involves looking and fondling, and attempts at intercourse are uncommon. The paedophile is most frequently middle-aged, often with marital or relationship problems, while older men are more likely to be socially isolated and may abuse alcohol. Occasionally, immature adolescents engage in sexual activity with pre-pubertal children just a few years younger than themselves. The child is often known to the adult as either a relative or friend, and in many cases is an active participant, through either interest or fear. Most commonly, girls are aged between 7 and 10 and boys between 11 and 14.

Incest

Incest involves sexual intercourse with a parent, sibling, child or grandchild, and is an imprisonable offence. **Father–daughter** and **brother–sister** relationships are the most common, although many cases go undetected, so that the prevalence is generally thought to be much higher than was previously acknowledged. The development of an incestuous relationship is more likely in socially isolated families living in overcrowded conditions (e.g. parents and children sharing beds). In father–daughter incest, there may be a history of paternal alcohol abuse, and it is sometimes evident that the wife overtly or covertly colludes with her husband's behaviour. There is a high rate of psychiatric morbidity among victims, and treatment might involve both individual and family work (*see* Chapter 13).

Exhibitionism

This is defined as purposeful exposure of the male genitals to unwilling females, without being a preliminary to sexual intercourse. The offence committed is known as **indecent exposure** and is the commonest form of sexual misdemeanour in England and Wales, with approximately 3000 convictions each year. The vast majority of offenders are aged between 15 and 25 years and fall into two categories:

1. the first group are shy and inhibited men, who struggle to suppress the urge to expose themselves, before finally capitulating. They derive little, if any, pleasure from their behaviour, the penis remaining flaccid throughout the act, and later experience an overwhelming sense of guilt and shame
2. the second group are more assertive with psychopathic inclinations,

and are therefore likely to have a worse prognosis. They generally expose themselves in a state of great excitement, with an erect penis, and often masturbate while deriving sadistic pleasure from the reaction of the witness.

The victim chosen is nearly always a total stranger, and the act is usually carried out in a public place, with the risk of being caught a seemingly important feature. Attempts at physical contact are rare, and although the woman may be temporarily distressed by the incident, she seldom suffers long-term psychological trauma.

The **aetiology** of exhibitionism is unclear, although a disturbed parent–child relationship in the early years is perhaps important. When exhibitionism occurs for the first time late in life, the possibility of dementia, functional psychosis or alcohol abuse should be considered. Such behaviour can also be a feature of mental retardation and brain damage. In many cases, appearance in court is an effective deterrent, since those who are convicted rarely re-offend.

Fetishism

In fetishism, inanimate objects or parts of the body that do not usually have sexual connotations become the preferred or sole focus of sexual interest. Nearly all fetishists are male, most of whom are heterosexual. Common objects of desire include rubber clothing, stiletto shoes, female lingerie and parts of the body, such as the nose and the feet. Sexual arousal is usually obtained by physical or genital contact with the fetish.

As with other sexual deviations, the **cause** of fetishism is uncertain. However, learning theory suggests that the disorder arises from sexual arousal at an early age becoming inadvertently associated and then paired with the fetish object. An illustrative example is that of a man who had a fetish for broom handles. He traced the association back to early childhood when his mother often played with him while she did the housework, which involved touching his genital region with the tip of the broom handle in a game of 'tag'.

Transvestism

Transvestism is a disorder of **gender role behaviour** which usually begins before puberty and involves the habitual wearing of clothes of the opposite sex (**cross-dressing**). Most transvestites are **heterosexual** males and some become sexually aroused when cross-dressing (fetishistic transvestism). They may wear their wife's clothing, often in secret, or sometimes resort to theft to obtain female apparel, such as stealing underwear from washing lines. Discovery frequently provokes a strong feeling of revulsion in the wife, and the relationship may end if she is unable to come to terms with her husband's deviant behaviour. However, some spouses do adjust to the idea, and even help their husbands to choose and buy female clothing.

A minority of men and most female transvestites are **homosexual**, and sometimes the disorder is associated with transsexualism (*see below*). These individuals do not usually become sexually excited by their behaviour, cross-dressing either to relieve anxiety or to fulfil some fantasy within a homosexual relationship.

Transsexualism

Transsexualism is a rare disorder of **gender identity** in which the individual is certain of having been born into the wrong sex. The majority of transsexuals are male and can date their discordant feelings back to childhood or early puberty.

Transsexuals have a profound distaste for the external evidence of their anatomical sex, which becomes intensified at the time of puberty. Many are transvestites who also adopt gestures and behaviour appropriate to the opposite sex, and some go on to demand hormonal or surgical treatment to alter their physical appearance (*see below*). Most transsexuals have fantasies or relationships which are predominantly homosexual, although their general level of interest in sex is low. However, heterosexual liaisons are not uncommon, and up to one-third may marry, but most later divorce.

The feeling of being 'trapped' in the body of the wrong sex can lead to depressive episodes and suicide attempts. Transsexuals tend to have an unsettled lifestyle in which alcohol abuse is frequent, relationships are often unstable and their work record is generally poor.

The **aetiology** of the disorder remains unknown, although animal studies have postulated that hormonal abnormalities can influence gender identity in the prenatal period. Despite this, transsexuals have no detectable endocrine disturbance and they are chromosomally normal. Because gender identity is firmly established by the age of 5, environmental factors may contribute to the development of transsexualism, where accidental or deliberate assignment to the opposite sex occurs at an early age.

Other Sexual Deviations

Sadism is sexual gratification derived from inflicting pain on others, e.g. by whipping or beating. **Masochism** is sexual satisfaction obtained by being subjected to pain, humiliation or acts of cruelty. Varying degrees of both types of behaviour are encountered within many relationships, although extreme cases are rare. **Voyeurism** is sexual arousal and gratification obtained by watching others copulate, or by secretly observing women undressing or in the nude ('peeping Tom'). Men who indulge in this behaviour do so in preference to other forms of sexual activity, although they are usually heterosexual in orientation. They are frequently solitary and inadequate individuals, and may take unnecessary risks of being caught while carrying out voyeuristic activities. **Bestiality** involves sexual activity with animals. It tends to occur mainly among farm and agricultural workers in rural areas. **Necrophilia**, which is sexual gratification derived from having intercourse with a dead body, is extremely rare.

The Management of Sexual Deviation

Treatment should only be offered if the deviation is unlawful, harmful to others or causing the individual suffering. Furthermore, the subject must consent to treatment and be motivated to change. Once any underlying psychiatric disorder has been excluded, a therapeutic plan should be established, aimed at either reducing the aberrant behaviour or helping the person to adjust to his deviation.

Counselling is directed towards reducing distress and exploring the subject's feelings and attitudes towards his behaviour, the problems it causes and how they can be reduced. **Behavioural methods** aim to modify deviant activities by the use of techniques such as aversion therapy and covert sensitisation, which are also employed to reduce arousal in response to abnormal fantasies (*see* Chapter 13). Techniques of this kind may be of help to the exhibitionist who repeatedly offends, and in minimising fetishistic behaviour. Other procedures aim at increasing 'normal' arousal by replacing deviant imagery with heterosexual fantasies (orgasmic conditioning), while social skills training is designed to enhance the individual's confidence in developing adult heterosexual relationships.

Drugs are sometimes administered to male sex offenders to reduce libidinal drive. Cyproterone acetate, an antiandrogenic substance, produces fewer side-effects than female hormones such as oestradiol, but is probably not as effective. Oestrogens are also administered to transsexuals prior to **surgical sex reassignment**. Strict criteria are applied before embarking on this form of radical treatment, in that the subject must be well-motivated, psychologically stable and have lived as a member of the opposite sex for at least 2 years prior to surgery being undertaken.

SUMMARY

1. **Sexual dysfunction** is the repeated failure either to achieve or to enjoy 'normal' sexual intercourse. It occurs in both sexes, with men usually complaining of performance difficulties and women more likely to present with lack of desire or enjoyment. Problems specific to the male include

erectile impotence and premature, delayed or absent ejaculation. Disorders occurring in women include vaginismus, dyspareunia, anorgasmia and frigidity. Loss of desire and sex phobia may occur in either sex.

2. Psychological factors are the commonest cause of sexual dysfunction in younger age groups, although a multifactorial aetiology is more likely in middle-aged and elderly patients. A comprehensive assessment of both partners must be undertaken before embarking on treatment. The latter may include educative measures and strategies aimed at improving communication within the relationship. Behavioural techniques are employed to treat specific dysfunctions, as well as to reduce anxiety and inhibitions, and increase confidence and pleasure. Combined methods may be used which include sensate focusing, graded exposure and biofeedback. Dynamic psychotherapy, drugs or surgery can be helpful in certain instances.

3. **Sexual deviation** is said to exist when a person displays or engages in recurrent sexual behaviour which departs from that generally considered to be normal. Some practices may also be harmful, and cause suffering to either the self or others. Deviations which might come to the attention of the psychiatrist include homosexuality, paedophilia, incest, exhibitionism, fetishism, transvestism and transsexualism. Where indicated, treatment involves counselling and/or behavioural techniques which are aimed at modifying the aberrant behaviour or helping the individual to adjust to his deviation. Drugs are occasionally used to reduce libidinal drive in male sex offenders, or administered to transsexuals prior to surgical sex reassignment.

REFERENCES AND FURTHER READING

Bancroft, J. (1974). *Deviant Sexual Behaviour: Modification and Assessment.* Oxford: Clarendon Press.

Cole, M. (1985). Sex therapy — a critical appraisal. *British Journal of Psychiatry*; **147**: 337–51.

Green, J., Miller, D. (1985). Male homosexuality and sexual problems. *British Journal of Hospital Medicine*; **33**: 353–55.

Kaplan, H. S. (1974). *The New Sex Therapy.* New York: Brunner/Mazel.

Masters, W. H., Johnson, V. E. (1966). *Human Sexual Response.* Boston: Little, Brown.

Masters, W. H., Johnson, V. E. (1970). *Human Sexual Inadequacy.* Edinburgh: Churchill Livingstone.

Rooth, F. G. (1980). Exhibitionism: an eclectic approach to its management. *British Journal of Hospital Medicine*; **23**: 366–70.

Wilson, G. D. (1981). Sexual deviations. *British Journal of Hospital Medicine*; **26**: 8–14.

20 PSYCHIATRIC DISORDERS SPECIFIC TO WOMEN

This chapter is concerned with psychiatric disorders which are associated with menstruation, pregnancy and childbirth.

PREMENSTRUAL TENSION AND THE MENOPAUSE

Many women feel tense, irritable and mildly depressed for a few days prior to the onset of a period, and there may be accompanying symptoms of breast tenderness and abdominal distension. In most cases, the symptoms resolve rapidly once menstruation begins, but in some women they are sufficiently distressing for medical help to be sought. There is no clear evidence that hormonal treatment is effective in this condition, although diuretics and mild analgesics may be of help in relieving physical discomfort.

Physical problems which occur at the time of the menopause are sometimes accompanied by feelings of anxiety and depression. Although hormone replacement therapy is widely used to treat somatic complaints such as 'hot flushes' and sweating, its effect on psychological symptoms is uncertain. Major life changes at this time (such as the loss of child-bearing capacity and children leaving home) are just as likely to result in mood disturbance as any reduction in oestrogen levels.

PREGNANCY

Depending upon the circumstances, pregnancy is perhaps unique among 'life events' in being able to evoke feelings ranging from great joy to total despair. Psychological disturbance during this time will be influenced not only by the woman's perspective of her condition, but also by her social circumstances, the state of her physical health and any predisposition to develop psychiatric disorder.

In general, pregnancy has an ameliorating effect on major mental illness, so that women suffering from chronic conditions, such as schizophrenia or bipolar affective illness, are probably less likely to

378

relapse during this time. However, minor disturbances of mood and feelings of tension are common, particularly in the late stages of pregnancy, when worries about the delivery or the baby being abnormal may occur.

Unwanted Pregnancy

Since the passing of the 1967 Abortion Act, termination of pregnancy in England and Wales has been permissible on therapeutic grounds if its continuation would involve risk to the life of the woman, her physical or mental health, or that of any existing children. In each case, the risk must be greater than if the pregnancy were terminated. A fourth indication is that if the child were born, there would be a substantial risk that it would suffer from mental or physical abnormality resulting in serious handicap.

The majority of therapeutic terminations are carried out on the grounds of risk to the mental health of the mother, due to the stress of an unwanted pregnancy. In most cases, psychiatrists are not involved in the assessment, certification being made by the obstetrician and general practitioner. However, symptoms of anxiety and depression frequently occur in women prior to therapeutic abortion, although in the majority they rapidly resolve afterwards. Even so, persistent feelings of guilt, leading to the development of a depressive illness, are sometimes encountered in those who were ambivalent about the termination (e.g. due to coercion by a parent or boyfriend), or had terminations on medical grounds. Therefore, counselling should be available to all women referred for therapeutic abortion, so that conflicts of this type can be detected early on, and dealt with prior to termination.

Stillbirth

Stillbirth is an emotionally painful experience, accentuated by the lack of a 'real child' to mourn. The mother should be given an opportunity to see or hold the dead baby, and in many units a photograph is provided. After the delivery she should be nursed on a gynaecological rather than a postnatal ward and given every opportunity by the staff to express her grief (see Chapter 7). Anticipatory guidance in dealing with the emotional problems likely to be experienced on returning home (e.g. explaining the loss to others, giving away clothes and toys, and meeting friends with young babies) can also be helpful in minimising the risk of a subsequent depressive illness.

PSYCHIATRIC DISORDERS IN THE PUERPERIUM

A connection between childbirth and mental illness was recognised by the physicians of Ancient Greece, although it is only in the last 100 years that the association has been scientifically evaluated. It is well established that there is an increased prevalence of psychiatric disorder among women during the puerperium (the 6–8 week period following childbirth) when compared with age-matched, non-puerperal controls. Disorders which occur at this time are puerperal psychosis, postnatal depression and the 'maternity blues'.

Puerperal Psychosis

The weight of current opinion holds that the clinical features of psychoses in the puerperium do not differ to any great extent from those occurring at other times, and neither DSM III-R nor ICD 9 recognise its existence as a discrete entity. (Similarly, there will be no specific category for puerperal psychosis in ICD 10.) Consequently, disorders of this type are classified according to the recognised diagnostic categories of psychotic illness, i.e. schizophrenic, affective or organic.

Some authorities dissent from this viewpoint, claiming that the concept of puerperal psychosis is worth retaining, because of the marked occurrence of severe and unexpected mental illness developing abruptly during the first few weeks after childbirth in healthy women with no previous psychiatric history. This is supported by several studies which have shown that the rate of admission of women to mental hospitals in the first month postpartum is dramatically higher than at any time during pregnancy.

The incidence of puerperal psychosis is low, with only one or two women affected in every 1000 deliveries. It is commoner among those having their first baby (primiparous women).

AETIOLOGY

Despite a great deal of research, very little is known about the cause of puerperal psychosis. There is often a family history of mental illness, although a more direct genetic influence has been inferred from the observation that women whose own mothers had a history of puerperal psychosis have a sixfold increased risk of developing the condition themselves. An association with bipolar affective illness is suggested by a similarity in the clinical presentation of the disorders, and the high rate of puerperal relapse in women with a history of affective illness. No clear aetiological link has been established with any psychological or environmental factors, although a biological cause might seem likely in view of the dramatic physiological changes which occur at this time. However, no significant endocrine or biochemical abnormality has been detected in these women which distinguishes them from other postpartum females. Non-puerperal episodes of psychosis occur in 50% of these women at some time in the future, which may indicate that many have a lifelong tendency to develop major mental illness.

CLINICAL FEATURES

The onset is often sudden, characteristically between the third and fourteenth day following childbirth, and is usually preceded by 24–48 hours of insomnia, restlessness and sometimes confusion. Clinically, the disorder most frequently resembles an **affective illness**, with features of mania (often accompanied by confusion and disorganised speech) or psychotic depression (where delusions may focus on the health and well-being of the baby). Less commonly, a **schizophrenic-like illness** develops, in which auditory hallucinations and other first rank symptoms are demonstrated.

> Staff on a postnatal ward became concerned about the behaviour of a 24-year-old woman who had given birth 3 days previously. She had been observed repeatedly checking her baby as he lay in his cot, and had muttered vaguely to the nurses about 'something being wrong'. A routine examination by the paediatrician failed to reassure her that all was well, and later on in the day she was found wandering around the ward, scrutinising other babies in a similar fashion to her own. She told a nurse that she was alarmed that her baby's body was dramatically expanding and contracting in size, and wanted to see if other infants were similarly affected. Despite being given a sedative, she slept very little that night, and by the next morning she had become markedly overactive, constantly repeating that she wanted to see 'a vicar, God and the Man in the Moon'. Physical examination showed no evidence of infection or other organic dysfunction, and following a psychiatric assessment, mother and infant were transferred to the local psychiatric unit.

MANAGEMENT

Although hospital admission is frequently required to treat the mother's illness, every effort needs to be made to ensure that she remains with and continues to play a part in the care of her baby. Only if the mother is extremely disturbed should separation be considered, and as soon as her symptoms are under control, she should be reunited with her child. Statistically, the risk of suicide or infanticide is rare. Nevertheless, careful enquiries must always be made to determine if the mother harbours any delusional ideas which might result in harm to her baby or herself.

In some areas, **mother and baby units** have been established which cater specially for mentally ill mothers and their infants in an environment simulating domestic living conditions as closely as possible. Many women with puerperal psychosis continue to relate well to their babies during their illness, and providing they are carefully supervised by appropriately trained nurses, they can carry out many of the tasks necessary in caring for their infant. This facilitates bonding and allows the mother to feel more competent in coping with her child when she is ready to leave hospital. Where no specialist facility exists, it is common practice to admit both mother and baby onto an acute psychiatric ward. In either case, the continuing involvement of the father and other children should be encouraged. As her mental state improves, individual or group psycho-therapy may be of benefit in helping the patient to come to terms with her new role and responsibilities as a mother.

The choice of physical treatment will depend upon the clinical presentation of the condition. With the generally high standards of obstetric care practised in the UK, organic psychoses (which were mainly due to infection) are now extremely rare. However, the possibility of infection should always be borne in mind, and where necessary, treatment with antibiotics started as soon as possible. Depressive psychoses can be treated with a MARI antidepressant (sometimes given in combination with a neuroleptic drug) or ECT (*see* Chapter 5). Manic symptoms respond well to lithium and neuroleptics, while schizophrenic-like illnesses are best treated with neuroleptics alone. However, due attention must be given to the mother's desire to breast feed and the subsequent risk to the infant with certain forms of drug treatment, especially lithium (*see* p. 248).

PROGNOSIS

The short-term prognosis is generally favourable, the majority of patients being well enough to leave hospital within 2–3 months. However, there is a one in five risk of recurrence following further childbirth, and 50% of these women will suffer a non-puerperal psychotic episode at some later stage in their lives.

Postnatal Depression

Most studies indicate that about 10% of women become significantly depressed after childbirth. The diagnosis may be missed for two important reasons. First, transient mood disturbances ('the blues') are very common postpartum, and if sustained depressive symptoms do develop, they often evolve insidiously and may be overlooked or considered a 'normal' reaction to the responsibilities of motherhood. Second, anxiety and irritability are frequently prominent and may mask the true nature of the condition. Some authorities suggest that postnatal depression should only be diagnosed where symptoms have persisted for more than 2 weeks.

AETIOLOGY

Postnatal depression is thought more likely to develop when there is a previous history of psychiatric disorder, depression during pregnancy or severe postpartum blues. Ambivalence towards the baby (as with an unwanted pregnancy) and a previous history of miscarriage also predispose towards its occurrence. Other associated factors include a recent stressful life event (which may not be related to the birth) and chronic stressors such as long-term marital difficulties, housing problems or physical ill-health. There is no definite evidence that hormonal factors influence the onset or perpetuation of depression in the puerperium.

CLINICAL FEATURES

The onset is usually during the first 4 weeks postpartum (although sometimes the illness may take up to 6 months to develop fully), so that symptoms are most evident after the mother and baby return home from hospital. Feelings of depression are often overshadowed by anxiety regarding the baby, and the mother may present to her general practitioner or health visitor with fears or complaints about the infant's health which subsequently prove to be groundless. Fatigue and exhaustion can aggravate the situation and result in feelings of guilt and inadequacy concerning her ability to cope with being a wife and mother.

Somatic symptoms, such as anorexia, nausea and sleep disturbance, are common and may lead the mother to assume that she is physically unwell. Loss of libido and marital discord are frequently encountered and, unaware that his wife is ill, the husband may withdraw his support at a time when it is much needed.

A 34-year-old man visited his general practitioner asking for something to help him sleep. He complained of feeling run down, which he attributed to problems within his marriage. The family had only recently moved into the area, and since the birth of their second child 3 months previously, his wife had seemed unable to re-establish a routine in her life. Whereas beforehand she had been a happy and capable woman, she now appeared to be constantly irritable, and complained about the impossibility of coping with the children and running the home. Despite having a busy and demanding job, he had tried hard to offer his wife extra help and support around the house. However, she seemed unappreciative of his efforts, and he felt totally displaced from her affections.

The doctor arranged to see the couple together the following evening, but the next morning, the wife attended surgery on her own, looking tense and exhausted. She had talked with her husband the night before and had come to ask for help, as she felt she could no longer cope. She felt intensely guilty about the problems in her marriage, which she believed were entirely her fault. Furthermore, she was constantly worried that her new baby was not eating enough, and that she was not giving her 2-year-old child sufficient attention. Further questioning by the doctor elicited that she was sleeping poorly and had lost her appetite. After a brief physical examination to exclude any obvious organic cause, the general practitioner considered that the woman's symptoms were attributable to postnatal depression.

MANAGEMENT

Early recognition and treatment is essential, in order to reduce the risk of bonding difficulties between mother and baby, as well as to prevent marital breakdown. Primary health care workers, in particular general practitioners and health visitors, should be aware of the variable presentation of postnatal depression, since most cases can be managed in the community, provided support is adequate. More recently, an easily administered 10-item self-report scale has been developed for the detection of postnatal depression, which may prove to be of great benefit in helping doctors and community workers identify the disorder.

Any social precipitants (such as accommodation problems or marital difficulties) need to be identified and appropriate intervention undertaken. Unless symptoms are mild or resolve rapidly, antidepressant treatment should be instituted without delay. It is advisable to continue the medication for at least 6 months after symptoms have resolved in order to prevent a relapse. If no initial response occurs, ECT may need to be considered, although its administration will depend upon the clinical features of the illness (*see* Chapter 5). Both the woman and her spouse should be offered support and practical advice where needed, so as to enable them to adjust to their new circumstances. With this aim in mind, regular visits by the health visitor, community psychiatric nurse or general practitioner can be of great benefit.

PROGNOSIS

With early treatment, the prognosis is generally good and full recovery can usually be expected within a few months, although in some cases, symptoms may persist for up to a year.

The Maternity Blues

Transient episodes of weeping and depression occur in 50–70% of recently delivered women and are known as the 'maternity blues'. The peak onset is between the third and sixth day following childbirth, at which time lability of mood, irritability, feelings of depersonalisation, insomnia and headache may be evident. Short-lived negative feelings towards the baby can also occur.

There is often a striking association between the onset of weeping and the rapid weight loss which takes place in the first few days after delivery, although the significance of this finding is not clearly understood. No correlation has been found between the large hormonal changes which occur at this time and the alterations in mental state. Similarly, there is no

Table 20.1

Comparison of the main psychiatric disorders occurring in the puerperium

	Puerperal psychosis	Postnatal depression	Maternity blues
Percentage of births affected	0.1–0.2%	10%	50–70%
Onset after delivery	3rd–14th day	Within first month	3rd–6th day
Main clinical features	Prodromal period of insomnia, restlessness, confusion. Affective symptoms more common than schizophrenic	Depressive symptoms may be masked by anxiety, irritability. Feelings of guilt or inadequacy, insomnia and fatigue, anorexia and nausea, decreased libido, marital discord	Labile mood, transient episodes of weeping, irritability and insomnia, minor somatic symptoms, transient negative feelings towards the baby
Management	Hospitalisation of both mother and baby usually necessary. Antidepressants, lithium, neuroleptics, ECT all have a place in management. Supportive psychotherapy	Early recognition important. Antidepressants, ECT. Identification and resolution of social, interpersonal or environmental precipitants. Supportive psychotherapy	None besides reassurance and explanation
Prognosis	Good. Full recovery within 2–3 months. 1 in 5 risk of recurrence following further pregnancies, 50% risk of further non-puerperal episode of psychosis	Good with early treatment. Recovery usual within a few months, but symptoms may persist for up to a year	Very good. Resolution of symptoms usually rapid and complete

evidence that psychological or social factors play a significant role in the development of the blues.

The symptoms are usually short-lived, so that no intervention is required other than reassurance and explanation. However, the blues may occasionally be severe, and in rare instances, progress to a postnatal depression.

SUMMARY

1. Minor psychiatric disturbances (such as mild depression and anxiety) are common **premenstrually** and at the time of the **menopause**. Their causation is uncertain, and there is no clear evidence that hormonal treatment is effective in resolving psychological symptoms occurring at such times.
2. **Pregnancy** generally has an ameliorating effect on major mental illness, although minor psychiatric disturbances are common in the third trimester. The majority of therapeutic terminations are carried out on the grounds of risk to the mental health of the mother. Symptoms of anxiety and depression are common prior to termination, but in the majority of cases, resolve rapidly afterwards. Counselling may help to prevent more serious psychiatric sequelae, and is also important following a stillbirth.
3. **Puerperal psychosis** is a rare condition of unknown aetiology, with an overall incidence of 1–2 cases per 1000 deliveries. It is more common among primiparous women. The onset of the disorder is characteristically between days 3 and 14 postpartum, and is often preceded by a period of insomnia and confusion. Symptoms most frequently resemble those of manic or depressive illnesses, and less commonly schizophrenia. Hospital admission is usually required, which in some areas may be to a specialised mother and baby unit. Every effort should be made to keep mother and baby together, in order to facilitate bonding and maintain the mother's confidence in caring for her child. Treatment will depend upon the clinical presentation, with antidepressant drugs, ECT, lithium and neuroleptics all having a place in management. As the mental state improves, supportive psychotherapy is often helpful in assisting the mother to come to terms with her new role and responsibilities. The short-term prognosis is good, although there is a one in five risk of recurrence following further childbirth, and 50% of women suffer a non-puerperal psychotic episode at some later stage in their lives.
4. **Postnatal depression** occurs in about 10% of women following childbirth. Associated factors include a past history of psychiatric disorder, depression during pregnancy, ambivalence towards the baby, a recent adverse life event and chronic stress. Depressive symptoms are often masked by anxiety and irritability, and the presentation may be atypical, with the mother expressing concern about her marriage, the

baby's health or an inability to cope with domestic responsibilities. Early recognition is important to prevent bonding difficulties and marital breakdown. Unless symptoms are very mild or transient, antidepressant treatment should be commenced without delay and continued for at least 6 months after recovery, to prevent a relapse. Most cases can be managed at home, although hospital admission is occasionally necessary. ECT is sometimes required in those who do not respond to antidepressants. Support and practical advice from community health care workers is often helpful in assisting all members of the family to adjust to their new roles and circumstances. With early treatment, the prognosis is generally good, although symptoms can sometimes persist for up to a year.

5. The **maternity blues** occur in 50–70% of women postnatally, the main features of which are transient episodes of weeping and lability of mood. In nearly all cases, symptoms resolve spontaneously, so that no treatment other than explanation and reassurance is usually necessary.

REFERENCES AND FURTHER READING

Brockington, I. F., Kumar, R., eds (1982). *Motherhood and Mental Illness*. London: Academic Press.

Cox, J. L., Holden, J. M., Sagovsky, R. (1987). Detection of postnatal depression — development of the 10-item Edinburgh postnatal depression scale. *British Journal of Psychiatry*; **150**: 782–86.

Kumar, R., Robson, K. (1978). Neurotic disturbance during pregnancy and the puerperium. Preliminary report of a prospective study of 119 primiparae. In *Mental Illness in Pregnancy and the Puerperium* (Sandler, M., ed.) pp. 40-51. Oxford: Oxford University Press.

Pitt, B. (1968). 'Atypical' depression following childbirth. *British Journal of Psychiatry*; **114**: 1325–35.

21 SLEEP DISORDERS

INSOMNIA

Many people complain of difficulty in sleeping or of feeling tired the following day. Sometimes, no clear cause can be established, but in other cases, insomnia arises as a result of stress, a change in normal routine, or is attributable to excessive consumption of alcohol, caffeine or other stimulant drugs. Occasionally, insomnia is the presenting or prominent feature of a psychiatric or physical illness. Sleeplessness is a common complaint among the elderly (since the amount of time spent asleep diminishes with age) and is more likely to occur in females than males.

The pattern of sleep disturbance may be helpful in establishing the underlying cause of insomnia. For example, **anxiety states** are associated with difficulty in falling asleep (early insomnia), as well as a tendency to awaken repeatedly throughout the night. In contrast, **depressive illnesses** are characterised by early morning wakening (*see* p. 75), which is also observed in anorexia nervosa. In **manic** and **hypomanic episodes** there is a reduced need for sleep, so that those affected often sleep no more than 1 or 2 hours per night.

Where insomnia is a symptom of a physical or psychiatric illness, treatment of the primary disorder often leads to resolution of the problem. Similarly, sleeplessness resulting from anxiety or worry requires an assessment of current difficulties, and the formulation of plans to overcome them. In other cases, where no clear precipitant is established, a change in bedtime routine may be helpful. For example, advising the subject to refrain from alcohol or caffeine in the few hours before bedtime, and to have a warm malted milk drink prior to retiring, may help to induce sleep. Taking regular exercise and avoiding going to bed at irregular times may be equally beneficial. Hypnotic drugs, such as short-acting benzodiazepines, are occasionally needed, but should only be prescribed for brief periods in order to avoid dependence.

THE HYPERSOMNIAS

Problems of excessive sleep or daytime drowsiness are much less common than insomnia, and may be a feature of the following disorders:

1. **Narcolepsy**: typified by episodes of uncontrollable sleep during the day, frequently accompanied by cataplexy (in which the individual suddenly collapses due to loss of muscle tone). Associated features in this rare syndrome include sleep paralysis (a sensation of being awake but unable to move) and hypnagogic hallucinations (which occur at the onset of sleep). The onset of the narcoleptic syndrome is frequently in the teenage years and usually continues throughout life. A family history is often present, and the condition is more common among males. No treatment is totally effective, although tricyclic antidepressants or amphetamines may help reduce the frequency of attacks.

2. **Sleep drunkenness**: a disorder in which the subject is unable to awaken fully for several hours after rising, during which time he is irritable and confused. It is the commonest cause of hypersomnia and may respond to mild stimulant drugs such as caffeine.

3. **Sleep apnoea**: most commonly occurs in obese men under the age of 40. It is characterised by upper respiratory obstruction during sleep, in association with excessive snoring and nocturnal motor restlessness, which is followed by daytime drowsiness. Symptoms usually resolve with loss of weight, but when the periods of apnoea are severe and persistent, pulmonary hypertension can develop.

4. **Kleine-Levin syndrome**: an extremely rare condition, probably arising from a hypothalamic disorder, in which prolonged episodes of hypersomnia occur in association with increased appetite and hypersexuality.

OTHER DISORDERS OF SLEEP

Night terrors most commonly occur in young children, who appear to awaken an hour or two after going to sleep in a state of panic or extreme distress. Typically, the child screams out in terror, sits up or gets out of bed, but does not respond to attempts to comfort him. The episode may last for a few minutes prior to a return to normal sleep, and the child has no recollection of events the following day. Although the subject seems to be awake, night terrors have been demonstrated to occur during deep (slow wave) sleep. The phenomenon is sometimes accompanied by **sleep-walking** or associated with **nocturnal enuresis**, both of which also take place during slow-wave sleep. In contrast, **nightmares** are a feature of rapid eye movement (dream) sleep and often occur at times of anxiety or stress.

REFERENCES AND FURTHER READING

Hallstrom, C. (1983). Which hypnotic — if any? *British Journal of Hospital Medicine*; **30**: 188–92.
Oswald, I. (1984). Insomnia. *British Journal of Hospital Medicine*; **31**: 219–24.

22

TRANSCULTURAL PSYCHIATRY AND PSYCHIATRIC DISORDERS AMONG IMMIGRANTS

Transcultural psychiatry is concerned with the influence of culture on the epidemiology, clinical presentation, course and prognosis of mental disorders, as well as with the diverse theories of causation and treatment which exist in different societies.

Psychiatric disorder is recognised in both primitive and developed communities across the globe, and there is reasonable conformity world-wide in distinguishing between mental health and illness when the latter results in gross derangement of mental processes or behaviour. However, lesser degrees of disturbance may be considered within normal limits by some cultures, although not by others. For example, a study conducted by the World Health Organisation (using a standardised format for the examination of the mental state) showed close agreement in the diagnosis of schizophrenia in several centres across the world. On the other hand, cultural factors can greatly influence the manner in which an individual responds to stress or displays emotion, and either may be readily misinterpreted as a sign of mental illness if the psychiatrist is unfamiliar with that person's cultural background. Certain unusual conditions which are considered to be culture-specific are discussed in Chapter 23.

Because many areas of the UK now have large ethnic communities, local psychiatric services are increasingly involved in dealing with the behavioural, social and psychological problems of such groups. A knowledge of how clinical disorders can be modified by cultural effects is therefore essential if diagnostic accuracy is to be maintained and appropriate help offered.

DEPRESSION

People from Western cultures who are depressed will often start by describing their symptoms in emotional terms, and further questioning is frequently necessary to elicit somatic features such as insomnia, loss of appetite or diminished libido. In contrast, people from the Indian subcontinent who become depressed will usually emphasise their physical symptoms, and on direct questioning may deny any disturbance of mood.

This can arise because the unsophisticated subject sees no connection between his somatic problems and his emotions, and therefore considers it inappropriate to discuss such matters with the doctor. Furthermore, certain dialects have no words which approximate to 'low mood', 'depression' or other synonyms commonly used in English. Consequently, in the absence of any demonstrable organic pathology, these symptoms are often considered to be hypochondriacal in nature. Another variant is found in men of West Indian origin, who may complain about impotence or low sex drive when they are depressed. Depression in ethnic groups may also be a consequence of uncommon physical conditions such as thalassaemia, parasitic infestation, vitamin deficiency or tuberculosis, and these should be borne in mind when considering the cause.

SCHIZOPHRENIA

When standardised diagnostic criteria are used, schizophrenia is found to exist worldwide, with only a few minor variations in its prevalence (*see* Chapter 8). Schizophrenic patients originating from Third World countries are said to display catatonic features more frequently than those from developed societies. Care must be taken when diagnosing schizophrenia in those from other cultures, because ideas and behaviour which might be considered abnormal by Western standards, may be understandable in the context of the individual's social and cultural background. For example, beliefs which are likely to be considered delusional in the UK, such as possession by evil spirits, are widespread in certain areas of Asia, Africa and the Caribbean.

PSYCHOGENIC PSYCHOSES

People from non-Western cultures are more prone to react to stress by the development of excitable behaviour or transient symptoms such as hallucinations, thought disorder or delusional beliefs, which are indistinguishable from those found in the major psychoses. Those of Afro-Caribbean origin occasionally respond to stressful situations by acting in a wild, chaotic and aggressive manner, to which the term 'West Indian psychosis' is sometimes applied. Although their behaviour may closely resemble features of mania or other psychoses seen in the indigenous population, symptoms of a psychogenic psychosis characteristically abate spontaneously once the source of stress is removed, or the subject is placed in a different environment.

HYSTERIA

Hysterical disorders are discussed in Chapter 4, and although seen in all cultures, they may be especially florid in patients of Asian, African or Caribbean origin, sometimes taking the form of trance-like states or grossly disabling symptoms.

PSYCHIATRIC DISORDERS IN IMMIGRANTS

Several studies have shown that the rate of psychiatric disorder among immigrants is higher than that in the indigenous population, and sometimes greater than that in their country of origin. Two hypotheses have been advanced to account for these findings; the theory of **social causation** proposes that the stress of migration is a precipitant of psychiatric disorder in predisposed individuals. The second theory, that of **social selection**, postulates that people prone to certain psychiatric conditions (such as schizophrenia) have a tendency to migrate. However, other research has shown that migration is not necessarily associated with increased rates of mental illness, and in some cases (such as with Irish immigrants to the UK), the prevalence of psychiatric disorder is actually less than that in their country of origin.

Although no definite conclusions can be drawn, it is possible that the development of mental illness in predisposed immigrants is influenced by stress factors operating before, during and after migration.

Stress Factors Occurring Before and During Migration

The **attitude** of the original society towards migration may have some bearing on the development of subsequent psychiatric problems in migrants. For example, where it is seen as a sign of ambition and is admired, there may be a lower rate of mental illness in those who leave, than in cases where migration is viewed as an act of desertion.

The **circumstances** of migration are also likely to be of significance. For instance, the effect on migrants will probably be different if they are expelled from their country of origin for political reasons, than if they leave because of a desire to escape impoverishment. Where migration is seen as temporary and contact with the home country is maintained, there may be less stress than where the move is permanent without hope of return. Other circumstances which might contribute to the development of psychiatric problems include illegal immigration and obstructed migration (such as with those who are refused permission to leave a country for ideological reasons).

Stress Factors Occurring After Migration

Irrespective of their cultural background, a number of stresses are common to all immigrants, which may well lead to an increase in psychiatric morbidity. Many migrants have moved away from their homelands in order to improve their social standing, but because of financial impoverishment, they are often forced to live in **deprived** inner city areas where bad housing, overcrowding and high levels of unemployment are common. Such an environment is likely to encourage **racial hostility** and **prejudice**, which act as further sources of stress.

Loneliness and **social isolation** are frequent problems in immigrant communities, particularly among men who migrate on their own in order to establish a home before sending for their families. Similar problems can occur with the elderly migrant whose spouse dies and with young women who do not work, but instead remain at home to raise their children. The sense of isolation may be compounded by **language difficulties**, which create a barrier to social integration. An additional source of stress for some skilled migrants is the refusal of their adopted society to recognise their professional qualifications, so that they are forced to undertake menial and poorly paid work instead. The resultant **frustration** of financial and occupational ambitions may lead to a lack of self-confidence and a predisposition to anxiety, depression or other psychiatric disorder. Further strain might be created by the need to send money to relatives overseas who are dependent upon the immigrant's financial success.

First generation immigrants may find that their own **cultural** and **religious beliefs** are discordant with those of their children, who have adopted the views of the society in which they were born and raised. This can create **family conflict** and stress, particularly within the context of matrimony and sexual morals. For example, Asian parents may wish to arrange a marriage for their daughter in line with their own customs, and difficulties can arise if she expresses a desire to choose a partner for herself. Moral behaviour in many Western societies is often considered unacceptably lax by the standards of certain Eastern religions. Strict rules of behaviour laid down by parents may cause children to rebel against their authority, thereby undermining the stability of the family.

Management

Effective management of psychiatric disorders among immigrant groups and ethnic minorities can only be achieved by attempting to understand the presenting problem in the context of the individual's personal, cultural and social background. Once the diagnosis has been established, treatment should proceed along conventional lines. Where possible, use should be made of trained interpreters to overcome language barriers, rather than family members or friends who may relay information inaccurately.

> A 54-year-old Bengali man, residing in the UK, was admitted to the psychiatric ward of a hospital in London because he appeared to be clinically depressed. His command of English was very poor, and several interviews were conducted with his son acting as interpreter, in an attempt to establish the cause of his distress. The father spoke for lengthy periods in response to the doctor's questions, but on each occasion they were translated by the son as 'the ravings of an old man'. Subsequently, an independent interpreter told the ward staff that the patient had been made redundant from his job 6 months beforehand, and had felt unwell ever since. His misery was compounded by the reaction of his family, who no longer treated him with any respect, and among whom he had become a figure of ridicule.

If hospitalisation is necessary, close contact with family and friends is particularly important in non-English speaking patients, in order to avoid problems of loneliness and isolation. In addition to dealing with psychiatric problems in the index patient, help and support should also be provided for other family members where appropriate.

SUMMARY

1. **Transcultural psychiatry** is concerned with the study of mental disorder in different cultures. Major psychiatric disorder is recognised worldwide with some degree of conformity, although cultural factors can greatly influence the manner in which an individual displays emotion or responds to stress. Consequently, the latter can be readily misinterpreted as signs of mental illness if knowledge of cultural norms is poor. Psychiatric disorders can also be modified by cultural effects. A familiarity with differing modes of presentation is important when dealing with patients from ethnic communities, in order to maintain diagnostic accuracy and offer appropriate help.

2. Several (but not all) studies have shown that the rate of **psychiatric disorder among immigrants** is generally higher than that in the indigenous population. This may be related to stress factors operating before, during or after migration. These include the circumstances of migration, the degree of social deprivation and isolation experienced in the adopted country, and the extent of integration into local community life.

3. Effective **management** of psychiatric disorders among immigrants and ethnic minorities relies on an understanding of the presenting problem in the context of the individual's personal, cultural and social background. Where possible, use should be made of trained interpreters to overcome language barriers.

REFERENCES AND FURTHER READING

Cochrane, R. (1977). Mental illness in immigrants to England and Wales. An analysis of mental hospital admissions 1971. *Social Psychiatry*; **12**: 25–35.

Lipsedge, M., Littlewood, R. (1979). Transcultural psychiatry. In *Recent Advances in Clinical Psychiatry-3* (Granville-Grossman, K. L., ed.) pp. 91–134. Edinburgh: Churchill Livingstone.

London, M. (1986). Mental illness amongst immigrant minorities in the United Kingdom. *British Journal of Psychiatry*; **149**: 265–73.

Ødegaard, O. (1932). Emigration and insanity. *Acta Psychiatrica et Neurologica Scandinavica*; supplement 4.

World Health Organization (1973). *The International Pilot Study of Schizophrenia, Volume 1*. Geneva: WHO.

23 UNCOMMON PSYCHIATRIC SYNDROMES

A number of interesting, but relatively rare, psychiatric syndromes exist, which may occur in isolation, or as part of another mental disorder. Some of the conditions have been described universally, while others are culture-bound.

CAPGRAS SYNDROME

The central feature of this condition is a delusional belief held by the subject that a person close to him (most commonly a spouse) has been replaced by an exact double. The majority of recorded cases have been females, and the symptom is often part of a paranoid disorder such as schizophrenia, although it can also occur in affective and organic psychoses. Treatment is of the underlying illness, but despite this the belief often persists, so that prognosis tends to be poor.

FOLIE À DEUX

This disorder involves the 'transfer' of delusional beliefs between two (or sometimes more) people, who have usually lived together in close proximity for a considerable length of time. Psychotic symptoms initially develop in the dominant member of the pair, and these gradually become adopted by the other, who is characteristically passive and suggestible. Folie à deux between mother and daughter or between two sisters are the types most commonly described, and often the pair live in isolation, having little contact with the outside world. Separating the couple usually results in the spontaneous resolution of symptoms in the passive member, and appropriate treatment can then be given to the other person.

MORBID JEALOUSY (OTHELLO SYNDROME)

Shakespeare's character Othello epitomises the psychopathology of this condition, in which the subject (usually male) holds delusional beliefs of infidelity directed towards his spouse or sexual partner. Those who develop this syndrome may have suspicious or obsessional premorbid personalities, although the onset of the delusion is frequently sudden and explosive. The subject commonly accuses his partner of having been unfaithful, citing trivial or totally improbable evidence accumulated over a period of time to substantiate his claims. He may submit her to a relentless and prolonged ordeal, ceaselessly interrogating her for hours on end, repeatedly examining underwear or bed clothing for seminal stains, and even resorting to violence in an attempt to extract a confession. Around 5% of cases end in homicidal acts, so that the gravity of this condition should not be underestimated.

Separation of the couple is often necessary to protect the spouse, sometimes by compulsory detention of the patient in hospital. Although it can occur in isolation, morbid jealousy more commonly arises as part of another psychiatric disorder, such as schizophrenia, alcohol abuse or a depressive illness. The response to treatment is variable depending upon the underlying pathology, but even when full recovery ensues, the condition has a tendency to recur.

DE CLÉRAMBAULT'S SYNDROME

Otherwise known as 'pure erotomania', this disorder usually occurs in females and is characterised by the subject's delusional belief that a man, often famous or of high social standing, is in love with her. In reality, she is not personally acquainted with him, and his position in life is such that he is totally inaccessible as an object of love. Nevertheless, the woman frequently considers her life incomplete without her 'suitor' and, as a consequence, she may crave an intimate relationship with him. 'Victims' of this unrequited passion may be royalty, politicians, show business personalities, doctors or priests. The man is often relentlessly pursued and pestered by the subject, so that his life and that of his family become intolerable. Hospitalisation of the patient is sometimes necessary to prevent further harassment and treatment with neuroleptic drugs may be helpful. However, the condition commonly follows a chronic course and prognosis is usually poor.

COTARD'S SYNDROME

The main feature of this syndrome is a false belief held by the subject that some person or object no longer exists. Such nihilistic delusions can encompass convictions that he or his family are dead, the world has been destroyed, or parts of his body do not function or are no longer present. Beliefs of this type are sometimes associated with delusions of ruination, poverty and guilt. Cotard's syndrome is more common in females and is most likely to develop in the setting of a severe depressive illness, although it has also been described as occurring in schizophrenia and organic states. Treatment is of the underlying condition.

EKBOM'S SYNDROME

This disorder is characterised by delusions of infestation, in which the individual believes that his body or his immediate surroundings are overrun with insects or parasites. It sometimes occurs as an encapsulated symptom, but is more frequently part of a paranoid or depressive illness.

GANSER SYNDROME

Sometimes referred to as 'prison psychosis', Ganser syndrome is thought to be an example of an hysterical dissociative state (*see* p. 67). It is characterised by the giving of approximate answers to elementary and well-known questions, such as 'How many legs does a dog have?' Answer: 'Five'; or 'How many days in the week are there?' Answer: 'Eight'. Other features include apparent clouding of consciousness (in which there is impairment of concentration, attention and memory), anxious mood, conversion symptoms and pseudohallucinations. Its sudden onset in relation to stressful events has led some authorities to the conclusion that the presentation is a skilful form of malingering rather than a dissociative state. This is said to account for its seemingly increased frequency among certain groups who might profit from such behaviour (e.g. prisoners). Whatever the cause of the symptoms, recovery is usually rapid and spontaneous once the source of stress is removed.

COUVADE SYNDROME

This condition derives its name from the ancient ritual of 'couvade', in which the husband confined himself to bed and imitated labour pains during his wife's delivery. The syndrome occurs during a woman's pregnancy, when her partner may develop symptoms of anxiety, vomiting, abdominal distension (due to excessive air swallowing) and pain. Treatment is usually effected by simple reassurance and the prognosis is good.

MÜNCHAUSEN SYNDROME

This disorder is named after the eighteenth century fictional character Baron Münchausen, who was renowned for his travels and recounting of fantastic stories. The syndrome is most common in young men and involves the persistent simulation of illness, resulting in frequent hospital admissions. Three characteristic features are described: pathological lying, exaggeration of symptoms and wandering from one hospital to another. The individual often willingly subjects himself to various investigations and treatments, some possibly invasive, following which he is likely to discharge himself against medical advice. 'Patients' may be detected by their use of various aliases in casualty departments, evidence of multiple laparotomy scars, or through inappropriate requests for narcotic analgesia.

Illness is simulated in a number of ways which can include swallowing foreign bodies or emetics, using animal blood to mimic haemorrhage, traumatising the skin to produce the appearance of disease, or pretending to suffer from an extensive variety of physical or psychiatric symptoms. Some consider the syndrome as a manifestation of a severe psychopathic personality disorder, while others have postulated hysterical mechanisms to account for the behaviour. Treatment is usually difficult and ineffective, mainly because those concerned rarely stay in one place long enough to be engaged in a therapeutic relationship.

Münchausen syndrome 'by proxy' (Meadow's syndrome) is a recently described variant in which a parent (most commonly the mother) repeatedly seeks medical attention for her child using non-existent symptoms or deliberately induced signs as an excuse. For example, episodes of fictitious rectal bleeding may be described, or the child given an emetic to cause vomiting.

GILLES DE LA TOURETTE SYNDROME

Features of this disorder include multiple motor tics (most frequently facial) associated with uncontrollable utterances, which are often of an obscene nature (coprolalia), as well as echopraxia and echolalia. Most cases have an onset in late childhood, occurring mainly in boys of normal intelligence, although the condition tends to run a life-long course. Symptoms are worse under conditions of stress, but cease during sleep and can be voluntarily modified. Although the aetiology remains unknown, behavioural modification can help to reduce the frequency of tics, while treatment with haloperidol may also be beneficial in controlling abnormal movements and coprolalia.

CULTURE-BOUND SYNDROMES

A number of unusual psychiatric disorders are specific to certain cultural groups.

Latah most commonly occurs in Malaysian women and is thought to be a form of hysteria. The subject enters a trance-like state in reaction to a stressful event, following which features of automatic behaviour are exhibited, associated with echolalia and echopraxia. Similar disorders are described among inhabitants of Arctic regions, where they are known as **Myriachit** (Siberia) and **Piblokto** (Eskimos).

Amok is an hysterical fugue state which occurs in men from South-East Asia. A period of social withdrawal develops in reaction to stress, and is followed by an outburst of frenzied and violent behaviour, during which homicidal acts may occur or suicide is attempted.

Koro is a condition primarily affecting young men in South China or Malaysia. It is thought to be an acute anxiety reaction in which the individual expresses the fear that his penis is shrinking into his abdomen, and that as a result he will die. Treatment is said to involve tying a piece of string around the phallus (preferably held by a female relative) in order to prevent its disappearance!

Windigo occurs in North American Indians and is regarded as a form of depressive psychosis. The subject has a delusional belief that he has turned into a cannibalistic monster, and subsequently may attempt to act on this conviction.

Possession states are most commonly seen among primitive cultures in Third World countries. The sufferer believes that he is possessed by an alien spirit, which may cause his demise (**voodoo death**). Because of the widespread cultural belief in such powers, it is debatable as to whether or not such ideas can be considered delusional. **Glossolalia** ('speaking in tongues') is an interesting variant of possession characterised by spontaneous nonsensical speech which the subject does not seem to knowingly initiate, and is often attributed to divine influence. It is probably a dissociative phenomenon.

REFERENCES AND FURTHER READING

Asher, R. (1951). Münchausen's syndrome. *Lancet*; **i**: 339–41.
Christodoulou, G. N. (1977). The syndrome of Capgras. *British Journal of Psychiatry*; **130**: 556–64.

Enoch, M. D., Trethowan, W. H. (1979). *Uncommon Psychiatric Syndromes*, 2nd edn. Bristol: Wright.

Leff, J. (1981). *Psychiatry Around the Globe: a Transcultural View*. New York: Marcel Dekker.

O'Shea, B., McGennis, A., Cahill, M., Falvey, J. (1984). Münchausen's syndrome. *British Journal of Hospital Medicine*; **31**: 269–74

Singer, H. S. (1982). Tics and Tourette syndrome. *Johns Hopkins Medical Journal*; **151**: 30–35.

24

PSYCHIATRY
AND THE LAW

Most people in need of psychiatric care readily accept help, and if this entails inpatient treatment, they enter hospital on a voluntary basis with the freedom to leave of their own volition. Occasionally, however, a person's mental state or behaviour may give others cause for concern, while the subject remains adamant that he neither wants nor needs psychiatric help. Of course, not everyone seen under such circumstances proves to be mentally disordered, but of those who are, some will need to be compulsorily detained in hospital under the provisions of the Mental Health Act, either in the interests of their own health or safety, or for the protection of others.

Mental health legislation is also concerned with mentally disordered people who appear before the courts in violation of either criminal or civil law. This area is the remit of the **forensic psychiatrist**, who specialises in the assessment and treatment of the mentally abnormal offender, although many general psychiatrists are also involved in such work.

MENTAL HEALTH LEGISLATION

From earliest times, punishment played an important part in the treatment of mental illness, being used to drive out or kill evil spirits held responsible for the affliction. In 1714, Parliament passed a law allowing for the insane poor to be locked up if they were thought dangerous. Containment was achieved by chains, and corporal punishment was administered to coerce the patient into obedience.

Mechanical restraint remained the main form of treatment in 'madhouses' until the end of the eighteenth century, at which time a more humane approach was introduced at a few progressive institutions, where 'lunatics' were freed from their chains. During the nineteenth century, further reforms were introduced to improve the care of the mentally ill in England and Wales. These included the building of asylums by County Authorities and Government acceptance of financial responsibility for the admission of people to these institutions. However, it was not until 1915 that an Act of Parliament enabled the voluntary admission of psychiatric patients to mental hospitals.

The Mental Health Act of 1959 was a progressive piece of legislation which extended the rights of psychiatric patients so that they could receive treatment at any suitable hospital, and not just an asylum. Where possible, voluntary (informal) admission was seen as a priority, and throughout the course of the next decade the mental hospital population fell rapidly as patients were discharged back into the community.

In time, certain aspects of the 1959 Act proved unsatisfactory, and a growing concern with civil rights led to Parliament passing new legislation embodied in **The Mental Health Act 1983** for England and Wales. (Scotland has its own Act — the Mental Health (Scotland) Act 1984 — which has similar provisions for the detention of both civil and offender patients.) The main improvements were that it reduced the periods for which patients could be compulsorily detained in hospital and increased access for appeal against detention. The position on consent to treatment was clarified, and the conditions of patient care were safeguarded by the establishment of a new overseeing body, the Mental Health Act Commission. In addition, there were new provisions for the assessment and treatment of mentally abnormal offenders.

THE 1983 MENTAL HEALTH ACT

The Act is mainly concerned with the care and treatment of mentally disordered patients detained in hospital and those placed under guardianship. Various sections deal with compulsory admission procedures, the rights of patients to appeal against detention, and consent to treatment. Compulsory admission is only possible when the patient is suffering from one of four forms of **mental disorder**, which are defined in the Act. The powers of the courts are also specified when dealing with mentally disordered offenders (*see later*).

Definitions of Mental Disorder

Mental disorder is defined by the Act as one of the following:

1. mental illness
2. mental impairment
3. severe mental impairment
4. psychopathic disorder.

Mental illness is undefined, and remains a matter for clinical judgement in each case. **Mental impairment** and **severe mental impairment** (also known as mental retardation) refer to states of arrested or incomplete development of mind which include significant or severe impairment of intelligence and social functioning, and are associated with abnormally aggressive or seriously irresponsible conduct. (The distinction between the two is simply a matter of degree.) It is not possible to detain somebody in hospital who is mentally retarded, unless the behaviour which is part of their condition justifies the use of those powers (*see also* Chapter 18). **Psychopathic disorder** is defined as a persistent disorder or disability of mind (i.e. one which has existed for a considerable period of time) which results in abnormally aggressive or seriously irresponsible conduct. Evidence of significant impairment of intelligence may or may not be present (*see also* Chapter 3).

For the purposes of the Act, promiscuity, sexual deviance, other immoral conduct and dependence on alcohol or drugs alone are not considered forms of mental disorder. Although it is not permitted to detain someone in hospital simply because they abuse drugs or alcohol, if they are suffering from an associated mental disorder, such as depression or delirium tremens, then detention is possible provided other conditions are met.

Compulsory Admission Procedures

Compulsory admission to hospital of a person suffering from mental disorder may be necessary under certain circumstances, when their condition is in need of assessment or treatment. Details of formal admission procedures and the sections of the Mental Health Act which deal with the detention of voluntary inpatients are shown in Table 24.1.

Section 2 is a 28-day order allowing for the compulsory admission to hospital of an individual suffering from mental disorder for the purposes of assessment, which may be followed by treatment. **Section 3** is a 6-month order permitting the compulsory admission to hospital of an individual suffering from mental disorder in order to provide treatment. An application for invoking either of these orders is founded upon the written **medical recommendations** of two doctors, one an approved specialist and the other usually being the patient's general practitioner. Having both examined the subject, they must agree that a mental disorder is present of a nature or degree warranting hospital detention, which is necessary in the interests of the person's health or safety or for the protection of others. For patients detained under Section 3, the type of mental disorder must be specified, and in the case of psychopathic disorder or mental impairment, the treatment must be considered likely to alleviate or prevent a deterioration of the condition. Once the documentation has been completed, an **application** is made by the nearest relative or an approved social worker acting on his behalf to the managers of the admitting hospital. As soon as possible after admission, the patient should be informed of his legal status while detained, his right of appeal to a Mental

Health Review Tribunal, those who have the power to discharge him, and his position with regard to consent to treatment.

Section 4 is a 72-hour order used to admit a patient to hospital as an emergency and detain him for assessment. It only requires one medical recommendation by any registered doctor, as well as an application by the nearest relative or social worker. The grounds for detention are the same as those for Section 2, but it should only be implemented if an undesirable delay would be involved in obtaining the second medical recommendation (as required under Section 2).

Compulsory detention of those who are already in hospital as informal patients can be made under Sections 2 or 3, should this become necessary. An informal inpatient undergoing assessment or treatment (for either psychiatric or non-psychiatric conditions) can also be detained under **Section 5(2)** if, in the opinion of the responsible medical officer or his nominated deputy, an application for admission under Section 2 or 3 ought to be made. The patient may then be detained in hospital for up to 72 hours following the provision of a written report to the managers by the doctor.

Informal inpatients who are already being treated for mental disorder may require *immediate* restraint from leaving hospital, for their own health and safety or for the protection of others. Under **Section 5(4)**, an **approved nurse** can detain the patient for up to 6 hours where it is not possible for a doctor to attend immediately in order to implement Section 5(2).

Section 136 empowers a **police officer** to remove to a place of safety (such as a hospital) any person found in a public place who appears to be suffering from mental disorder, and is in need of immediate care and control in his own interests or for the protection of others. The duration of this order is up to 72 hours, during which time the detained person should be assessed by a doctor. Following this, alternative arrangements will be made, such as discharge home. informal admission to hospital or compulsory detention under Sections 2 or 3.

Section 135 empowers a police officer or other authorised person acting on a magistrate's warrant to enter premises to remove to a place of safety a person believed to be suffering from mental disorder, who is being ill-treated, neglected, or not under proper control, or who lives alone and is not able to care for himself. Detention is for up to 72 hours.

Guardianship

The purpose of guardianship is to ensure that, where necessary, mentally disordered people aged 16 or over receive proper care and protection while living in the community. The guardian may be named as the local social services authority (or an individual nominated by them) and has the following powers which require the patient to:

Table 24.1 Compulsory admission procedures

Section:	2	3	4	5 (2)	5 (4)	136
Duration*	28 days — not renewable	6 months — renewable	72 hours — not renewable	72 hours — not renewable	6 hours — not renewable	72 hours — not renewable
Purpose	Admission for assessment or assessment followed by treatment	Admission for treatment	Emergency admission for assessment	Compulsory detention of informal patients	Compulsory detention of informal patients	Removal to a place of safety
Grounds for detention	Mental disorder of a nature or degree which warrants detention in hospital for assessment, or assessment followed by treatment; detention is in the interest of the subject's own health or safety or for the protection of others	Mental disorder (the type being specified) of a nature or degree which warrants detention in hospital for treatment. In the case of psychopathic disorder or mental impairment, such treatment is likely to alleviate or prevent a deterioration of the condition;	As for Section 2, except that urgent detention is necessary, and complying with the provisions of Section 2 would involve undesirable delay	It appears that application for compulsory detention under Sections 2 or 3 ought to be made; the patient may be under psychiatric or non-psychiatric care at the time	Patient is suffering from mental disorder to such a degree that immediate restraint from leaving the hospital is necessary, for his health and safety or for the protection of others; it is not practicable for a doctor to attend immediately to detain under Section 5 (2)	A person found in a public place appears to be suffering from a mental disorder, and is thought to need immediate care and control in his own interests or for the protection of others
Medical recommendations	By two doctors, one of whom must be 'approved' as having special experience in the diagnosis or treatment of mental disorder (usually the consultant psychiatrist or his deputy), and the other who preferably has had previous acquaintance with the patient. Both doctors must have personally examined the patient within 5 days of each other and must state in writing their reasons why compulsory detention is necessary		By one doctor, who preferably has had previous acquaintance with the patient, and has seen him within the 24 hours preceding the recommendation	Responsible medical officer or his nominated deputy	None	None

continued overleaf

Table 24.1 *Continued*

Section	2	3	4	5 (2)	5 (4)	136
Application	By the nearest relative or an approved social worker acting on his behalf to the managers of the admitting hospital. The applicant must have seen the patient within 14 days prior to the date of the application		As for Sections 2 and 3, except that the applicant must have seen the patient within the 24 hours preceding the application	By the responsible medical officer or his nominated deputy to the hospital managers	By a registered mental nurse in writing to the hospital managers	By a police officer, who should remove the person to a designated place of safety (e.g. hospital)
Power of discharge	Responsible medical officer, hospital managers, nearest relative (can be overruled by RMO) or Mental Health Review Tribunal (MHRT)		Responsible medical officer or the hospital managers	Responsible medical officer only		Responsible medical officer or the hospital managers if the person is in hospital
Appeal to MHRT	Yes, by patient within the first 14 days of detention	Yes, by patient at any time during 6-month period. If section is renewed and no appeal has been made, then the case is automatically reviewed by MHRT	None	None	None	None

* The duration of detention shown for each section is a maximum, and the order can be terminated at any time beforehand, if it is considered appropriate to do so.

1. reside at a specified place
2. attend at specified places and times for medical treatment, occupation, education or training
3. allow certain specified people, such as doctors and approved social workers, access to his residence.

The duration of guardianship is for 6 months in the first instance; medical recommendation, application and renewal require the same procedures as for Section 3.

Mental Health Review Tribunals

Where a patient has the right of appeal against a compulsory order (*see* Table 24.1), his case will be heard by a Review Tribunal which will receive evidence from the detainee, his relatives and professionals involved in the case. The Tribunal members include an independent psychiatrist, a solicitor or other legally qualified person, a lay member and a secretary. After considering all the information made available, the Tribunal will either uphold the order or revoke it. The patient may be legally represented at the hearing.

The Mental Health Act Commission

This multidisciplinary body consists of doctors, lawyers, nurses, psychologists, social workers and lay members appointed by the Secretary of State. In addition to fulfilling administrative duties, such as appointing doctors to give second opinions, it also protects the interests of detained patients by regularly reviewing their care, and establishing a code of practice relating to treatment.

Mentally Abnormal Offenders

The Mental Health Act is also concerned with offenders who appear before the court for imprisonable offences (other than murder), and are either suspected or known to suffer from mental disorder.
Provision exists for:

1. remanding an accused person appearing before a Crown Court or convicted before a Magistrates' Court to hospital for up to 12 weeks for preparation of a report on his mental condition (**Section 35**)
2. remanding an accused person awaiting trial or sentencing before the Crown Court to hospital for up to 12 weeks for treatment (**Section 36**)
3. ordering hospital admission or reception into guardianship for 6 months of a person found guilty before a Crown Court or

Magistrates' Court (**Section 37**). If it is not certain that hospital admission is appropriate, an interim hospital order can be made (**Section 38**) lasting for 12 weeks and renewable every 28 days for up to 6 months. Where it is necessary to protect the public from serious harm (e.g. if the nature of the offence is very grave), an order restricting the date of discharge may be imposed by the Crown Court, either for a finite period, or more commonly without limit of time (**Section 41**)

4. transferring sentenced prisoners or those held on remand to hospital for treatment (**Sections 47 and 48**).

The assessment and treatment of mentally disordered offenders may be provided in ordinary psychiatric hospitals, or in the case of those who present a serious risk to the public, at a **Special Hospital**. These institutions (four in England, and one in Scotland) provide conditions of special security for patients considered to be too dangerous to be cared for elsewhere. **Interim secure units** are for detainees who require treatment in an environment of intermediate security between an ordinary and Special Hospital.

Consent to Treatment

A patient (whether voluntary or detained) is deemed capable of giving **informed consent** to treatment if he understands its nature, purpose and likely effects. In most instances, voluntary patients can only be treated with their consent, while detained patients can withdraw their consent at any time. In certain cases, treatment may be given even though the patient refuses or is incapable of giving consent. The Mental Health Act deals with four categories of psychiatric treatment:

1. TREATMENT FOR WHICH CONSENT IS NOT REQUIRED

(a) General treatments such as nursing care.
(b) Medication (oral or parenteral) given to patients detained under Section 2.
(c) Medication (oral or parenteral) given to patients detained under Sections 3, 36, 37 or 41 during the first 3 months of their detention, and thereafter (except Section 36), providing a concurring second medical opinion is obtained (*see below*).

2. TREATMENT FOR WHICH THE ISSUE OF CONSENT IS SET ASIDE

Urgent treatment (which is not irreversible or hazardous) can be given without consent to a detained patient* when it is immediately necessary to save life, prevent serious deterioration of health, alleviate serious suffering or prevent the patient behaving in a manner which is dangerous to himself or others.

3. TREATMENT FOR WHICH CONSENT OF THE PATIENT IS REQUIRED *OR* A SECOND MEDICAL OPINION MUST BE OBTAINED

This applies to ECT given at any time or medication (oral or parenteral) given after the first 3 months of detention under Sections 3, 37 or 41. If a detained patient refuses or is incapable of giving informed consent, a second opinion is required. This is provided by a doctor appointed by the Mental Health Act Commission, who will consult with the responsible medical officer and two other people professionally concerned with the patient, one of whom must be a nurse, and the other neither a doctor nor a nurse. If the Commission doctor is of the opinion that the treatment is necessary and likely to alleviate or prevent a deterioration of the patient's condition, he will certify that it may be given.

4. TREATMENT FOR WHICH CONSENT OF THE PATIENT IS REQUIRED *AND* A SECOND OPINION MUST BE OBTAINED

This covers psychosurgery or hormone implants given to reduce male sexual drive. If the patient refuses or is incapable of giving informed consent, the treatment cannot be given. Where the patient consents to the treatment (whether he is informal or detained), the Commission will send a doctor and two other non-medical persons to consider the validity of the patient's consent. If all three agree that the consent is valid, they will issue a certificate to this effect, following which the Commission doctor must take steps to establish the appropriateness of the treatment (*see above*).

---

* Urgent treatment given to detained patients under 72-hour orders, Section 35 or on conditional discharge is not covered by the Mental Health Act. As in the case of voluntary patients, it is administered under the auspices of Common Law.

PSYCHIATRIC ASPECTS OF CRIME

Delinquency

Nearly one-half of all crime committed in the UK is carried out by people aged between 10 and 21 years, the majority of whom are male and not suffering from any form of mental disorder. Subcultural influences such as peer pressure, social deprivation, substance abuse and an unstable family background, are the most important factors in the development of delinquent behaviour. However, of the minority who repeatedly offend (recidivists), a significant proportion are deemed to have severely deviant personalities or a history of psychiatric disturbance due to organic or functional illness.

The initial aim of management is to identify and treat any underlying psychiatric disorder. Psychotherapy may be helpful in changing antisocial attitudes and enhancing self-image, although custodial placement is often necessary to provide boundaries for acceptable behaviour.

Violent Behaviour and the Assessment of Dangerousness

Acts of violence occur in all age groups, but are most prevalent among young men. As with delinquent behaviour, social and cultural factors are important determinants, especially with regard to the disinhibiting effects of alcohol. However, acts of violence can occur in the context of all forms of mental illness, when abnormalities of mood, thought content or perception are sometimes the reasons for aggressive behaviour. Certain situations can precipitate violence in predisposed individuals, especially those with psychopathic or explosive personalities, who often have a low tolerance for stress.

The concept of **dangerousness** needs to be considered when assessing the likelihood of further violent behaviour. The best predictor is a past history of repeated violence; other indicators include a lack of remorse, persistent use of alcohol or drugs, evidence of sadistic fantasies and pastimes, and a family background of violence or child abuse. Consideration also needs to be given to the circumstances of the offence and the events which led up to it (especially the role of the victim), as well as the offender's personality and mental state at that time.

Homicide

Murder is defined as unlawful killing with 'malice aforethought', whereas **manslaughter** is a similar act without guilty intent (such as a 'hit and run' road traffic accident). **Infanticide** is a separate offence relating to the unlawful killing of a child under the age of 12 months by its mother. All three crimes are categories of **homicide.** There are approximately 500 murders each year in England and Wales, most of the perpetrators being male and the majority of the victims female. Alcohol is involved in nearly one-half of all cases and 75% of murder victims either know or are closely related to the killer. It is thought that between 10 and 30% of murderers commit suicide after the crime. Approximately one-half of those found guilty of murder are deemed to be mentally disordered on account of psychopathic personality disorder, depressive illness, paranoid psychosis or mental impairment.

Rape

Rape is 'sexual intercourse with a woman who at the time did not consent to the act, the man knowing that she did not consent, or being reckless as to whether or not she consented'. The prevalence of rape is difficult to determine because many cases are never reported, but it is thought to be on the increase. Most rapists are young and unmarried, often with a previous record of non-sexual offences and, in the majority of cases, are not mentally ill. However, abnormal personality traits are frequently encountered, particularly those involving aggressive, antisocial and sadistic tendencies. Otherwise shy and inhibited men may rape as a consequence of frustrated sexual impulses. About one-third of rapists are previously known to their victim, and a proportion of acts are committed under the influence of alcohol. In most cases, there is some degree of additional violence, ranging from intimidation and threats to severe brutality. Of convicted rapists, 80% receive prison sentences and the vast majority do not re-offend. Other sexual offences (paedophilia, incest and indecent exposure) are discussed in Chapter 19.

Arson

Arson is defined as the unlawful damage or destruction of property by fire. The majority of arsonists are young men; in some cases a political or financial motive may be apparent, or there is intention of self-harm or revenge. Other acts of fire-setting are committed by mentally disordered individuals suffering from schizophrenia, affective disorders, drug- or alcohol-induced states, organic brain disease or mental impairment. A third rare group, almost exclusively male, are known as **pyromaniacs,** who commit repeated acts of arson without any apparent motive. Some admit to release of tension by their behaviour, while others become excited or sexually aroused by watching a fire. Management is difficult and is primarily aimed at treating any underlying psychiatric disorder, although in pyromania the prognosis is poor.

Shoplifting

This is a relatively common offence which, in older age groups, is mainly committed by women, although under the age of 21 males predominate. Transient shoplifting in adolescence is thought by some to be a 'normal' phase of development, while habitual offenders are either 'professionals' (who consider it their livelihood) or compulsive shoplifters (who steal indiscriminately, but find the experience emotionally gratifying). Psychiatric disorder is uncommon, although the offence can occur in the setting of an affective illness, eating disorder or alcohol abuse. Shoplifting is also sometimes a reaction to emotional stress and constitutes a 'plea for help', particularly among middle-aged women. Management should initially involve treating any identifiable psychiatric disorder, while behaviour modification may be of use in those who shoplift compulsively.

Criminal Responsibility and Psychiatric Defences

Individuals who are charged with certain serious criminal offences, and are suspected or known to be mentally disordered, may have to stand trial. In order to secure a conviction, the prosecution must prove that the accused committed the offence (**actus reus**) and was capable of acting other than he did, this forming the basis of guilty intent (**mens rea**). If both are demonstrated to the court's satisfaction, then **criminal responsibility** is proven. Any accused person over the age of 14 is presumed to be fully responsible for his actions, unless shown otherwise.

Although *actus reus* is rarely disputed, in many cases where the accused is mentally disordered, guilty intent at the time of the offence is questionable and various **psychiatric defences** may be put forward:

1. UNFIT TO PLEAD

The question of whether an individual accused of a serious crime is fit to plead can be raised by the judge or counsel. In order to be able to do so, he must be capable of:

(a) understanding the nature of the charge against him
(b) appreciating the significance of his plea
(c) instructing counsel
(d) following the course of the trial
(e) challenging a juror.

The issue is decided by a jury, and if found unfit, the individual is usually admitted to a Special Hospital, until such time as the Home Secretary decides he is fit to plead.

2. 'NOT GUILTY BY REASON OF INSANITY' (SPECIAL VERDICT)

This plea is usually applied when the accused is charged with murder, but is now rarely used. It was first introduced following the trial of Daniel McNaughton, a paranoid schizophrenic, who shot dead the Prime Minister's secretary in 1843 while labouring under delusions of persecution. Also known as **McNaughton's rules**, the Special Verdict states that an individual was 'labouring under such a defect of reason from disease of the mind, as not to know the nature and quality of the act he was doing, or if he did know it, that he did not know what he was doing was wrong. If the plea is successful, the person is usually sent to a Special Hospital, the time of release being decided by the Home Secretary.

3. DIMINISHED RESPONSIBILITY

This defence can only be used if the charge is murder, and states that the person was 'suffering from such abnormality of mind as substantially impaired his mental responsibility for his acts . . .'. If the plea is successful, the charge of murder is reduced to one of manslaughter, sentencing being at the discretion of the judge.

4. AUTOMATISM

Rarely, criminal acts are judged to have taken place during an automatism (*see* p. 175), as a result of which the defendant is not held responsible for his behaviour.

5. AMNESIA

Although this is not in itself a defence, the underlying cause might be so judged (e.g. a post-traumatic state).

Mental Disorder in the Prison Population

Psychiatric disturbance is frequent among prisoners, and one study conducted in an English gaol found that nearly one-third of all detainees suffered from some form of mental disorder. The commonest conditions were alcohol and drug dependence, mental retardation and psychopathic personality disorder, although functional psychoses and organic conditions (such as epilepsy) were also more prevalent than in the general population. The reasons for this finding remain unclear, although various explanations have been put forward. These include suggestions that the mentally disordered are more inclined to break the law or be apprehended, or that psychotropic drugs increase the likelihood of criminal behaviour. The stress of imprisonment may act as a precipitant of mental disorder in predisposed individuals.

CIVIL LAW

This deals with the individual's rights and responsibilities in relation to other people, and may concern the psychiatrist in a number of ways.

Testamentary capacity refers to the ability of an individual to make a valid will, in that the testator must be of 'sound disposing mind'. To do this, he should know the nature and extent of his property, the persons having a claim on it, and the relative strengths of their entitlement. In addition, he must be able to express himself clearly and without ambiguity, understand the nature of the act of making a will and its effects, and not be influenced by any abnormal mental state which might distort his judgement. The psychiatrist may be asked for an opinion in the event of testamentary capacity being questioned because of suspected mental disorder. Even if this is found to be present, it does not automatically preclude the person from making a valid will, provided his condition does not interfere with the criteria listed above. Therefore, someone suffering from early dementia or a paranoid psychosis may still be of 'sound disposing mind'.

Contracts made by persons of unsound mind are not necessarily binding if it is shown that the agreement would not have been entered into but for the presence of insanity. Consequently, a marriage may be nullified if the point in question can be proven in the Divorce Court. **Torts** refer to civil actions, such as libel, slander and trespass, and when brought against a person of unsound mind, are likely to result in only minimal damages being awarded by a court.

The **Court of Protection** is sometimes called upon to manage the affairs and property of mentally disordered persons, when they are unable to do so themselves. Application to the court is usually by a relative or close friend, and must be supported by medical evidence of incapacity. A Receiver is then appointed, with powers to act on behalf of the individual concerned.

SUMMARY

1. The **1983 Mental Health Act** is mainly concerned with the care and treatment of mentally disordered patients detained in hospital, and the powers of the courts when dealing with mentally abnormal offenders. The

four forms of mental disorder defined by the Act are mental illness, mental impairment, severe mental impairment and psychopathic disorder. Various sections of the Act give details of compulsory admission procedures, guardianship orders, the rights of appeal against detention, consent to treatment and the detention of mentally disordered offenders. The functions of the Mental Health Act Commission are also outlined.

2. Most **delinquent behaviour** is not attributable to mental disorder, although a number of recidivists are deemed to have deviant personalities or a history of psychiatric disturbance. Acts of **violence** are occasionally the result of mental illness, although social and cultural factors (especially alcohol) are the usual precipitants. The concept of **dangerousness** needs to be considered when assessing the likelihood of further violent behaviour, the best predictor of which is a past history of repeated acts of aggression, although other factors must also be taken into account. There are approximately 500 **murders** per annum in England and Wales, nearly half being committed under the influence of alcohol. Most of the perpetrators are male and the majority of their victims female. Approximately 50% of those convicted of murder are found to be mentally disordered. Most **rapists** are young and unmarried, and the majority are not found to be mentally ill, although abnormal personality traits are commonly encountered. Intimidation or violence are frequently used to force the victim into submission. **Arson** is a crime predominantly committed by young men. It may be clearly motivated (e.g. financial gain or revenge), carried out as a result of mental disorder, or apparently motiveless and used as a means of releasing tension or creating sexual arousal. **Shoplifting** is a relatively common offence, which occasionally occurs as a result of psychiatric disorder or as a reaction to emotional stress.

3. **Criminal responsibility** rests upon proving that an accused person carried out an unlawful act (*actus reus*), as well as demonstrating guilty intent (*mens rea*) at that time. Where the latter is questioned due to mental disorder, various psychiatric defences may be presented which include unfitness to plead, automatism, diminished responsibility and not guilty by reason of insanity. Psychiatric disturbance is frequently encountered among **prisoners**, although the reasons for this remain unclear.

4. The psychiatrist may be asked for an opinion with respect to certain aspects of **civil law**, such as an individual's testamentary capacity, the validity of contracts entered into by mentally disordered persons, and the ability of such a person to handle his own affairs.

REFERENCES AND FURTHER READING

Bluglass, R. (1979). The psychiatric assessment of homicide. *British Journal of Hospital Medicine*; **22**: 366–77.

Bowden, P. (1978). Rape. *British Journal of Hospital Medicine*; **20**: 286–90.

Fisher, C. (1984). Psychiatric aspects of shoplifting. *British Journal of Hospital Medicine*; **31**: 209–12.

Gunn, J. (1979). Forensic psychiatry. In *Recent Advances in Clinical Psychiatry-3* (Granville-Grossman, K. L., ed.) pp. 271–95. Edinburgh: Churchill Livingstone.

Hamilton, J. R. (1983). The Mental Health Act, 1983. *British Medical Journal*; **286**: 1720–25.

Her Majesty's Stationery Office (1983). *The Mental Health Act 1983*. London: HMSO.

Scott, D. (1978). The problems of malicious fire raising. *British Journal of Hospital Medicine*; **19**: 259–63.

Scott, P. D. (1977). Assessing dangerousness in criminals. *British Journal of Psychiatry*; **131**: 127–42.

GLOSSARY

(Cross-referenced terms are shown in italics)

AA (*see Alcoholics Anonymous*).

Abreaction a method of bringing about the unrestrained expression of emotion to relieve mental distress. The process can be facilitated by lowering levels of arousal using suggestion, *hypnosis*, or an intravenous sedative drug.

Accident neurosis *see post-traumatic stress disorder*.

Acting out in *psychotherapy*, the conveyance of feelings in actions rather than words.

Actus reus a legal term for the performance of an unlawful act (*see also mens rea*).

Acute confusional state a term sometimes used synonymously with *acute organic reaction*.

Acute intermittent porphyria an inherited defect of haemoglobin metabolism, resulting in the excessive formation of the metabolite, porphobilinogen. Gastrointestinal and neurological symptoms may occur spontaneously, or can be precipitated by infection or certain drugs. Psychiatric complications include lability of mood, perplexity, *delirium* and schizophrenic-like psychoses.

Acute organic reaction a disorder in which the central clinical feature is impairment in the level of consciousness. The onset of the condition is usually rapid and it tends to run a fluctuating course, lasting at most a few weeks. Impaired consciousness can be further distorted by perceptual abnormalities and changes in mood, when the disorder is known as a *delirium*. Evidence of underlying structural brain damage is uncommon. In most cases, the disorder resolves spontaneously or is potentially reversible, although some can progress to a chronic irreversible stage (*see also organic psychiatry*).

Acute schizophrenia a disorder often characterised by the *positive symptoms of schizophrenia* (Schneider's *first rank symptoms*, other *delusions* and *hallucinations, thought disorder, catatonic* symptoms and *incongruity of affect*). The term 'acute' signifies symptom content as well as the course of the illness (*see also chronic schizophrenia*).

Adoption studies studies concerned with children who have been reared since early infancy by non-related adoptive parents. They are a useful method of determining the influence of genetic factors in the causation of mental disorders (*see also twin studies*).

Aetiology the science of the causation of disease.

Affect emotion which is expressed in observable behaviour, such as general manner or tone of voice (*see also mood*).

Affective disorder disorder of *affect* or *mood*, especially those involving depression and elation.

Affective personality a disorder of mood control persisting throughout life which includes: depressive personality — a tendency to gloominess and pessimism, unwarranted worrying, constant misery and diminished capacity for enjoyment; hyperthymic personality — persistent optimism and cheerfulness (irrespective of the circumstances), rashness and lack of judgement; cyclothymic personality — a tendency to alternate between depressive and hyperthymic forms.

Agnosia 'perception stripped of meaning'. The defect cannot be explained by sensory impairment, mental deterioration or disorders of consciousness and attention. It usually results from parietal lobe dysfunction, and can be tested for by demonstrating an inability to recognise objects visually (visual agnosia) or by touch (astereognosis), familiar faces (prosopagnosia), sounds (auditory agnosia), the position of an object on the skin (topognosia), numbers or letters written on the skin (agraphognosia), disability caused by disease (anosognosia) and certain parts of the body (such as finger agnosia).

Agoraphobia literally 'a fear of the market place'. It is clinically used in a wider context to include individuals who become anxious or afraid in crowds, when they travel on public transport or in lifts, go shopping or leave the safety of their own homes. The fear is often heightened in situations which cannot be easily left, such as a crowded room.

Agraphognosia *see agnosia.*

Akathisia an *extrapyramidal motor disturbance* associated with the administration of *neuroleptic drugs* which involves motor restlessness, particularly in the legs. There may be an accompanying psychological sense of tension.

Al-anon an affiliated group of *Alcoholics Anonymous* which provides support for the families of problem drinkers.

Alcohol dependence syndrome (alcoholism) characterised by (1) narrowing of the drinking repertoire, (2) increased tolerance to alcohol; (3) prominence of drink-seeking behaviour; (4) repeated withdrawal symptoms; (5) relief or avoidance of withdrawal symptoms by further drinking; (6) subjective awareness of loss of control over drinking; and (7) reinstatement after abstinence.

Alcoholic blackouts total loss of memory for specific events during heavy bouts of drinking, even though at the time the subject may appear fully conscious, and is behaving and conversing normally. Amnesia also occurs with very high levels of blood alcohol, when consciousness is grossly impaired.

Alcoholic hallucinosis an uncommon condition associated with alcohol abuse, in which *auditory hallucinations* occur in a setting of clear consciousness. They often commence with simple sounds such as buzzing, gradually evolving into voices which may be in the second or third person. The content is usually deprecatory or threatening and paranoid delusions can develop.

Alcoholics 'those excessive drinkers whose *dependence* on alcohol has attained such a degree that it shows noticeable disturbance or an interference with their bodily and mental health, their personal relationships and smooth economic functioning, or who show prodromal signs of such a development. They therefore require treatment.'

Alcoholics Anonymous (AA) a 'self-help' organisation for *dependent drinkers* and those with alcohol-related problems. The philosophy of 'AA' has now spread worldwide and promotes a policy of total abstinence from alcohol, while encouraging members to adopt an approach of 'one day at a time' in order to overcome their problems. Simple advice and mutual support are offered at group meetings which members are encouraged to attend on a regular basis.

Alexithymia a mechanism of unconsciously communicating distress to relatives or doctors by way of physical symptoms in those who have difficulty in expressing their feelings verbally.

Alzheimer's disease a disorder arising from a primary degenerative process within the brain. It is the most frequently encountered form of *presenile dementia*, with an age of onset between 40 and 60 years and a female to male ratio of 2:1. The pathological changes, clinical features and prognosis are otherwise almost identical to those of *SDAT*.

Ambitendency a feature of *catatonia* characterised by the subject making a series of hesitant and incomplete movements when expected to perform a voluntary action (e.g. repeatedly extending and withdrawing the hand when the examiner offers to shake hands).

Amentia a synonym for *mental retardation*.

Amitriptyline a *monoamine reuptake inhibitor* antidepressant which belongs to the *tricyclic* group.

Amok an hysterical *fugue* state which occurs in men from South-East Asia. A period of social withdrawal develops in reaction to stress, and is followed by an outburst of frenzied and violent behaviour, during which homicidal acts may occur or suicide is attempted.

Amotivational syndrome described in association with chronic *cannabis* abuse, resulting in a persistent loss of drive and apathy.

Amphetamine psychosis a disorder related to amphetamine abuse in which paranoid delusions and hallucinations occur. The illness is sometimes indistinguishable from *acute schizophrenia*, but usually abates as the effects of the drug wear off.

Amphetamines a group of drugs which are central nervous system stimulants and are widely abused for their 'mood-elevating' properties. They produce psychological, but not physical dependence.

Anal stage (of personality development) – according to Freud, the phase which begins around the second year of life, at which time pleasure is derived by the act of retaining or expelling faeces.

Analytical psychology a school of thought founded by the Swiss psychiatrist Carl Jung, who was an early follower of Freud, but later split from him to form his own movement.

Anankastic personality see *obsessional personality*.

Anhedonia an inability to experience pleasure from normally enjoyable activities or pursuits, which is characteristically a symptom of *depression*.

Anima according to Jung, the unconscious feminine side of the man's *persona*.

Animus according to Jung, the unconscious masculine side of the woman's *persona*.

Anorexia nervosa a disorder most commonly affecting females, the central psychopathology of which is a morbid fear of fatness. As a consequence, high-calorie foods (especially carbohydrates) are avoided, which in turn leads to substantial weight loss, resulting in a body weight more than 25% below normal. Associated endocrine changes also occur, producing amenorrhoea in females and loss of libido and impotence in males.

Anorgasmia in women, the persistent inability to achieve orgasm despite adequate desire and arousal.

Anosognosia *see agnosia.*

Anterograde amnesia in the case of trauma, the memory impairment occurring between injury and the return of normal, continuous memory (*see posttraumatic amnesia*). It may also occur in other organic conditions, such as *Korsakoff's psychosis.*

Anticholinergic drugs medication sometimes used to counter the *extrapyramidal* effects of *neuroleptic drugs.*

Antidepressant a drug prescribed mainly for the treatment of *depression*, although certain compounds may be useful in the management of *anxiety states, phobias, obsessive-compulsive neurosis* and childhood bed-wetting.

Antipsychotic drugs used in the treatment of *functional* and *organic psychoses* (*see also neuroleptic drugs*).

Anxiety an emotional state with the subjectively experienced quality of fear.

Anxiety state a disorder in which *anxiety* increases to the point where, by reasonable standards, it is out of proportion to a provoking stimulus and is said to be 'pathological'. Anxiety states may be generalised and persistent or occur in the form of unpredictable *panic attacks.*

Anxiolytic a drug used to lower arousal in *anxiety states.*

Approved doctor (practitioner) for the purposes of the *Mental Health Act 1983*, one who is approved by the Secretary of State as having special experience in the diagnosis or treatment of *mental disorder.*

Approved social worker for the purposes of the *Mental Health Act 1983*, one who is appointed by a local social services authority as having appropriate competence in dealing with persons who are suffering from *mental disorder* (*see psychiatric social worker*).

Apraxia the inability to perform voluntary movements in the absence of motor or sensory deficit. It can manifest as dressing apraxia (inability to dress oneself), constructional apraxia (inability to copy or construct three-dimensional figures), ideomotor apraxia (the inability to copy a complex task, such as striking a match) and ideational apraxia (the inability to execute complex instructions — 'show me how you would light a cigarette').

Archetypes according to Jung, aspects of the *collective unconscious* can enter the conscious mind in the form of symbols or archetypes, which then influence thought and behaviour.

Arson the unlawful damage or destruction of property by fire (*see also pyromaniac*).

Arteriosclerotic dementia *see multi-infarct dementia.*

Assertiveness training a behavioural treatment which can be of help to those who lack confidence and have difficulty in expressing themselves in a variety of social situations (*see also social skills training*).

Asthenic personality characterised by features which may include lack of willpower, side-stepping responsibility, undue compliance with the wishes of others and over-dependence on other people.

Athetosis slow, writhing involuntary movements, usually most prominent in the fingers and hands, although the face, neck and feet may be involved.

Attachment the normal tendency of a young child to seek close contact with particular individuals, and to feel secure in their presence (*see also bonding*).

Attention the ability to focus on a current situation.

Audible thoughts the repetition (in the form of *auditory hallucinations*) of thoughts which have occurred a short time before, so that the individual experiences voices speaking his thoughts aloud. It is a *first rank symptom of schizophrenia*, and the experience is also sometimes referred to as thought echo.

Auditory agnosia *see agnosia*.

Auditory hallucinations false perceptions which occur in the absence of any external stimulus, in the form of voices, music or noises (*see also hallucinations*).

Aura a phase sometimes experienced immediately before an epileptic attack, which may involve *perceptual abnormalities*, mood changes and feelings of unreality, including the phenomenon of *déjà vu*.

Autism, infantile a syndrome which has a recognised onset before the age of 30 months, and affects two to four children in every 10 000. Those affected demonstrate autistic aloneness, impaired communication and difficulty in coping with change (a desire for sameness). Additional features may include abnormal body movements and self-mutilation. Most autistic children are intellectually impaired with an IQ below 70, and the prognosis is generally poor.

Autochthonous delusion *see primary delusion*.

Automatic obedience a feature of *catatonia* characterised by a robot-like response to all commands, however silly and irrespective of the consequences. Asking a patient to hold out his hand and then pricking it with a pin would not deter him from endlessly repeating the action if requested.

Automatism the performance of simple or complex actions in a state of clouded consciousness, so that the subject is unaware of his behaviour. It is most commonly a feature of epilepsy.

Autonomic nervous system the division of the nervous system controlling involuntary functions.

Aversion therapy a behavioural technique which aims to reduce maladaptive behaviour by associating it with an unpleasant experience, such as pain or a noxious smell.

Barbiturates a group of drugs which are central nervous system depressants, widely used in the past as *sedatives* and *anxiolytics*, but now mainly as a substance of abuse.

Behaviour therapy a method of treatment which is aimed at improving a patient's functioning and well-being by a direct change in behaviour.

Bell and pad enuresis alarm a device used in the treatment of nocturnal *enuresis*. It consists of two mesh or foil pads separated by a sheet, each of which is connected to a buzzer. When urine starts to be voided, the circuit is completed and a bell sounds, waking the child and his parents.

Benzamide derivatives a group of drugs (including Sulpiride) which confer a theoretical advantage over other *neuroleptic drugs*, in that they selectively block D2 (dopamine) receptors with only minimal activity at D1 sites. Consequently, they should produce antipsychotic actions without the development of extrapyramidal side-effects, although this has yet to be confirmed in practice.

Benzodiazepines a group of drugs which are central nervous system depressants.

In addition to their *anxiolytic* and *hypnotic* effects, they are muscle relaxants and have anticonvulsant properties. They are used in the treatment of *anxiety states*, insomnia, for the control of epileptic fits and in alcohol withdrawal.

Bereavement the normal human condition in the period following loss.

Bestiality sexual activity with animals.

Beta-blockers drugs (such as propranolol) used in the treatment of *anxiety states* where physical symptoms are prominent and distressing.

Bilateral ECT administration of the treatment by application of the electrodes to both sides of the head (*see also ECT*).

Bingeing a bout of uncontrolled eating in which the subject regards the quantity of food consumed as excessive (*see bulimia nervosa*).

Biofeedback the process of bringing involuntary physiological responses, such as heart rate, muscle tension and blood pressure, under voluntary control.

Biological features of depression physical symptoms and changes which can occur in a *depressive illness*. They include alterations in sleep pattern, changes in weight, appetite and bowel habit, variations in the level of activity and a reduction in sexual energy.

Bipolar affective disorder a condition in which the individual has experienced at least one episode of *depression* and one episode of *mania*. Repeated episodes of mania without depression are also classified as bipolar affective disorders (*see unipolar affective disorder; see also manic-depressive psychosis*).

Blackouts *see alcoholic blackouts.*

Blunting (flattening) of affect a reduction in the normal variation of emotional expression, most commonly seen in *chronic schizophrenia*.

Bonding the development of emotional ties between mother and infant (*see also attachment*).

Borderline personality characterised by features which may include feelings of emptiness and boredom, impulsive or unpredictable behaviour, a poor sense of identity, instability of mood, a tendency to self-mutilation, unstable and intense relationships, poor control over anger and aggression, and intolerance of being alone.

Briquet's syndrome (somatisation disorder) — a variant of *hysteria*, characterised by the development of multiple, persistent physical complaints, for which there is no demonstrable organic basis. The condition is thought to be confined to women, who most commonly describe cardiac, respiratory and menstrual problems. The onset is said to be before the age of 30, and the disorder is thought to run a life-long, fluctuating course.

Bulimia nervosa a disorder almost exclusively of women, in which individuals report frequent *bingeing*, which they compensate for by self-induced vomiting, diuretic or laxative abuse and dieting. Body weight is often normal or above normal, and many women continue to menstruate. Bulimics are highly sensitive to changes in their weight or shape (*see also anorexia nervosa*).

Buspirone (BuSpar) an *anxiolytic* drug which is structurally unrelated to the *benzodiazepines*, producing little sedation and no obvious *dependence* with long-term use.

Butyrophenones a group of *neuroleptic drugs* which are structurally unrelated to the *phenothiazines*, but nevertheless block dopamine receptors and have potent antipsychotic actions. They include *haloperidol* and droperidol. Indications and unwanted effects are similar to those of the phenothiazines, except that sedation is usually less marked and postural hypotension is uncommon. Extrapyramidal side-effects tend to be pronounced, especially in the elderly.

CAGE questionnaire sometimes used for the identification of alcohol abuse among general and psychiatric hospital patients.

Cannabis a stimulant drug derived from the hemp plant *Cannabis sativa* (*see also hashish* and *marijuana*). It is widely taken for recreational purposes on a regular or intermittent basis, making it the most commonly abused illicit drug in the UK and North America. The effects are highly variable, but generally include a sense of relaxation, sociability and well-being.

CAPE *see Clifton assessment procedure for the elderly.*

Capgras syndrome a rare *psychosis*, in which the characteristic feature is a delusional belief held by the subject that a person close to him (most commonly a spouse) has been replaced by an exact double. It may occur as a feature of another illness, such as *schizophrenia.*

Carbamazepine an anticonvulsant drug which is also used in the treatment and prophylaxis of *bipolar affective disorders.*

Castration anxiety during the Oedipal phase, the child's fear that his desire for his mother will be punished by the father castrating him (*see also Oedipus complex*).

Catalepsy a feature of *catatonia* characterised by the maintenance of posture in unusual or awkward positions which have arisen spontaneously or are created by the examiner (e.g. moving the arm up the back, which then remains there). In the case of the latter, passive movement is often accompanied by a characteristic sensation of resistance in the muscle, known as waxy flexibility (likened to bending a soft wax rod).

Cataplexy *see narcolepsy.*

Catastrophic reaction an explosive display of emotion in response to demands beyond the subject's capabilities. Most commonly seen in *dementia.*

Catatonia a collective term for a number of abnormalities of speech, movement and posture which include *ambitendency, automatic obedience, catalepsy, cooperation, echolalia, echopraxia, mannerisms, negativism, perseveration, stereotypies, stupor* and *verbigeration.* Their causation is unclear, but they probably represent a disorder of voluntary muscle control. Catatonic phenomena can occur in *affective disorders,* some *organic reactions* and *schizophrenia.*

Catatonic schizophrenia a form of the illness in which catatonic symptoms are a prominent feature.

Catharsis the ventilation of strong emotion which sometimes produces temporary symptomatic relief.

CAT scan *see computerised axial tomography.*

Child abuse in which a child (under the age of 18) has been subjected to physical violence, sexual abuse or neglect by parents or caregivers.

Child guidance clinic a clinic which deals with problems concerning the child and/or the family. Based in the community, referrals are received from various sources including general practitioners, health visitors, social workers and parents. It is usually staffed by a multidisciplinary team which can include a child psychiatrist, educational psychologist, child psychotherapist and social worker.

Chlormethiazole (Heminevrin) a derivative of vitamin B_1 (Thiamine). Its short half-life makes it a popular *hypnotic* for use in the elderly. Because of its anticonvulsant properties, it is often prescribed to minimise or prevent alcohol withdrawal symptoms.

Chlorpromazine a *neuroleptic drug* belonging to the *phenothiazine* group, which is used extensively in the treatment of psychoses, and for the control of excitement and violent behaviour.

Chorea brief, rapid, jerky movements which are aimless and uncoordinated, but may resemble fragments of goal-directed behaviour.

Chronic grief in *bereavement*, grief which is expressed in full from the outset, and goes on for an abnormal length of time.

Chronic organic reaction an acquired global impairment of cerebral function, which occurs in a setting of clear consciousness. Characteristically, the disorder has a gradual onset and tends to run a progressive, irreversible course. Structural brain damage is frequently present. Impairment of intellect is the central feature (resulting in defects of memory, attention, thinking and comprehension), although other mental functions (mood, personality and social behaviour) are usually affected simultaneously, and may sometimes be the prominent or presenting features. Chronic organic reactions are also known as *dementias*.

Chronic schizophrenia a disorder which is characterised by the *negative symptoms of schizophrenia* (lack of initiative, slowness of action, poverty of speech, social withdrawal, lack of self-care and blunting of emotional expression), which can result in the development of a *defect state* and a permanent change in personality.

Clanging a pattern of speech sometimes seen in *mania* or *schizophrenia*, in which sound rather than meaning governs the choice of words.

Classical conditioning a very simple form of 'learning', in which a subject is taught to associate a response already known, with a new stimulus. Pavlov achieved this by consistently ringing a bell each time food was presented to a dog. In time, the animal came to associate the bell with the food, and eventually salivated in response to the bell alone.

Clifton assessment procedure for the elderly (CAPE) a brief method for evaluating mental and behavioural competence in the elderly. Using scores obtained from tests of basic skills (such as orientation, counting, reading and drawing) and observations of behaviour, subjects can be graded to indicate their level of disability and the degree of care they are likely to need.

Clinical psychologist a member of the *multidisciplinary* team who is concerned with assessment and treatment in a number of areas, including estimation of intellectual functioning, behavioural techniques for the treatment of specific disorders, and the implementation and supervision of *rehabilitation* programmes.

Closed group a *psychotherapy* group in which all members start and finish treatment at the same time.

Clouding of consciousness slight impairment of clarity of thinking, attention, awareness or memory, which may not be apparent unless specifically tested for.

Cocaine a stimulant drug derived from the leaves of the coca shrub. Many of its psychoactive properties are similar to those of *amphetamines*. An increase in energy and sense of well-being are usually experienced, along with elevation of mood and a decreased need for food and sleep.

Cocaine 'bug' *tactile hallucinations* sometimes arising as a result of cocaine abuse, in which the subject experiences a sensation similar to insects crawling on his body.

Cognitive state the aspect of the mental state which deals with the faculties of knowing and perceiving. It includes orientation, memory, concentration, powers of reasoning and other intellectual capabilities.

Cognitive theory of depression hypothesis which proposes that the lowered mood occurring in depressed individuals results from 'automatic' negative thoughts, in which the person sees himself, the world around him and the future unfavourably.

Cognitive therapy treatment based on cognitive theory and used in the management of depression. It involves a relearning of responses to situations, so that negative ways of thinking which lead to depressive feelings are avoided.

Collective unconscious according to Jung, that part of the psyche which holds the beliefs and experiences of all mankind (*see also archetypes*).

Coma a state of unconsciousness in which there is no response to external stimuli, absent reflexes, no spontaneous movement (other than those of respiration) and no sign of mental activity.

Community psychiatric nurse (CPN) a nurse whose main activity is the support and continuing care of mentally ill patients living in the community. The CPN is concerned with supervising treatment (especially depot neuroleptics) following discharge from hospital, providing support and advice to patients (and their families) in the community, assessing the need for psychiatric intervention in those referred by general practitioners, and recognising early signs of relapse.

Compensation neurosis *see post-traumatic stress disorder.*

Compliance with regard to treatment, acting in accordance with the instructions of a therapist.

Compulsions (or rituals) obsessional motor acts, which although voluntary, are performed with reluctance since they are regarded as absurd and alien to the personality. The act is therefore carried out with a sense of compulsion, coupled with a desire to resist. If resistance is attempted, anxiety mounts and can only be reduced by yielding (*see also obsessions*).

Computerised axial tomography (CAT scan) a procedure in which X-ray transmission readings are taken through the body at several angles, and are then processed by a computer to produce a series of pictures showing transverse slices of the part under examination.

Concentration the ability to sustain a focus of *attention.*

Concrete thinking a form of schizophrenic *thought disorder* which represents an inability to deal with abstract ideas.

Conditioning a form of learning which results in the formation of new links between stimuli and responses.

Conduct disorder a disorder of childhood in which persistent and extreme acts of antisocial behaviour occur, resulting in suffering to the child or his care givers.

Confabulation a falsification of memory. It occurs in those whose minds are devoid of a store of recent memories, who thereby automatically draw on more distant recollections (*see senile dementia* and *Korsakoff's psychosis*).

Confusion a state which indicates that someone is unable to think with his usual clarity and distinctiveness. It can occur in *both* organic and non-organic disturbances and may be due to: (1) impairment of consciousness in *acute organic reactions*; (2) loss of intellectual capacity, powers of reasoning or memory in *chronic organic reactions*; (3) poor attention and concentration in manic or depressive psychoses; (4) preoccupation with an inner world of fantasy in schizophrenic illnesses; (5) a response to sudden or strong emotional experiences.

Conscious mind   according to Freud's topographical model, that part of the mind containing present awareness.

Consciousness   a state of awareness of the self and the environment.

Constructional apraxia   *see apraxia.*

Conversion symptoms   hysterical phenomena, so named by Freud, who saw them as resulting from psychological energy which had been 'converted' into physical symptoms, thereby providing relief from some intolerable stress and avoiding conflict. They are often suggestive of neurological disease and include seizures, paralysis, anaesthesia and blindness (*see also hysteria and dissociative states*).

Cooperation (Mitmachen)   a feature of *catatonia* in which the body can be placed in any position without resistance from the patient, even though he has been instructed to oppose all movements. The part slowly returns to its resting position once the examiner desists from his actions. **Mitgehen** is an extreme form of cooperation in which the patient moves his body in the direction of the slightest pressure by the examiner, e.g. touching the patient lightly under the chin results in full extension of the neck.

Cotard's syndrome   a rare *psychosis*, the central feature of which is a false belief held by the subject that some person or object no longer exists. It most commonly occurs in the setting of a *depressive illness*. (*see also nihilistic delusion*).

Counselling services   an aspect of preventive psychiatry for those groups at high risk of developing mental disorder, such as the bereaved, divorced and the unemployed. Counsellors who are specially trained may offer their services at community 'drop-in' centres, or hold groups at hospitals or general practice surgeries.

Countertransference   the therapist's feelings towards the patient. In most forms of *dynamic psychotherapy*, these are not deliberately or overtly revealed, but by acknowledging and exploring the feelings that the patient evokes in him, the therapist can use the countertransference to understand more about the therapeutic relationship (*see also transference*).

Couple therapy   a form of treatment which is indicated when conflict arises within a relationship and results in emotional, sexual or behavioural problems in one or both partners.

Court of protection   a legal body sometimes called upon to manage the affairs and property of mentally disordered persons, when they are unable to do so themselves.

Couvade syndrome   a disorder associated with *hysteria*, occurring during a woman's pregnancy, when her partner may develop symptoms of anxiety, vomiting, abdominal distension (due to excessive air swallowing) and pain.

Covert sensitisation   a form of *aversion therapy* which relies on imagination. The subject is encouraged to think about the undesirable behaviour, and immediately associate it with a mental picture of something unpleasant.

'Crack' a highly purified form of *cocaine*, which is inexpensive and extremely addictive.

Cretinism (congenital hypothyroidism) an inherited disorder transmitted by an autosomal recessive gene, which if untreated, results in *mental retardation*. Clinical features include apathy, a protruding tongue, a characteristic cry, an umbilical hernia, yellow puffy skin and a low body temperature.

Creutzfeldt-Jakob disease a very rare form of *presenile dementia* which is thought to be caused by a transmissible viral agent.

Cri du chat syndrome a rare disorder resulting from the deletion of the short arm of chromosome 5, so named because of the characteristic cat-like cry made by these children at birth. The condition gives rise to severe *mental retardation*, spasticity, microcephaly, stunted growth and facial abnormalities. Survival beyond infancy is rare.

Crisis intervention an approach to community psychiatric treatment which utilises the crisis experienced by the patient to bring about change and the development of more effective coping strategies for the future.

Cross-dressing *see transvestism.*

Cycloid psychosis a term originating from Scandinavia, and used to describe a *functional psychosis* which shares features of both affective and schizophrenic illnesses. Characteristically, the condition has a sudden onset, in which fluctuations of mood are associated with paranoid delusions and episodes of ecstasy. Other features such as perplexity, anxiety or changes in the level of activity may also be evident. The prognosis is generally good, and personality deterioration does not usually occur.

Cyclothymic personality *see affective personality.*

Day centre a local authority facility which, in addition to providing company, offers leisure activities, meals and (in some cases) a sheltered working environment for those unable to obtain open employment. Day centres are suitable for people suffering from chronic mental illness who require little medical supervision, but are nevertheless in need of a supportive and stimulating environment to prevent relapse.

Day hospital intended for those who require more than outpatient supervision (but for whom inpatient care is unwarranted), and for the continuing rehabilitation of patients recently discharged from hospital. Day hospitals provide an opportunity for observation and assessment, as well as for the treatment of all categories of adult mental illness.

De Clérambault's syndrome a rare *psychosis* which usually occurs in females and is characterised by the subject's delusional belief that a man, often famous or of high social standing, is in love with her. It may occur as a feature of another illness such as *schizophrenia* (*see also erotic delusion*).

Defect state features of personality deterioration which sometimes occur in *chronic schizophrenia*, and may handicap the individual in every aspect of life including work, leisure and relationships (*see also negative symptoms of schizophrenia*).

Defence mechanisms hypothetical concepts which help the understanding of certain psychological symptoms or behaviour occurring in response to internal conflicts or external stress. They are employed automatically, without any degree of conscious awareness, and act by distorting reality in some way, thereby protecting the *ego*. They form a part of normal mental activity to help cope with the everyday pressures of life. Defence mechanisms include *denial*, *displacement*, *identification*, *introjection*, *projection*, *rationalisation*, *reaction formation*, *regression*, *repression* and *sublimation*.

Déjà vu   a sudden feeling of familiarity with a place or situation which the individual knows he has not previously encountered (*see also aura*).

Delayed ejaculation   that which occurs despite adequate stimulation and a sustained erection. It may result from psychological difficulties, certain medication or organic disease.

Delayed grief   an abnormal reaction to loss, in which *denial* and anger may suppress feelings of sorrow and despair.

Delirium   an *acute organic reaction* in which consciousness is impaired and also distorted by *perceptual abnormalities* and changes in mood.

Delirium tremens   an *acute organic reaction* characterised by a fluctuating level of consciousness and perceptual abnormalities, which occurs as a result of alcohol withdrawal in some *dependent drinkers*.

Delusion   a false belief which is unshakeably held, even in the face of evidence to the contrary, and is out of keeping with the individual's social and cultural background.

Delusional mood   a conviction held by the subject that there is something going on around him which concerns him, but he does not know what it is. It can precede a *delusional perception or a* sudden delusional idea, and often dissipates following their occurrence.

Delusional perception   a *first rank symptom of schizophrenia*, in which a normal perception is followed by an abnormal and false interpretation of that perception (a *primary delusion*), which is immediate, overwhelming and usually self-referential.

Delusion of control   a false belief held by the subject that his own thoughts, actions, feelings, impulses or sensations are being interfered with by some outside force or influence.

Delusion of guilt   a false belief held by the subject that he has committed a wicked act or performed some moral transgression, which in reality is trivial or non-existent, but for which he feels he ought to be punished. It is most commonly associated with a *depressive illness*.

Delusion of jealousy   a false belief held by the subject concerning the supposed infidelity of his spouse or partner, with highly dubious or improbable evidence being offered in support of his allegations (*see Othello syndrome*).

Delusion of reference   a false belief held by an individual that other people, events or objects have a particular and unusual meaning specifically for him. He may believe that people in the street take special notice of him, or that he sees reference to himself on the television, in the newspapers or on advertising hoardings. When the individual realises that the feelings originate within himself, they are known as ideas of reference.

Delusion of worthlessness   a false belief held by the individual that he is unworthy of help or beneath contempt. It usually occurs in the setting of a *depressive illness*.

Dementia   a term used as a synonym for *chronic organic reaction* (an acquired global impairment of memory, intellect and personality, in a setting of clear consciousness), and also as a label for a group of specific degenerative cerebral conditions, the *presenile* and *senile dementias*.

Dementia praecox a now redundant term first used by Kraepelin to describe illnesses in which disorders of thinking, emotional blunting, delusions and hallucinations seemed to progress to a dementia-like state. Disorders of this kind correspond closely to the modern-day concept of *schizophrenia*.

Denial a *defence mechanism* reflected by behaviour which suggests a failure to consciously acknowledge some wish, threat or unpleasant reality, even though the person is acquainted with the necessary facts.

Dependence a compulsion to take a drug following its repeated administration (*see also physical dependence* and *psychological dependence*).

Dependent drinkers those in whom signs or symptoms of alcohol withdrawal develop when they stop drinking (*see also dependence*).

Depersonalisation an experience in which the subject feels 'as if he is no longer real', which has an associated unpleasant quality. It is *not* a delusional belief, because the person is aware of the nature of the change he experiences (*see also derealisation*).

Depixol *see flupenthixol decanoate.*

Depot preparation a *neuroleptic drug* suspended in an oily base, which is then injected deep into muscle. The drug is gradually released into the bloodstream over the course of a few weeks, thereby maintaining adequate serum levels to ensure a therapeutic effect.

Depression a term widely used by patients and doctors variably to describe an isolated symptom, a normal reaction to adverse circumstances, a transient or sustained disturbance of *mood*, and a collection of signs and symptoms which constitute an illness.

Depressive illness an *affective disorder* in which a persistent lowering of *mood* occurs, from which the sufferer cannot be distracted. There may be accompanying changes in bodily function (early morning wakening, weight and appetite loss, *diurnal mood variation*, and loss of libido). Psychomotor function (the speed at which people think and move) may also be affected, along with the content of thoughts (such as ideas or *delusions of guilt, hopelessness,* illness, *persecution,* suicide and *worthlessness*) and perception (*hallucinations* and *illusions*).

Depressive neurosis (neurotic depression) a term used to describe a less severe form of depression which has no organic basis, and results from stress factors acting on a predisposed personality, so that the sufferer does not lose touch with external reality. Sometimes used synonymously with *reactive depression*.

Depressive personality *see affective personality.*

Derailment a form of *thought disorder*, in which there is an inability to maintain a consistent train of thought. It may be a feature of *schizophrenia*.

Derealisation a feeling of unreality which relates to the environment ('as if' the world is not real). As with *depersonalisation*, it is *not* a delusional belief, since the individual has insight into the nature of the experience.

Dexamethasone suppression test (DST) used as a putative biological marker for the diagnosis of *depressive illness*. When the synthetic hormone dexamethasone is injected, the normal response is for the production of cortisol by the body to be reduced for some hours; i.e. dexamethasone suppresses plasma cortisol levels. However, when dexamethasone is given to depressed patients with raised cortisol levels, a significant number (approximately two-thirds) fail to undergo suppression (positive DST).

Diagnostic formulation a unique profile of the patient, summarising the salient features of the history and the current mental state, possible aetiological factors, the personality structure and the diagnosis or differential diagnosis. In addition, consideration is given to further investigations or information necessary to determine immediate and long-term management, as well as the likely prognosis.

Diazepam a drug belonging to the *benzodiazepine* group.

Dichotomous thinking a common feature of *bulimia nervosa*, in which the subject tends to view certain aspects of herself or her behaviour in uncompromisingly positive or negative terms.

Diminished responsibility a psychiatric legal defence which can only be used if the charge is murder, and which states that the person was 'suffering from such abnormality of mind as substantially impaired his mental responsibility for his acts'. If successful, the charge is reduced to one of *manslaughter*.

Diphenylbutylpiperidines a group of *neuroleptic drugs* which are derivatives of the *butyrophenones* and include *pimozide*. They have a longer duration of action than the parent compounds and fewer unwanted effects.

Directive sex therapy behavioural techniques for treating *sexual dysfunction* which aim to reduce anxiety and inhibitions, as well as increase confidence and pleasure. Combined methods are often used, including a form of *biofeedback*, *exposure treatment* and *sensate focusing*.

Disintegrative psychosis a childhood disorder which is distinguished from *infantile autism* in that the onset of symptoms is after the age of 30 months, and follows a period of 2–3 years of normal development. The clinical picture is one of rapid and progressive social withdrawal and intellectual deterioration, associated with loss of speech. The prognosis is poor.

Displacement a *defence mechanism* involving the transfer of feelings linked with a particular person or situation onto someone or something else.

Dissociative states hysterical phenomena which are sudden but temporary alterations in the normally integrated functions of consciousness and (sometimes) motor behaviour. They include *fugue states*, *hysterical amnesia*, *multiple personality* and *somnambulism*.

Disulfiram a drug used in the treatment of alcohol dependence. If taken with alcohol, the subject experiences headache, nausea, vasodilatation and feels generally unwell (*see also aversion therapy*).

Diurnal mood variation daytime variation in mood. In the case of a depressive illness, feelings of sadness and despair are most marked in the morning.

Dopamine a biogenic amine and neurotransmitter. Dopamine receptors in the brain are aggregated into four main systems (the *mesolimbic*, nigrostriatal, hypothalamic–pituitary and medullary pathways), all of which are blocked by *neuroleptic drugs* (*see dopamine hypothesis*).

Dopamine hypothesis a theory which proposes that *schizophrenia* is due to an excess and overactivity of the neurotransmitter *dopamine* in the *mesolimbic pathway* of the brain.

Double-bind theory an outmoded hypothesis which proposes that abnormal and illogical thinking in *schizophrenia* is due to a parent repeatedly conveying two or more conflicting messages simultaneously. A double-bind is created, and the only way it can be resolved is by the subject's retreat into illogical ways of thinking.

Down's syndrome a disorder which is responsible for approximately one-third of all severe cases of *mental retardation*, occurring once in every 600 live births. It most commonly results from an extra chromosome (trisomy) at position 21, but in 5% of cases, the additional chromosome becomes translocated to one of another pair at positions 13, 15, or 22. Clinical features include a small round head, short stature, characteristic facial appearance (slanting palpebral fissures, small nose and ears, protruding tongue), shortened digits, an abnormal palmar crease, and congenital cardiac and bowel defects.

Dream work Freud saw dreams as expressions of conflicts and wishes buried in the unconscious mind. The unconscious material often becomes intermixed and incorporated with events and happenings of the previous day. The actual (or manifest) dream content was thought to be the result of modified or disguised unconscious material, the latter referred to by Freud as the latent dream content. He used *free association* to reveal the unconscious or real meaning underlying the actual dream.

Dressing apraxia *see apraxia.*

Drowsiness impairment of *consciousness* with lack of attentiveness and awareness, which is usually obvious on direct observation.

Drug any substance that is taken into a living organism and modifies one or more of its functions.

Drug abuse persistent or occasional excessive use of a drug which is out of keeping with accepted medical practice.

DSM III (Diagnostic and Statistical Manual of Mental Disorders) a *multiaxial classification* of mental disorder adopted by the American Psychiatric Association currently in its 3rd edition. It relies upon *operational criteria* (rather than descriptive definitions) for diagnostic consistency.

DSM III-R a revised and updated version of DSM III published in 1987.

Dynamic psychotherapy a form of treatment using talking and listening, that aims to bring about change by detecting and resolving underlying psychological conflicts which are the root cause of disturbed personal relationships and the unpleasant symptoms which often accompany them (*see also psychotherapy*).

Dyscalculia *see Gerstmann's syndrome.*

Dysgraphia *see Gerstmann's syndrome.*

Dysmnesic syndrome *see Korsakoff's psychosis.*

Dyspareunia pain on sexual intercourse, which may be superficial or deep. Superficial pain can result from psychological causes, inadequate lubrication, scarring, inflammation and other lesions of the vulva or vagina. Deep dyspareunia is more likely to be associated with pelvic disease.

Dysphasia partial failure of the comprehension and/or expression of language in either its spoken or written form (*see expressive* and *receptive dysphasia*).

Dysthymic disorder a term used in DSM III-R as an alternative to *depressive neurosis.*

Dystonia an involuntary contraction of skeletal muscle, which is an *extrapyramidal motor disturbance* associated with the use of *neuroleptic drugs*, and most commonly affects muscles of the head and neck.

Echolalia speech characterised by the subject repeating what is said to him. It may be a feature of *catatonia.*

Echopraxia the imitation of a simple action which the subject sees performed by somebody else, e.g. clapping, foot tapping. It may be a feature of *catatonia.*

Eclectic an approach to the practice of psychiatry which embraces various models of causation and management in a non-doctrinaire fashion.

ECT (Electroconvulsive therapy) a physical treatment used primarily in the management of *depression*, in which seizures are induced by the passage of an electrical current through the brain.

Educationally subnormal (ESN) the term used by educationalists for those with an IQ of 50–70 (*see also severely educationally subnormal*).

Edward's syndrome a rare disorder arising from an extra chromosome (trisomy) at position 17–18, resulting in severe *mental retardation*. Clinical features are similar to those of *Patau's syndrome*.

Ego according to *psychoanalytical theory*, one of the main elements involved in developing personality; that aware part of the 'self' whose function is to test reality (*see also id* and *superego*).

Ego defence mechanisms *see defence mechanisms*.

Ekbom's syndrome a rare *psychosis*, characterised by delusions of infestation, in which the individual believes that his body or his immediate surroundings are overrun with insects or parasites. It sometimes occurs as an encapsulated symptom, but is more frequently part of a *paranoid* or *depressive illness*.

Elective mutism a rare disorder of childhood in which there is a persistent refusal to talk in certain situations, particularly at school, while speaking freely in others (such as the home).

Electra complex female equivalent of the *Oedipus complex*.

Electroencephalograph (EEG) a record of the spontaneous electrical activity of the brain, obtained via electrodes attached to the scalp.

Encapsulated delusion a *delusion* that has no significant effect on the subject's behaviour or sense of well-being.

Encephalitis lethargica a form of epidemic encephalitis, common after the First World War. The acute phase was marked by daytime drowsiness and visual disturbance, following which many sufferers were left with residual features of Parkinsonism, as well as undergoing personality changes or developing schizophrenic-like illnesses.

Encopresis (*faecal soiling*) defaecation in inappropriate places (notably clothing or receptacles) beyond an age at which bowel control is expected — about 4 years old.

Encounter groups use either talking or actions to facilitate the expression of emotions in a setting where open communication and self-awareness are encouraged.

Endogenous depression a *depressive illness* whose causation is supposedly attributed to internal physiochemical changes rather than to environmental influences (*see reactive depression*). Sometimes used synonymously with *psychotic depression*.

Enuresis repeated involuntary urination beyond an age at which continence is expected. It may occur during sleep (nocturnal enuresis) and/or during waking hours (diurnal enuresis).

Epidemiology the study of how specific disorders are distributed throughout populations, and the factors which influence that distribution.

Epiloia *see tuberous sclerosis*.

Erectile impotence the inability to achieve or sustain an erection, despite adequate desire and stimulation.

Erotic delusion a false belief of being loved or admired by someone, who in reality is remote and inaccessible, such as a person of high standing or public renown (*see also de Clérambault's syndrome*).

Excessive drinkers men who regularly consume more than 21 units, or women who consume more than 14 units of alcohol/week. Even though their drinking may not affect their personal relationships or functioning at work, they are at increased risk of developing many of the physical complications associated with prolonged heavy drinking, as well as becoming dependent on alcohol.

Exhibitionism the purposeful exposure of the male genitals to unwilling females, without being a preliminary to sexual intercourse. The offence committed is known as indecent exposure.

Existential awareness the individual's appreciation of issues of 'ultimate concern', such as death, isolation and loneliness, which are inherent in existence.

Explosive personality characterised by features which usually include a tendency to outbursts of anger or violence and poor emotional control in the absence of any other antisocial behaviour.

Exposure a behavioural treatment based on the principle of encouraging the subject to re-enter situations which provoke anxiety and to remain in them until the fear subsides (*see also phobia, graded exposure* and *flooding*).

Expressive dysphasia a disorder of the expression of language, in either its spoken or written form, resulting from a lesion in Broca's area of the brain. Comprehension is unaffected.

Extrapyramidal motor disturbance produced by abnormalities in the basal ganglia and cerebellum. Symptoms may involve the loss of ability to coordinate or move muscles, as well as the development of new phenomena such as abnormal movements and postures. Extrapyramidal symptoms encountered in psychiatric patients are usually side-effects of psychotropic medication (especially *neuroleptic drugs*) and include *akathisia, dystonia, pseudo-parkinsonism* and *tardive dyskinesia*.

Faecal soiling *see encopresis*.

Family therapy the treatment of the family as a unit, rather than dealing with the problems of its members individually.

Fetal alcohol syndrome a disorder occurring in infants born to women who drink heavily during pregnancy. Characteristic features include low birth weight, short stature, microcephaly and mental retardation, as well as abnormal facies (small eyes, prominent forehead, maxillary hypoplasia and a short upturned nose). Poor muscle tone and incoordination can also occur. The full features of the syndrome are not always present.

Fetishism a *sexual deviation* in which inanimate objects, or parts of the body that do not usually have sexual connotations, become the preferred or sole focus of sexual interest.

Fictive goals according to Adler, impossible ambitions which provide a means of obtaining power by a 'retreat into illness' and the subsequent development of 'adult neurosis'. Superiority is gained by using symptoms to control others, or to provide an excuse for not living up to impossible ambitions.

Fight and flight a form of *resistance* encountered in *group therapy*, in which members either become withdrawn or aggressive.

Finger agnosia *see Gerstmann's syndrome*.

First-pass metabolism a process whereby a significant proportion of a drug taken orally is inactivated during its passage from the gut through the liver, before reaching the general circulation. First-pass metabolism is avoided when compounds are given intramuscularly or intravenously.

First rank symptoms (of schizophrenia) Schneider, a German psychiatrist, defined a number of symptoms which he considered to be of first rank importance in making the diagnosis of *schizophrenia*, in the absence of 'coarse brain disease' (i.e. organic disorders or drug intoxication). They are *audible thoughts*, *auditory hallucinations* arguing about the subject in the third person or commenting on his actions, *delusional perception*; *'made' actions*, *feelings* and *impulses*; *somatic passivity*, *thought broadcast*, *thought insertion* and *thought withdrawal*.

Fitness to plead in order to stand trial, the defendant must be able to understand the nature of the charge against him, appreciate the significance of his plea, instruct counsel, challenge a juror and follow the evidence presented in court.

Flashback a recurrence of the drug experience some length of time after an *hallucinogen* was last taken, often creating a feeling of disorientation and distress.

Flattening of affect *see blunting of affect*.

Flight of ideas a lack of coherent goal-directed thinking, with abnormal associations between thoughts, characteristically found in *mania* and *hypomania*.

Flooding a behavioural treatment used in the management of *phobias*, which involves exposure to the feared stimulus without using a graded approach and with no attempt to reduce anxiety by relaxation.

Flupenthixol decanoate (Depixol) a *neuroleptic drug* belonging to the *thioxanthene* group, administered as a *depot preparation*.

Fluphenazine decanoate (Modecate) a *neuroleptic drug* belonging to the piperazine group of *phenothiazines*, administered as a *depot preparation*.

Folie à deux a rare disorder which involves the 'transfer' of delusional beliefs between two (or sometimes more) people, who have usually lived together in close proximity for a considerable length of time.

Forensic psychiatry a term applied to aspects of psychiatry involving criminal and civil law, as well as those legislative procedures which deal with the assessment and treatment of mentally abnormal offenders.

Formulation *see diagnostic formulation*.

Fragile X syndrome a disorder accounting for about 10% of *mental retardation* in males (although it is less common in females), resulting from fragmentation or detachment of the terminal portion of the long arm of the X chromosome. Some of those affected are noted to have large floppy ears, macro-orchidism and prognathism, although the fragile X anomaly has also been demonstrated in otherwise normal individuals.

Free association a mode of thinking encouraged in *dynamic psychotherapy* (in order to obtain access to unconscious psychological conflicts), in which the subject reports spontaneously whatever comes to mind, irrespective of its content.

Frigidity a disorder of sexual arousal characterised by a failure of vaginal lubrication, despite adequate stimulation.

Fugue amnesia accompanied by wandering, which may be a feature of an hysterical *dissociative state*, a *depressive illness* or epilepsy.

Functional psychosis a *psychosis* in which no demonstrable physiological disturbance (such as infection) or alteration in the structure of the brain or other body organ (e.g. a tumour) consistently occurs. Functional psychoses include *schizophrenia* and the *affective disorders* (compare with *organic psychosis*).

GABA the inhibitory neurotransmitter gamma-amino butyric acid.

Gain *see primary gain* and *secondary gain*.

Ganser syndrome a rare disorder which is thought to be an example of an hysterical *dissociative state*. It is characterised by the giving of approximate answers to elementary and well-known questions, apparent clouding of consciousness (in which there is impairment of concentration, attention and memory), anxious mood, *conversion symptoms* and *pseudohallucinations*.

Gaucher's disease an inherited disorder of lipid metabolism transmitted by an autosomal recessive gene. It is due to a deficiency of the enzyme cerebroside-glucosidase. Clinical features include *mental retardation*, splenomegaly, nerve palsies, pathological fractures and skin pigmentation.

General paresis of the insane (GPI) a form of neurosyphilis which may develop up to 25 years after the initial infection. Pathological changes comprise thickening of the dura mater, cerebral atrophy and inflammatory and degenerative changes of the cerebral cortex. Psychiatric manifestations may include *depression*, *mania*, personality changes of a frontal lobe type (apathy and disinhibition), paranoid psychosis and a slowly progressive *dementia*.

Genital phase (of personality development) according to Freud, the phase which begins during early adolescence and eventually results in the development of mature sexual relationships.

Gerstmann's syndrome a rare disorder of the dominant parietal lobe, resulting in dyscalculia (impairment of numerical skills), dysgraphia (impairment of the ability to write), finger agnosia (inability to recognise or name digits) and left–right disorientation.

Gilles de la Tourette syndrome a rare disorder characterised by multiple motor tics (most frequently facial) associated with uncontrollable utterances often of an obscene nature (coprolalia) as well as *echolalia* and *echopraxia*.

Glossolalia ('speaking in tongues') a form of *possession state* characterised by spontaneous nonsensical speech, which the subject does not seem to knowingly initiate and often attributed to divine influence. It is probably a *dissociative* phenomenon.

GPI *see general paresis of the insane.*

Graded exposure a form of *exposure* treatment used in the management of *phobias*, which involves exposing the subject to the feared stimulus one step at a time.

Grandiose delusion a false belief held by the subject that he possesses exceptional powers or talents, or that he is a person of great importance, sometimes with a special purpose or mission in life. It is most commonly seen in the context of *mania* and *hypomania*.

Grasp reflex a clinical sign indicative of a lesion in the prefrontal cortex. Drawing a finger across the subject's palm results in it being grasped firmly.

Grief the emotional reaction to a loss.

Grimacing a feature of *catatonia* characterised by the maintenance of a fixed facial expression in which the subject rounds his lips and protrudes them, so that they resemble an animal's snout ('Schnauzkrampf').

Group home a form of *sheltered accommodation* which offers ordinary residential housing for 4–8 people, who live together on a permanent basis and benefit from mutual support.

Group therapist acts as a conductor or facilitator (but not a leader) to help create an atmosphere of honest communication in a psychotherapy group, while encouraging interaction between group members. The therapist is also responsible for selecting patients, establishing ground rules and making practical arrangements, dealing with disruptive processes, promoting cohesion and maintaining an awareness of the aims of the group.

Group therapy psychotherapy with two or more people. Group therapy may be purely supportive in its aims or more dynamically orientated. Small groups usually consist of 6–10 people who meet regularly to pursue a common purpose, and include one or two therapists who act as facilitators or conductors. The group may comprise inpatients on a hospital ward or outpatients who meet at a specified time, usually once a week. Large groups consist of 20 or more members (*see also small group psychotherapy and large group psychotherapy*).

Guardianship an order of the *Mental Health Act 1983* which if invoked, ensures that, where necessary, mentally disordered people aged 16 or over receive proper care and protection while living in the community. The guardian is empowered to ensure that the patient resides at a specified place, attends for medical treatment, work or education, and allows certain specified people (such as doctors or social workers) access to his residence. A guardianship order is for 6 months in the first instance.

Guided mourning a structured approach to facilitate grief, in which a spouse or close relative may be encouraged to visit the grave, alter the arrangement of the contents of rooms, and handle photographs and possessions of the deceased. This aims to provoke 'grief work' and to 'confirm' the reality of the change in circumstances. It may be useful in cases of *delayed grief.*

Gustatory hallucination a false perception of taste arising in the absence of an external stimulus.

Guthrie test a routine screening procedure used for detecting *phenylketonuria*, which is carried out between 6 and 14 days after birth. A small sample of blood taken from the baby's heel is introduced into a culture of *Bacillus subtilis*, to which an inhibitory substance has previously been added. The degree of culture growth is proportional to the level of phenylalanine present in the blood.

Half-life the time taken for half the amount of a drug to be eliminated from the body.

Hallucination a false perception which arises in the absence of any external stimulus, which is therefore not merely a distortion of a real perception. It is experienced as being located in the external world and has the same qualities of vividness, solidity and constancy as a real perception. As with the latter, it cannot be produced or dismissed at will. Hallucinations may be perceived as originating in the external environment, or emanating from within the subject's own body (compare with *illusions* and *pseudohallucinations*).

Hallucinogens a group of drugs characterised by their ability to produce distinctive alterations in thought, feeling, behaviour and perception (*see also LSD*).

Haloperidol a *neuroleptic drug* belonging to the *butyrophenone* group.

Hartnup disease an inherited disorder of protein metabolism transmitted by an autosomal recessive gene. It is due to defective renal transport of amino acids. Clinical features include *mental retardation*, photosensitive skin, ataxia, pellagra and weight loss.

Hashish a derivative of a clear sticky resin produced by the plant *Cannabis sativa*, which is then dried and compressed into blocks (*see also cannabis*).

Hebephrenic schizophrenia a subtype of the disorder which has an early onset, usually in the teens. Thought disorder and affective symptoms form a prominent part of the clinical picture.

Heroin (diamorphine) an *opioid* drug, first synthesised from morphine in 1874 in an attempt to find a non-addictive substitute for opium.

High-expressed emotion families families with a schizophrenic member in which relatives tend to be overinvolved with the life of the patient, and also express an excessive amount of critical comment (compare with *low expressed emotion families*). Environments of this type appear to increase the rate of relapse of the condition.

Histrionic (hysterical) personality characterised by features which may include egocentricity, insincerity, vanity, emotional shallowness, a tendency to dramatise situations, sexual immaturity and frigidity, a craving for excitement, flirtatiousness, attention-seeking, manipulative and dependent behaviour, as well as the capacity for self-deception and inconsistency.

Holistic referring to the 'whole person' with regard to mind and body (*see also psychosomatic medicine*).

Homicide unlawful killing which includes *infanticide*, *murder* and *manslaughter*.

Homocystinuria an inherited disorder transmitted by an autosomal recessive gene. It occurs once in every 50 000 live births, and is caused by a deficiency of the enzyme cystathionine synthetase, which results in raised blood levels of the amino acids homocystine and methionine. In addition to *mental retardation*, clinical features include dislocation of the lens of the eye, osteoporosis and other skeletal abnormalities, thromboembolism and epilepsy. Affected children characteristically have fair skin and hair, as well as a prominent malar flush. Mental retardation may be prevented by early treatment with a low methionine diet.

Homosexuality sexual attraction towards a person of the same sex.

Hospice a unit which specialises in dealing with the physical and psychological care of the dying.

Hunter's syndrome an inherited connective tissue disorder transmitted by a sex-linked recessive gene. It is due to a defect of the enzyme L-iduronosulphate sulphatase. Clinical features include *mental retardation*, gargoylism, short stature, deafness, hepatosplenomegaly and cardiac abnormalities.

Huntington's chorea a degenerative disorder of the brain characterised by a *presenile dementia* associated with abnormal choreiform movements. It is caused by a single autosomal dominant gene, although cases without a family history also occur, presumably due to spontaneous mutation.

Hurler's syndrome an inherited connective tissue disorder transmitted by an autosomal recessive gene. It is due to a defect of alpha-L-iduronidase. Clinical features include *mental retardation*, gargoylism, short stature, corneal opacities, hepatosplenomegaly and cardiac abnormalities (*see also Hunter's syndrome*).

Hyperactivity a term used in the USA to describe a disorder in which children are overactive in *specific* situations (typically at school) and show evidence of distractability, together with impulsive and excitable behaviour (*see also hyperkinetic syndrome*).

Hyperkinetic syndrome in the UK, a term applied to those children who demonstrate severe, pervasive overactivity (in two or more situations) that is excessive for the child's age and IQ, and is a handicap to development. In addition, there is evidence of marked inattentiveness and restlessness from direct observation by the diagnostician, and an absence of childhood autism or affective disorder (compare with *hyperactivity*). It is a rare condition affecting approximately 1 in 1000 children, characteristically before the age of six, the majority showing evidence of neurological dysfunction or *mental retardation*, although some are of normal intelligence.

Hypersomnia abnormally prolonged sleep.

Hyperthymic personality *see affective personality*.

Hypnagogic hallucinations false perceptions experienced just as the subject is falling off to sleep. They commonly take the form of hearing one's name being called, but are not necessarily an indication of mental illness (*see also narcolepsy*).

Hypnopompic hallucinations false perceptions experienced at the time of awakening.

Hypnosis a heightened state of focal awareness brought about by artificial means.

Hypnotic a drug which induces sleep.

Hypochondriacal delusion a false conviction of ill health, which is held despite reassurance from doctors or other professionals that it is groundless.

Hypochondriasis a disorder in which the sufferer displays excessive concern with his health in general, or an unrealistic interpretation of physical signs or sensations as being abnormal. This can lead to a preoccupation with the fear of having a serious disease. Hypochondriacal symptoms sometimes form part of a *depressive illness*.

Hypomania a less severe form of *mania*, such as the stage when the illness is developing.

Hysteria (Hysterical neurosis) a term applied to signs and symptoms of illness which occur in the absence of demonstrable physical pathology. The condition arises in response to stress and confers some advantage or *gain* to the individual. In contrast to malingering, symptoms are not created deliberately, but instead are constructed unconsciously around the person's own notion of the disorder gained from past experience, personal knowledge or by observing the behaviour of others. Symptoms are not attributable to overactivity of the autonomic nervous system. Hysterical features include *dissociative states* and *conversion symptoms*.

Hysterical amnesia an abrupt memory loss for a specific and often traumatic episode, although more commonly, the individual complains that he knows nothing of his earlier life It is a *dissociative state*.

Hysterical personality *see histrionic personality*.

ICD 9 (International classification of diseases, 9th edition) a classification system used in the UK and other countries, which attempts to standardise diagnosis by using descriptive definitions of the major syndromes, as well as giving some directives on differential diagnosis. It also provides a system of diagnostic coding which is understandable throughout the world.

ICD 10 (International classification of diseases, 10th edition) a uniaxial classification system, making use of both *operational criteria* and descriptive definitions, which will supersede ICD 9 in the early 1990s.

Id according to *psychoanalytical theory*, one of the main elements involved in developing personality; the unconscious part of the self which contains the instinctual drives (*see also ego* and *superego*).

Ideas of reference *see delusion of reference.*

Ideational apraxia *see apraxia.*

Identification a *defence mechanism* closely related to that of *introjection.*

Ideomotor apraxia *see apraxia.*

Idiot savant isolated areas of excellence, such as musical ability, drawing or feats of memory, sometimes seen in individuals who are otherwise severely handicapped (such as in *infantile autism*).

Illness behaviour the concept whereby an individual may learn to be 'unwell', if the illness state is repeatedly rewarded.

Illusions *sensory deceptions* which are misinterpretations of real external stimuli. For example, a red floral pattern on curtains may be mistaken for writhing snakes. They have the same qualities as normal perceptions, but tend to be more fleeting than *hallucinations.*

Imipramine a *monoamine reuptake inhibitor antidepressant* which belongs to the *tricyclic* group.

Implosion a behavioural technique involving maximal *exposure* in fantasy (compare with *flooding*).

Incest sexual intercourse with a parent, sibling, child or grandchild.

Incidence the number of new cases of a disorder which occur within a population over a certain period of time (compare with *prevalence*).

Incongruity of affect emotional expression which is inappropriate to the individual's current circumstances, e.g. laughing at sad news. It may be a feature of *schizophrenia.*

Indecent exposure *see exhibitionism.*

Individual psychology a school of thought founded by Adler, who was an early follower of Freud, but later split from him to form his own movement. Adler saw man's struggle for power and status (rather than the fulfilment of sexual needs) as the main determinant of adult character.

Industrial rehabilitation an important aspect of rehabilitation for patients recovering from mental illness, who either require help in returning to former employment or retraining if there has been a change in their level of functioning.

Infanticide the unlawful killing of a child under the age of 12 months by its mother.

Infantile autism *see autism, infantile.*

Informed consent a patient (whether voluntary or detained) is deemed capable of giving informed consent if he understands the nature, purpose and likely effects of the proposed treatment.

Insight the degree of correct understanding that an individual has as to the nature of his condition, its underlying cause, and its implications regarding treatment and outcome.

Insomnia a chronic inability to obtain the amount of sleep necessary for efficient daytime functioning.

Institutionalisation syndrome   the development of apathy, loss of interest and initiative, submissiveness, lack of individuality and deterioration of personal habits as a result of living in an unstimulating, authoritarian and impoverished environment.

Intellect   that aspect of cognitive function which involves memory, attention, thinking, reasoning and comprehension.

Intelligence   an individual's powers of reasoning and understanding, the level of which will have some bearing on behaviour in terms of its direction and purpose, and on the ability to maintain an independent existence in society.

Intelligence quotient   a score used for reporting intelligence test performance, originally derived from the ratio between mental and chronological age. In adulthood, the difference between the mental and chronological ages has little meaning, so that *IQ* scores (no longer a quotient) are instead calculated from tables in which a standard score of 100 (average intelligence) is assigned for each age group.

Interictal   the time interval between epileptic seizures.

Interim secure units   are for patients detained under the *Mental Health Act 1983* who require treatment in an environment of intermediate security between an ordinary and a *Special Hospital*.

Introjection   a *defence mechanism* in which the individual adopts the feelings, attitudes or behaviour of another person in order to deal with the anxiety of separating from them.

IQ   *see intelligence quotient.*

Kendrick battery   a two-part *psychometric test* used in the assessment of cognitive impairment. The first section is a test of recall of briefly perceived information. The subject is shown four cards with pictures of common objects for a short time, and is then asked to recount from memory as many as possible. The second section is a test of speed of information processing. This involves a digit copying exercise, in which the subject is required to copy numbers from a sheet as fast as possible.

Kleine-Levin syndrome   a rare condition, probably arising from a hypothalamic disorder, in which prolonged episodes of *hypersomnia* occur in association with increased appetite and hypersexuality.

Klinefelter's syndrome   a disorder arising from the presence of an extra sex chromosome (XXY karyotype), occurring in approximately 1 in 500 males. Those affected are infertile as a consequence of hypogonadism, and the absence of secondary male sex characteristics is associated with the development of female bodily proportions, although they are often tall. Klinefelter males tend to be timid and withdrawn, and although *mental retardation* is usually mild, other psychiatric disorders (particularly neuroses and personality disorders) are common.

Knight's move thinking   an aspect of *thought disorder* in which unclear or irrelevant answers to questions are given as the individual constantly wanders off the point.

Koro   a culture-bound syndrome, primarily affecting young men in South China or Malaysia. It is thought to be an acute anxiety reaction in which the individual expresses the fear that his penis is shrinking into his abdomen, and that as a result he will die.

Korsakoff's psychosis (dysmnesic syndrome)   a disorder characterised by impairment of *short-term memory* with preservation of other aspects of intellect. It results from damage to the posterior hypothalamus, the mamillary bodies and the floor of the third ventricle, which in the majority of cases, is due to *thiamine* deficiency in those who abuse alcohol. The ability to learn new information is therefore severely impaired, and an *anterograde amnesia* develops. There is also a period of *retrograde amnesia* which extends for weeks, months and occasionally longer before the onset of the illness. *Confabulation* is commonly present (*see also Wernicke's encephalopathy*).

La belle indifference a cheerful acceptance of disability sometimes seen in *hysteria*.

Labelling theory a hypothesis which regards diagnostic labelling as meaningless and antitherapeutic, serving only to increase an individual's difficulties when he is 'labelled' according to supposed disease entities.

Large group psychotherapy a form of *group therapy*, usually conducted with 20 or more people, which may be supportive or analytical in its approach. Many psychiatric wards begin the day with a meeting of all patients and staff members to allow the general problems of living together to be discussed. Staff can facilitate the ventilation of emotion and conflicts, point out how the group is functioning, and create a forum for social learning (*see also therapeutic community*).

Latah a culture-bound disorder which most commonly occurs in Malaysian women and is thought to be a form of *hysteria*. The subject enters a trance-like state in reaction to a stressful event, following which features of automatic behaviour are exhibited, associated with *echolalia* and *echopraxia*.

Latency period (of personality development) according to Freud, the phase during which interest in the body is replaced by increased attention to the acquisition of environmental skills.

Learned helplessness a theory, based upon the observation of behavioural changes in animals, which states that depressive disorders in man occur as a result of an acceptance by the individual that his actions will have no effect in altering the course of events.

Learning a relatively permanent change in behaviour that occurs as a result of practice.

Learning theory a system of ideas and principles which attempts to describe and predict the observed phenomena of learning in all organisms.

Lesch-Nyhan syndrome an inherited disorder transmitted by an X-linked recessive gene. It is due to a deficiency of the enzyme hypoxanthine transferase, which leads to an accumulation of uric acid in the tissues. In addition to being mentally retarded, affected children have a tendency to self-mutilate. Other clinical features include spasticity, cerebral palsy, choreoathetosis, anorexia and excessive thirst.

Leucotomy (Prefrontal) a now redundant surgical procedure which involved severing nerve pathways between the frontal lobe and the rest of the brain by inserting a specially curved blade (known as a leucotome) through burr holes in the skull.

Liaison psychiatry the work of the psychiatrist in the general hospital and other clinical areas where psychological problems occur in association with physical disorders.

Libido a hypothetical form of mental energy.

Life events potentially stressful events, such as marriage, bereavement or loss of a job, which may be related to the onset of psychiatric disorders.

Lithium a drug used in the treatment and prevention of *affective disorders.*

Long-term memory comprises 'recent' long-term memory (events of the last few days or weeks) and 'remote' memory, extending back months and years. Memories in long-term stores are 'permanent' but can be lost to *recall.*

Low expressed emotion families families with a schizophrenic member that are not overinvolved with the patient, nor express an excessive amount of critical comment. Consequently, they are associated with a reduced rate of relapse of the condition (compare with *high expressed emotion families*).

LSD (lysergic acid diethylamide) an extremely potent synthetic *hallucinogen*, which may produce psychological but not physical dependence.

Made acts a *first rank symptom of schizophrenia* in which the individual experiences his actions as being under the control of an external influence which he believes initiates and directs his movements throughout. He feels like a robot, the passive observer of his own actions.

Made feelings a *first rank symptom of schizophrenia* where feelings or emotions that are experienced are not recognised by the individual as his own, but are attributed to some external force and are believed to be imposed upon him.

Made impulses a *first rank symptom of schizophrenia* in which a person has the experience of being overcome by a sudden impulse that he believes is derived from some external influence, and on which he subsequently acts.

Major depressive episode a term used in DSM III-R to include melancholia (equivalent to *endogenous depression*) and severe forms of *unipolar affective illness.*

Major tranquillisers a synonymous term for *neuroleptic drugs.*

Mania an *affective disorder* in which a persistent elevation of *mood* or increased sense of well-being is associated with mental and physical overactivity. Occasionally, irritability (without evidence of euphoria) predominates. Although the mood is mainly cheerful, it may frequently be punctuated by periods of depression or anger, which can last from a few minutes to several hours. Accompanying changes may include a reduced need for sleep, disinhibited behaviour, racing thoughts, *flight of ideas*, distractability, *pressure of speech* and *grandiose* ideas or *delusions* (*see also hypomania*).

Manic-depressive psychosis a term applied by Kraepelin to describe *affective illness*. It was used whether the patient experienced only one episode of affective illness or many in the course of a lifetime, irrespective of severity, duration or symptom content. It therefore included *unipolar* and *bipolar affective disorders.*

Manic stupor an occasional feature of *mania*, where the subject presents as mute and motionless.

Mannerism an unusual performance of a 'goal-directed' motor act (such as proferring a clenched fist when shaking hands), or modifying an adaptive posture in a curious fashion (e.g. sitting cross-legged with one knee placed under the chin). It may be a feature of *catatonia.*

Manneristic speech characterised by alterations in the quality of speech (talking with a strange or stilted quality, e.g. sounding like a foreigner), the vocal tone (e.g. talking in a falsetto voice or 'through the nose'), or the mode of pronunciation (consistently mispronouncing words). It may be a feature of *catatonia*.

Manslaughter unlawful killing without guilty intent (such as a 'hit and run' road traffic accident) (compare with *murder*).

Maple syrup disease an inherited disorder of protein metabolism transmitted by an autosomal recessive gene. It is due to a deficiency of the enzyme ketoacid decarboxylase. Clinical features include *mental retardation*, epilepsy and spastic paresis.

Marijuana made from a dried mixture of the crushed leaves and flowering tops of the plant *Cannabis sativa* (*see also cannabis*).

Marital schism a dysfunctional marital relationship, formerly believed to be of aetiological significance in the development of *schizophrenia* among the offspring. Conflicting views held by the parents, and a lack of communication between them, lead to the development of divided loyalties in the child.

Marital skew a dysfunctional marital relationship, formerly believed to be of aetiological significance in the development of *schizophrenia* among the offspring. One partner habitually capitulates in the face of the other's idiosyncratic behaviour, the latter tending to dominate the family's mode of functioning.

Masochism sexual satisfaction obtained by being subjected to pain, humiliation or acts of cruelty (*see also sadism*).

Massed practice a behavioural technique which involves the subject repeatedly practising the unwanted behaviour until he is fatigued. It may be used in the treatment of *tics* and other habit disorders.

MAST questionnaire (Michigan alcohol screening test) sometimes used for the identification of alcohol abuse among general and psychiatric hospital patients.

Maternity blues transient episodes of weeping and depression which occur in 50–70% of recently delivered women.

Melancholia a term used in DSM III-R as a synonym for *endogenous depression*.

Mens rea a legal term for 'guilty intent' in association with the performance of an unlawful act (*see actus reus*).

Mental disorder as defined in the *Mental Health Act 1983*, either *mental illness*, *mental impairment*, *severe mental impairment* or *psychopathic disorder*.

Mental handicap a synonym for *mental retardation*.

Mental Health Act 1983 an Act of Parliament which is mainly concerned with the care and treatment of mentally disordered patients detained in hospital and those placed under guardianship. It also deals with compulsory admission procedures, the rights of patients to appeal against detention, and consent to treatment.

Mental Health Act Commission a multidisciplinary body, which in addition to fulfilling administrative duties with regard to the *Mental Health Act 1983*, also protects the interests of detained patients by regularly reviewing their care, and establishing a code of practice relating to treatment.

Mental Health Review Tribunal a patient who appeals against a compulsory detention order invoked under the *Mental Health Act 1983* may have his case considered by a Review Tribunal. After evaluating all the information made available, the tribunal will either uphold the order or revoke it.

Mental impairment as defined in the *Mental Health Act 1983* 'a state of arrested or incomplete development of mind which includes significant impairment of intelligence and social functioning, and is associated with abnormally aggressive or seriously irresponsible conduct' (*see also severe mental impairment* and *mental retardation*).

Mental retardation 'a condition of incomplete development of mind which is especially characterised by subnormality of *intelligence*'. It includes individuals in whom intellectual development is predictably impaired from conception by genetic influences, and those in whom it would otherwise have proceeded normally, but has become arrested at some stage due to environmental factors.

Mental state examination concerned with the subject's appearance and behaviour during a consultation, as well as an assessment of his speech, mood, thought content, perception, cognitive function and level of insight.

Mental subnormality a synonym for *mental retardation*.

Mesolimbic pathway one of the four main cerebral systems in which *dopamine* receptors are aggregated (*see also dopamine hypothesis*).

Methadone an *opioid* drug prescribed orally, often provided at a drug dependency unit as a substitute for *heroin*.

MID *see multi-infarct dementia*.

Mill Hill vocabulary test an *intelligence test* which is a two-part exercise of verbal ability involving recall and recognition of words. The first part assesses an individual's written expressive word knowledge. In the second part, the subject is required to select one word, from a choice of six to eight, which is closest in meaning to a target word.

Mini-mental scale a rating scale for the assessment of cognitive impairment in the elderly which is based upon various aspects of cognitive function, including *short-term memory*, *orientation*, visuo-spatial abilities, the capacity to respond to simple commands, as well as the ability to name and recognise common objects.

Minor tranquillisers a group of drugs, including the *benzodiazepines*, which are used for the treatment of insomnia, anxiety and other minor psychological disturbances.

Misuse of Drugs Act legislation introduced by the UK Parliament in 1971, which specified certain 'controlled' drugs (including *opioids*, *cannabis*, *cocaine*, *LSD* and *amphetamines*) and made it illegal to supply or possess them without a certified prescription, or to produce, import or export them without authority.

Mitgehen — *see cooperation*.

Mitmachen — *see cooperation*.

Mixed affective state an *affective disorder* in which, most commonly, a predominantly depressed mood and thought content occurs in association with manic behaviour. Occasionally, manic patients may present as mute and motionless (*manic stupor*). Other transition states between *mania* and *depression* are sometimes seen, when *mood*, behaviour and thought content alter independently of each other.

Modecate — *see fluphenazine decanoate*.

Modelling a behavioural technique which involves imitating behaviour demonstrated by the therapist.

Monoamine hypothesis a biochemical theory of the causation of *affective disorders*, which proposes that a deficiency of the monoamines, noradrenaline and serotonin (5–hydroxytryptamine), at certain strategic sites in the brain causes *depression*, while an excess results in *mania*.

Monoamine oxidase inhibitors (MAOIs)   antidepressant drugs which exert their effect by blocking the intracellular action of monoamine oxidase enzymes, so reducing the degradation of biogenic amines.

Monoamine reuptake inhibitors (MARIs)   antidepressant drugs (including tricyclic compounds) which exert their effect through increasing the concentration of biogenic amines at the neuronal synapse by blocking their reuptake.

Monosymptomatic (simple) phobia   a persistent irrational fear of particular objects, events or situations (such as spiders, dogs, heights and darkness), which leads to an overwhelming desire to avoid them.

Mood   a sustained emotion which, in the extreme, markedly colours the individual's perception of the world.

Morbid grief   a condition in which there is prolonged denial or repression of the expression of feeling, or where grief continues well beyond a time when it would be expected to have resolved (*see also delayed grief* and *chronic grief*).

Morbid jealousy   *see Othello syndrome.*

Mother and baby unit   a specialised unit catering for mentally ill mothers and their infants in an environment simulating domestic living conditions as closely as possible.

Mourning   the social expression of *grief.*

Multiaxial classification   a system of classification in which two or more sets of information are coded (*see also DSM III*).

Multidisciplinary team   a group of health care workers of various disciplines who meet regularly to discuss problems and exchange information about patients for whom they are mutually concerned, as well as to formulate plans for their management.

Multi-infarct dementia (MID)   a cerebral disorder caused by thromboemboli originating in extracranial vessels damaged by atherosclerosis. Deterioration tends to occur in a stepwise fashion, correlating with repeated episodes of cerebral infarction over a period of time. The mood is often labile and nocturnal confusion is a common feature, although characteristically, personality and insight are preserved until the later stages of the illness.

Multiple personality   a rare *dissociative state* in which the individual may have several different personalities, none of which has any apparent knowledge of the others.

Münchausen syndrome   a disorder named after the eighteenth century fictional character Baron Münchausen, which is most common in young men and involves the persistent simulation of illness, resulting in frequent hospital admissions. Three characteristic features are described: pathological lying, exaggeration of symptoms and wandering from one hospital to another. The individual often willingly subjects himself to various investigations and treatments, some possibly invasive, following which he is likely to take his own discharge against medical advice.

Murder   unlawful killing with 'malice aforethought'.

Narcissistic personality   characterised by features which may include an increased sense of self-importance, a desire for constant attention, a rich fantasy life, anger or indifference in response to criticism, selfishness, a disregard for others and egocentricity.

Narcolepsy a rare syndrome typified by episodes of uncontrollable sleep during the day, frequently accompanied by cataplexy (in which the individual suddenly collapses due to loss of muscle tone). Other features include sleep paralysis (a sensation of being awake but unable to move) and *hypnagogic hallucinations* (which occur at the onset of sleep).

Nearest relative for the purposes of the *Mental Health Act 1983*, this refers to the person first described in the following list (persons of the 'whole blood' taking preference over those of 'half-blood', as does the elder of two relatives of similar status): husband or wife, son or daughter, father or mother, brother or sister, grandparent, grandchild, uncle or aunt, nephew or niece. For the purposes of the Act, a person living with the patient for at least 6 months as a husband or wife can be considered as the nearest relative. Any other person needs to have resided with the patient for at least 5 years before he can be treated as a relative.

Necrophilia sexual gratification derived from having intercourse with a dead body.

Negative symptoms of schizophrenia those which are usually associated with the chronic phase of the illness (compare with *positive symptoms of schizophrenia*), often forming part of a *defect state*. They include lack of initiative and drive, slowness of action, poverty of speech, social withdrawal, blunting of emotional expression, deterioration of social behaviour and self-neglect.

Negativism a feature of *catatonia* characterised by apparently motiveless resistance to suggestion or interference, i.e. a refusal to carry out orders or follow instructions. Command negativism is when the patient carries out in a reflex fashion the exact opposite of what he is asked to do (e.g. when asked to remain seated, the subject stands up).

Neologism an occasional feature of schizophrenic speech, involving the use of a newly invented word, unknown to any language.

Neurofibrillary tangles helically paired, twisted filaments seen on microscopy in the cerebral tissue of patients suffering from *senile dementia* and *Alzheimer's disease*.

Neurofibromatosis (von Recklinghausen's disease) an inherited disorder transmitted by an autosomal dominant gene. The central clinical features are pigmented skin patches associated with multiple neurofibromata (tumours arising from cells of the nerve sheaths). Intracranial tumours can also develop, and in one-third of cases some degree of *mental retardation* is present.

Neuroleptic drugs compounds used in the treatment of *psychoses* and for producing sedation in violent or excitable patients. They induce a state of calmness without loss of consciousness (neurolepsis). Also known as major tranquillisers.

Neuroses a group of disorders that are a combination of symptoms in which there is no evidence of any organic brain disorder, sufferers do not lose touch with external reality, behaviour may be greatly affected but remains within socially acceptable limits and the personality is not grossly abnormal or disorganised. Neuroses include *anxiety states*, *hysteria*, *neurotic depression*, *obsessive-compulsive disorders*, *phobic states*, *hypochondriasis* and the *depersonalisation syndrome*.

Neurotic defence mechanisms *see defence mechanisms.*

Neurotic depression *see depressive neurosis.*

Neurotic symptoms these include anxiety, depression, obsessional thoughts and physical symptoms with no organic basis, which are a reaction to stress in everyday life. They are seen in psychodynamic terms as a resurfacing of conflicts which were not resolved in childhood. They may exist in isolation or develop together, and are usually mild. When they become more severe or exaggerated, the patient is said to be suffering from a *neurosis*.

Nicotinic acid a vitamin, deficiency of which can result in the development of *pellagra*.

Niemann-Pick disease an inherited disorder of lipid metabolism transmitted by an autosomal recessive gene. It is due to a deficiency of the enzyme sphingomyelinase. Clinical features are similar to those of *Tay-Sachs disease*.

Night terrors a condition which most commonly occurs in young children, who appear to awaken an hour or two after going to sleep in a state of panic or extreme distress. Typically, the child screams out in terror, sits up or gets out of bed, but does not respond to attempts to comfort him. The episode may last for a few minutes prior to a return to normal sleep, and the child has no recollection of events the following day.

Nihilistic delusion a false belief held by the subject that certain things, such as the world, his loved ones, his career, parts of his body or indeed his entire self, no longer exist. It most commonly occurs in the setting of a *depressive illness*, and is the central feature of *Cotard's syndrome*.

Nocturnal enuresis *see enuresis*.

Nominal aphasia an inability to name objects, while retaining an understanding of their function or purpose (compare with *agnosia*).

Non-fatal deliberate self-harm an intentional, self-inflicted, non-fatal act effected by physical means, drug overdosage or poisoning. It is done in the knowledge that it is potentially harmful and, in the case of drug overdosage, that the amount taken was excessive. It is also sometimes referred to as parasuicide.

Noradrenaline a biogenic monoamine neurotransmitter.

Normal pressure hydrocephalus a disorder resulting from an obstruction in the subarachnoid space, which prevents the normal circulation of cerebrospinal fluid. Characteristic features include the insidious onset of *psychomotor retardation*, urinary incontinence, an unsteady broad-based gait and progressive *dementia*, which can be prevented by early recognition and treatment.

Nurse of the prescribed class for the purposes of *Section 5(4)* of the *Mental Health Act 1983*, one who is a registered mental nurse (RMN) or a registered mental subnormality nurse (RMNS).

Object in analytical terms, any person who is emotionally significant to the subject.

Object relations theory concerned with the way in which the child's perceptions and fantasies about the relationships between important people or 'objects' in his life (such as between parents, or mother and child) become incorporated into the mind at an early stage of development. These mental constructs of prototypal relationships continue to have a bearing on the capacity of the individual to relate to others throughout life, to sustain emotional ties and to cope with separation.

Obsessional personality characterised by features which may include meanness, orderliness, rigidity of character, excessive cleanliness and a fondness for collecting things.

Obsessions recurrent ideas, thoughts, images or impulses which repeatedly enter the mind, and are persistent, intrusive and unwelcome. Although they are recognised as a product of his own mind, the individual regards them as absurd and alien to his personality. Attempts are sometimes made to ignore and resist them (*see also compulsions*).

Obstruction a feature of *catatonia* characterised by intermittent inability or difficulty in carrying out an action, which may be initiated and then stopped half-way. Reacting at the last moment is another feature of obstruction (e.g. despite asking a patient to sit down several times, each request is ignored. As the examiner turns away, the patient complies with the request).

Occupational therapy a method of treatment, in both physical and psychological medicine, concerned with the promotion and maintenance of maximum personal and functional independence for the patient, through the analysis and application of activities.

Oedipus complex named after the mythical Oedipus, who killed his father and married his mother, without knowing they were his parents. In boys, it represents a normal period of the developing personality, when sexual drives focused on the mother are accompanied by feelings of jealousy and resentment towards the father, who is seen as a rival for her affections (*see also castration anxiety*). The equivalent phenomenon in girls is known as the Electra complex.

Olfactory hallucination a false perception of smell in the absence of an external stimulus.

Open group a psychotherapy group with a regular turnover of members, those leaving being replaced by others.

Operant conditioning a procedure in which behaviour is increased or reduced in frequency by supplying or withholding reinforcement when the behaviour occurs.

Operational criteria employed in the *DSM III-R* classification of mental disorders to improve diagnostic accuracy. Strict criteria are specified (from a supplied list) for each diagnostic entity.

Opiates a group of drugs including opium, morphine and codeine, derived from the opium poppy (*see also opioids*).

Opioids a group of drugs which are central nervous system depressants and include both naturally occurring compounds derived from the opium poppy (*opiates*), and a number of synthetic derivatives e.g. *heroin*. They produce a sense of peace and tranquillity, and a relaxed detachment from the outside world. *Tolerance* and *dependence* develop rapidly.

Opposition a feature of *catatonia* characterised by opposition to attempts at passive movement by the examiner.

Oral stage (of personality development) according to Freud, the phase of development at which the infant obtains pleasure from sucking, so that in the absence of comfort derived from the breast or bottle, the thumb or other objects are placed in the mouth.

Organic psychiatry the study of those conditions in which mental disorder arises as a result of demonstrable structural disease of the brain or a physiological disturbance affecting cerebral function.

Organic psychosis a *psychosis* in which it is possible to demonstrate a physiological disturbance (such as infection) or alteration in the structure of the brain or other body organ (e.g. a tumour), which as a consequence produces mental disorder.

Organic reaction *see acute* and *chronic organic reaction.*

Orientation the individual's awareness of time, place and person.

Othello syndrome (Morbid jealousy) a rare *psychosis* characterised by a false conviction of infidelity concerning one's spouse or sexual partner. It may occur in isolation, in association with alcohol abuse or as part of another illness, such as *schizophrenia* (*see also delusion of jealousy*).

Overinclusiveness a form of schizophrenic *thought disorder* which represents a failure to maintain boundaries around topics, so that irrelevant information continually creeps in.

Overvalued idea an abnormal belief, often with a strong emotional content, which unlike a *delusion*, is held with almost total, but not absolute, conviction.

Paedophilia the condition of being sexually attracted to children, and sometimes indulging in sexual activity with them.

Pairing a form of *resistance* encountered in *group psychotherapy* in which two members of the group form an alliance which separates them from interacting with the others.

Pangs of grief episodes of acute distress experienced in the early stages of *bereavement*. Anxiety symptoms are often severe, and yearning or crying out is accompanied by an urge to search for the departed, to the exclusion of other activities.

Panic attack a sudden episode of *anxiety*, which is so severe that behaviour ceases to be rational and controlled.

Paradoxical intention a behavioural treatment which aims to reduce anxiety by encouraging the subject to carry out the very behaviour he fears.

Paranoia a *psychosis* in which logically constructed, systematised *delusions* of grandeur, persecution, jealousy or reference have developed in the absence of hallucinations or other schizophrenic symptoms (*see also paranoid state*).

Paranoid personality characterised by features which may include suspiciousness and mistrust of others, over-sensitivity to set-backs or criticism, absence of tenderness and sentimentality, a tendency towards jealousy and aggressiveness, excessive ideas of self-importance and self-reference, and argumentativeness.

Paranoid schizophrenia a form of the illness in which *hallucinations* and/or *delusions* of *any* type are prominent (it is *not* specific to delusions of persecution).

Paranoid state a *psychosis* (such as *paranoia* or *paraphrenia*) that is not classifiable as *schizophrenia*, an affective psychosis or an organic disorder, in which *delusions* of *reference, persecution, jealousy* or *grandeur* are the main symptoms. Personality and intellect are well preserved.

Paraphasias the use of ordinary words in unusual ways, which may be a feature of schizophrenic speech.

Paraphrenia a *psychosis* which frequently develops late in life, and is characterised by prominent *hallucinations* often associated with paranoid beliefs, but with preservation of personality and intellect (*see also paranoid state*).

Parapraxes slips of the tongue ('Freudian slip') or pen, misidentification of people and mislaying of objects seen by Freud as expressions of conflicts and wishes buried in the *unconscious mind.*

Parasuicide *see non-fatal deliberate self-harm.*

Parkinson's disease a common condition of the elderly, recognised clinically by the triad of bradykinesia, rigidity and tremor. Psychiatric problems, notably *depression*, are encountered in nearly half of all cases.

Partial delusion a false belief which is expressed with great conviction, but is not firmly held, and may therefore be amenable to reason. This can occur at a stage prior to the development of the full *delusion*, or in the recovery phase of an illness where *insight* is being regained.

Part III accommodation residential accommodation named after that part of the 1948 National Assistance Act which requires local authorities to provide such establishments for the care of the elderly.

Passivity experience a phenomenon in which the subject believes that actions, impulses, emotions, or sensations which he experiences are not his own, and are being imposed on him by some outside force or influence against his will (*see also first rank symptoms of schizophrenia*).

Patau's syndrome a rare disorder resulting from an extra chromosome (trisomy) at position 13–15. Clinical features include microcephaly, extra fingers and toes, defects of the eyes and mouth, as well as cerebral and cardiac abnormalities. The degree of *mental retardation* is severe, and survival beyond infancy is rare (*see also Edward's* and *Down's syndrome*).

Pathological gambling an inability to stop gambling once started, despite being aware of the adverse consequences of such behaviour. Interference with the psychological, social or economic functioning of the gambler and/or his family occurs.

Pathological intoxication highly irrational or aggressive behaviour which arises in certain individuals who have consumed relatively small amounts of alcohol. It may also occur in chronic heavy drinkers who have underlying physical damage to the central nervous system.

PCP *see phencyclidine.*

Pellagra a condition resulting from *nicotinic acid* deficiency, characterised by dermatitis, diarrhoea and *dementia*. During the acute stages, the individual may be emotionally labile and delirious.

Penile strain-gauge a device sometimes used in the assessment of *erectile impotence*. It consists of a loop of conductive material placed around the penis, which is connected to a pen recorder via a Wheatstone Bridge arrangement. Penile engorgement alters the resistance of the loop, thereby allowing a current to flow.

Perceptual abnormalities abnormal experiences including *sensory distortions* and *sensory deceptions*.

Persecutory delusion a false belief of being followed, picked on, defamed, poisoned or conspired against by others, who may or may not be known to the subject.

Perseveration (of action) a feature of *catatonia* characterised by the pointless repetition of a goal-directed action which is no longer appropriate, e.g. continuing to offer the hand after it has already been shaken.

Perseveration (of speech) characterised by the senseless repetition of words, which unlike stereotypies, are initially in context. For example, repeating an answer to a previous question: ('What is the name of the Queen?' – 'Elizabeth';

'What day is it today?' – 'Elizabeth'). It may be a feature of organic brain disease or *catatonia*.

Persona according to Jung, the outer layer of the personality, which is the exact opposite of feelings and sensitivities embodied in the underlying level of the personal unconscious (*see also anima* and *animus*).

Personality includes those aspects of a person's behaviour, thinking and emotional reactions which are enduring and predictable throughout a wide range of circumstances and life situations. Features of personality include an individual's persisting attitudes, values, feelings and intellectual capabilities.

Personality disorder a *personality* which is distorted by an exaggeration or imbalance of its constituent traits, resulting in behaviour which is identified as being maladaptive from an early age, and which causes suffering to the self, others or society in general (*see also affective, asthenic, borderline, explosive, histrionic, narcissistic, obsessional, paranoid, psychopathic* and *schizoid personalities*).

Personality trait a persisting characteristic or aspect of personality.

Peyronie's disease a rare idiopathic condition in which the development of fibrous tissue in the corpora of the penis prevents engorgement and erection.

Phallic stage (of personality development) according to Freud, the phase which occurs at around the ages of 2–5 years, when the focus of gratification and interest is transferred to the genitalia.

Phencyclidine (PCP, 'angel dust') a synthetic *hallucinogen*.

Phenothiazines a group of *neuroleptic drugs*, including chlorpromazine and trifluoperazine, which probably exert their antipsychotic effects by blocking *dopamine* receptors in the *mesolimbic pathway* of the brain. They also have antiemetic actions, as well as producing *extrapyramidal motor disturbance*.

Phenylketonuria (PKU) an inherited disorder transmitted by an autosomal recessive gene, which occurs once in every 12000 live births. It is due to a deficiency of the enzyme phenylalanine hydroxylase, and affected infants are unable to adequately convert the aminoacid phenylalanine to tyrosine. Unless the defect is detected shortly after birth, excessive phenylalanine accumulates in the bloodstream, resulting in irreversible brain damage and *mental retardation*. Associated clinical features include low birth weight, reduced pigmentation of the skin and hair, blue eyes, eczema and epilepsy (*see also Guthrie test*).

Phobia a fear which is out of proportion to the demands of the situation, so that it cannot be reasoned or explained away. It is beyond voluntary control, and leads to avoidance of the provoking stimulus (*see also agoraphobia, monosymptomatic* and *social phobia*).

Phobic anxiety *anxiety* that is experienced only in certain situations, such as crowds, which in reality are not dangerous or threatening.

Physical dependence characterised by a specific group of symptoms which occur after an individual stops taking a drug. The withdrawal symptoms which develop have a well-defined course and are unpleasant, but they can be stopped or prevented by further drug-taking (*see also dependence*).

Pick's disease an uncommon form of *presenile dementia*, which is probably transmitted by a single autosomal dominant gene. Characteristic pathological changes in the brain result in a proliferation of 'Pick's cells', and circumscribed frontal and temporal lobe atrophy occurs, although the parietal lobes are usually unaffected.

Pimozide (Orap)   a member of the *diphenylbutylpiperidine* group of *neuroleptic drugs.*

Place of safety   for the purposes of the *Mental Health Act 1983*, it refers to residential (*Part III*) *accommodation*, a hospital, a police station, a mental nursing home or any other suitable place where the occupier is willing to receive the patient temporarily.

Positive symptoms of schizophrenia   these include *thought disorder, delusions* and *hallucinations* (such as *first rank symptoms*), which are more often associated with the acute phase of the illness (compare with *negative symptoms of schizophrenia*).

Possession state   a condition most commonly seen in primitive cultures in which the subject believes that he is possessed by an alien spirit, which may have the power to cast a fatal spell (e.g. 'Voodoo' death).

Postictal   the period of time directly after an epileptic seizure.

Postnatal depression   a *depressive illness* which usually has an onset in the first four weeks post-partum.

Post-traumatic amnesia (PTA)   the memory impairment occurring after head injury up to the return of normal, continuous memory. It is sometimes referred to as anterograde amnesia, and is a good indicator of outcome following head injury. The longer its duration, the worse the prognosis.

Post-traumatic stress disorder   term applied to a constellation of physical and psychological symptoms which occasionally follow relatively trivial head (and other bodily) injuries, and are not attributable to any demonstrable organic pathology. In some instances, such as following an industrial injury or road traffic accident, victims may resort to litigation to obtain compensation for their disabilities, and it was for this reason that the disorder was initially termed 'compensation (or accident) neurosis'.

Pre-conscious mind   according to Freud's topographical model, that part of the mind in which unconscious mental activity is capable of recall (*see also unconscious mind*).

Preictal   the period of time prior to an epileptic seizure.

Premature ejaculation   the inability to control the ejaculatory reflex to the satisfaction of both partners (*see also squeeze technique*).

Presenile dementia   a dementing illness which has an onset before the age of 65. The presenile dementias include *Alzheimer's disease, Huntington's chorea, Pick's disease* and *Creutzfeldt-Jakob disease.*

Present state examination   a standardised interview schedule for examining the mental state, the results of which are interpreted by computer.

Pressure of speech   an increase in the quantity and rate of speech compared to that which is socially normal, so that the individual is difficult to interrupt. Usually a feature of *mania* or *hypomania.*

Prevalence   the total number of cases of a disorder, new and old, in a given population at any one time (compare with *incidence*).

Primary affective disorder   an affective illness which is not preceded by, or associated with, any other psychological or physical illness, except in the case of *mania* preceding *depression* or vice versa (compare with *secondary affective disorder*).

Primary care team community health care workers (such as general practitioners, health visitors and field social workers) who are the first line of referral for patients.

Primary delusion a false belief which appears suddenly in the mind fully formed like a 'brain wave', so that its development is not understandable in terms of previous thoughts or other experiences. It is also known as an autochthonous delusion (*see* *also delusional perception* and *secondary delusion*).

Primary gain mechanism whereby anxiety over a psychological conflict is excluded from consciousness.

Problem drinkers those in whom alcohol consumption is either continuously or intermittently out of control, thereby causing physical, psychological or social damage to themselves or other people.

Procyclidine (Kemadrin) a synthetic *anticholinergic drug* sometimes used to counteract the *extrapyramidal motor disturbance* associated with the use of *neuroleptic drugs*.

Programmed practice a form of *exposure* treatment (especially used in the management of *agoraphobia*) in which the individual is encouraged to seek out situations which would formerly have been avoided, and to practice ways of controlling anxiety symptoms should these develop during exposure.

Projection a *defence mechanism* in which unacceptable aspects of the self are attributed to someone else, so that they become more tolerable.

Pronominal reversal a disorder of speech, sometimes seen in *infantile autism*, in which the child may refer to himself as 'you'.

Pseudodementia any functional disorder (c.g. depression) in which there is apparent intellectual impairment resembling that of organic disease.

Pseudohallucination an ambiguous term which is used in two distinct ways. On the one hand, it is applied to a perception which is experienced in the 'mind's ear or eye', and is therefore a form of imagery. Although vivid, it lacks the substance of both normal perceptions and true hallucinations, and patients often retain some insight into its nature. Nevertheless, it cannot be produced or dismissed at will. The second use of this term is to describe an *hallucination* which the subject recognises as having no place in the external world. For example, this applies to phenomena which sometimes occur in the acute stages of *bereavement*, when the deceased's voice may be heard or his form seen by the spouse or other close relative.

Pseudoparkinsonism an *extrapyramidal motor disturbance* associated with the use of *neuroleptic drugs*, resulting in the development of symptoms similar to those of Parkinson's syndrome, namely stiffness and rigidity, tremor and bradykinesia.

Psilocybin a naturally occurring *hallucinogen* found in a number of species of wild mushroom.

Psychiatric history a systematic enquiry which contains details of events and symptoms experienced by the subject prior to the interview.

Psychiatric social worker a member of the *multidisciplinary team*, who provides a link between the hospital and community-based social services and agencies. In addition to performing social assessments and offering help with financial problems, the social worker also advises on welfare rights and accommodation difficulties. An *approved social worker* may be involved in making an application for the compulsory admission of a mentally disordered person to hospital under the *Mental Health Act 1983*.

Psychoanalysis   an intensive form of *dynamic psychotherapy*. It can continue for several years, with up to five sessions a week being held, during which time a detailed and intensive exploration is conducted into the subject's behaviour and psychological functioning.

Psychoanalytical theory   developed by Freud, in which all aspects of mental life (thoughts, emotions and resultant behaviour) are seen as being influenced by inborn psychological forces, which often come into conflict with each other and also collide with the demands of the environment.

Psychodrama   a form of therapy which allows individuals to re-enact, in a dramatic form, some emotionally painful experience or conflict from their past. Other group members portray the parts of significant people involved in the situation, and this re-enactment leads the patient to a greater understanding of the problem.

Psychogenic psychosis   the development of excitable behaviour or transient symptoms, such as *hallucinations*, *thought disorder* or *delusional beliefs*, in response to stress, which are indistinguishable from those found in the major psychoses. Characteristically, symptoms abate spontaneously once the source of stress is removed, or the subject is placed in a different environment.

Psychological dependence   craving for a drug in order to experience its psychic effects, or to avoid the discomfort of its absence (*see also dependence*).

Psychology   the scientific study of behaviour and mental processes.

Psychometric testing   psychological tests which measure various aspects of cerebral function.

Psychomotor function   the speed at which a person thinks and moves.

Psychoneuroses   a term applied by Freud to three specific syndromes: anxiety hysteria (now referred to as *phobic anxiety*), *obsessive-compulsive disorder* and *hysteria*. He attributed the development of these conditions to unconscious conflicts arising within the mind.

Psychopathic personality disorder   a disorder which is persistent from an early age and results in behaviour that is variably described as abnormally aggressive, antisocial, seriously irresponsible or inadequate. As a consequence of this, society is impelled to deal with such individuals. It is sometimes known as sociopathy.

Psychopathology   the study of abnormal mental states which relates either to their description (phenomenology) or mode of causation (psychodynamic psychopathology).

Psychosis   a psychiatric disorder in which there is impairment of mental functioning of such a degree that it interferes with the ability to meet the demands of everyday life and maintain adequate contact with reality. Distortion of the environment can occur through the individual harbouring abnormal beliefs which are demonstrably false (*delusions*), and experiencing deceptions and misinterpretations of his senses, known as *hallucinations* and *illusions*. Consequently, *insight* is diminished or lost (*see also organic* and *functional psychosis*).

Psychosomatic medicine   the study of the interrelationship between biological, psychological and social variables in health and disease. It also refers to the *holistic* approach to the practice of medicine, in which the mind and body are seen as a single unit. Clinical activities at the interface of medicine and psychiatry, which developed from this approach to medical practice, are termed *liaison psychiatry*.

Psychosurgery the destruction of normal or abnormal brain tissue in order to bring about changes in behaviour or emotions.

Psychotherapy a term which covers a number of different treatments, all of which use talking and listening to bring about relief from specific symptoms, or to help people adjust to and cope with the problems of everyday life (*see also supportive psychotherapy* and *dynamic psychotherapy*).

Psychotic depression an ambiguous term which may be used synonymously with *endogenous depression*, or to describe a *depressive illness* in which *delusions* and/or *hallucinations* are evident.

Psychotropic drug a drug which acts upon the mind.

Puerperal psychosis a severe and usually unexpected mental illness developing abruptly during the first 2 weeks after childbirth.

Puerperium the 6–8 week period following childbirth.

'Punch-drunk' syndrome results from repeated head injuries, such as those sustained by boxers, which cause a chronic progressive encephalopathy. The clinical features include ataxia, tremor, spasticity, a shuffling gait, personality changes and a progressive *dementia*.

Pyromaniac a person who commits repeated acts of *arson* without any apparent motive.

Rape 'sexual intercourse with a woman who at the time did not consent to the act, the man knowing that she did not consent, or being reckless as to whether or not she consented.'

Rationalisation a *defence mechanism* involving the unconscious offering of reasonable (but false) explanations for feelings or behaviour which would otherwise be unacceptable to the self.

Raven's progressive matrices a diagram completion test which assesses performance skills as a measure of *intelligence*. The subject is shown pictures of patterns in which a segment is missing, and is then asked to identify the missing piece from a selection of possible parts.

Reaction formation a *defence mechanism* in which true feelings or motives are obscured from the self by the individual thinking and behaving in an opposite manner.

Reactive depression a depressive state, the causation of which is supposedly related to environmental influences rather than internal physiochemical changes (sometimes used synonymously with *neurotic depression*).

Recall the retrieval of a stored memory into consciousness.

Receptive dysphasia a disorder of the comprehension of language, in either its spoken or written form, resulting from a lesion in the posterior part of the superior temporal gyrus.

Recidivist one who repeatedly breaks the law.

Recognition the process whereby information in the memory store is recognised as being relevant to the current situation (e.g. recognising a face as one that has been seen before).

Refsum's disease an inherited disorder of lipid metabolism transmitted by an autosomal recessive gene. It is due to a deficiency of the enzyme phytanic acid oxidase. Clinical features include *mental retardation*, blindness, deafness, cerebellar signs and ichthyosis.

Registration   the first step in the process of memory, which can be assessed by asking the subject to repeat back a sequence of digits that have been spoken slowly to him.

Regression   a *defence mechanism* resulting in the individual behaving in a manner which is representative of a younger age.

Rehabilitation   the process of minimising or preventing severe social disablement accompanying psychiatric disorder, and helping the individual to develop and use his talents to acquire confidence and self-esteem through success in social roles.

Relaxation training   a behavioural technique in which the subject learns to recognise and relieve muscular tension, and to control irregularities of breathing. By becoming 'physically relaxed', mental relaxation follows as a matter of course.

REM (rapid eye movement) sleep   a phase of sleep in which dreaming usually occurs, characterised by rapid movements of the eyes and low voltage, asynchronous fast waves on EEG (*see also slow wave sleep*).

Repression   a *defence mechanism* resulting in the exclusion from the conscious mind of unacceptable thoughts or feelings, which if allowed to reach awareness, would create conflict or tension.

Resistance   the opposition encountered in *dynamic psychotherapy* to bringing unconscious processes into the conscious mind.

Response prevention   a behavioural treatment used in the management of compulsive behaviour or rituals. The subject is instructed to desist from carrying out the unwanted behaviour (such as repeated hand-washing), while simultaneously being exposed to a situation which is likely to increase his need to perform the act, e.g. rummaging through a dustbin. Except in very severe cases, constant supervision does not appear to be necessary, merely telling the subject to refrain being sufficient to control the behaviour. The treatment will need to be carried out several times before the patient is able to cope with the resultant anxiety (*see also compulsions*).

Retention   the capacity to store memories.

Retrograde amnesia   in the case of trauma, memory impairment between the moment of injury to the head and the last clear memory before the incident. It may also occur in other organic conditions such as *Korsakoff's psychosis*.

Rituals   *see compulsions*.

Roth-Hopkins test   a rating scale for the assessment of cognitive impairment in the elderly which is based upon various aspects of cognitive function, including *short-term memory* and *orientation*.

Sadism   sexual gratification derived from inflicting pain on others, e.g. by whipping or beating (*see also masochism*).

Scapegoating   a form of *resistance* encountered in *group therapy* in which a group member is repeatedly verbally attacked by the others, thereby preventing the assailants from acknowledging comparable aspects of their own personalities.

Schizoaffective illness   a disorder in which symptoms of *mania* or *depression* are intermingled with those of *schizophrenia*. Illnesses in this category do not usually result in permanent damage to the personality.

Schizoid personality   characterised by features which may include introspectiveness, aloofness, detachment from socialising, lack of emotional warmth, a tendency to solitary existence, and a self-absorption with an inner world of fantasy.

Schizophrenia a term coined by Bleuler in 1911 which means literally 'split mind' and refers to a *functional psychosis* in which shattering or disintegration of the various mental functions occurs (including thinking, behaviour, perception and sometimes *mood*). (*See also acute schizophrenia* and *chronic schizophrenia.*)

Schizophrenogenic mothers women who were thought to influence the development of *schizophrenia* in their children through an abnormal relationship with them, which was both overprotective and hostile.

School refusal a persistent reluctance or inability to attend school due to fear.

SDAT *see senile dementia–Alzheimer's type.*

Secondary affective disorder an *affective disorder* which is preceded by another psychological illness, or associated with a physical illness (compare with *primary affective disorder).*

Secondary delusion a *delusion* which can be understood as developing from other psychological experiences. For example, the elated mood in *mania* may give rise to *grandiose delusions* of great wealth or fame (compare with *primary delusion).*

Secondary gain the additional advantage conferred by organic or hysterical symptoms of illness, such as the increased attention of others or the abrogation of responsibilities (*see also sick role).*

Section 2 (of the *Mental Health Act 1983*) a 28 day order allowing for the compulsory admission to hospital of an individual suspected or known to be suffering from *mental disorder* for the purposes of assessment, which may be followed by treatment.

Section 3 (of the *Mental Health Act 1983*) a 6 month order permitting the compulsory admission to hospital of an individual suffering from *mental disorder* in order to provide treatment.

Section 4 (of the *Mental Health Act 1983*) a 72 hour order used to admit a person suspected or known to be suffering from *mental disorder* to hospital in an emergency, and detain him for assessment.

Section 5(2) (of the *Mental Health Act 1983*) a 72 hour order allowing for the detention of an informal inpatient undergoing assessment or treatment for either psychiatric or non-psychiatric conditions, if, in the opinion of the responsible medical officer or his nominated deputy, an application for admission under Section 2 or 3 ought to be made.

Section 5(4) (of the *Mental Health Act 1983*) allows for the detention of an informal inpatient who is already being treated for *mental disorder* and requires *immediate* restraint from leaving hospital, for his own health and safety or for the protection of others. Under this order, a *nurse of the prescribed class* can detain the patient for up to 6 hours where it is not possible for a doctor to attend immediately in order to implement Section 5(2).

Section 136 (of the *Mental Health Act 1983*) empowers a police officer to remove to a *place of safety* (such as a hospital) any person found in a public place who appears to be suffering from *mental disorder*, and is in need of immediate care and control in his own interests or for the protection of others.

Semicoma a state in which the subject appears unconscious, but can be roused by painful stimuli. There may be evidence of uncoordinated movement.

Senile dementia–Alzheimer's type (SDAT) a disorder resulting from a primary degenerative process within the brain. It is the commonest form of *chronic organic reaction* encountered clinically, and is pathologically identical to *Alzheimer's disease*, although it occurs in an older age group.

Senile plaques seen on microscopy in the cerebral tissue of patients suffering from *senile dementia* and *Alzheimer's disease*. They are silver-staining and contain amyloid, and the number present appears to relate closely to the degree of cognitive impairment.

Sensate focusing a form of *directive sex therapy* which concentrates on the pleasurable aspects of sex (touching, cuddling and caressing), and aims to dispel fears about sexual performance or failure by initially forbidding intercourse. 'Giving pleasure to get pleasure' is axiomatic of this procedure, and graded exercises are prescribed which progress from non-erotic contact, through erotic and genital stimulation, to full sexual intercourse.

Sensory deceptions include *illusions*, *true hallucinations* and *pseudo-hallucinations*.

Sensory distortion a perceived alteration in either the intensity, quality or spatial form of a stimulus. For example, colours might appear more vivid, sounds louder or softer, and objects larger (macropsia) or smaller (micropsia).

Serotonin (5-hydroxytryptamine) a biogenic monoamine neurotransmitter.

Severe mental impairment as defined in the *Mental Health Act 1983*, 'a state of arrested or incomplete development of mind which includes severe impairment of *intelligence* and social functioning, and is associated with abnormally aggressive or seriously irresponsible conduct' (the distinction from *mental impairment* is simply a matter of degree) (*see also mental retardation*).

Severely educationally subnormal (ESN) (S) the term used by educationalists for those with an *IQ* below 50 (*see also educationally subnormal*).

Sex phobia an uncommon disorder, predominantly of females, which takes the form of a fear of sexual intercourse or of the genitalia of the opposite sex.

Sexual deviation habitual sexual activity which is outside the norm of the society concerned.

Sexual disorder sexual behaviour which causes suffering, in the form of psychological or physical discomfort, to the person or their partner, or is outside the range of that generally accepted as normal by the society concerned (*see also sexual dysfunction* and *sexual deviation*).

Sexual dysfunction the repeated failure either to achieve or to enjoy 'normal' sexual intercourse.

Shaping a behavioural technique which involves the gradual development of complex pieces of behaviour by reinforcement of the constituent parts.

Sheltered accommodation dwellings provided for mentally disordered people living outside of hospital, in the form of *group homes*, hostels, warden-controlled flats or board and lodgings. They should offer an acceptable social environment, protection from stress related to accommodation difficulties and help with some of the practical problems of daily living.

Short-term memory that part of the memory store in which information is held for a short period, before being lost or transferred to long-term storage. It can be assessed by testing the subject's ability to learn new information and repeat it after a few minutes.

Sick role   the exemption from normal social responsibilities during illness.

Simple phobia   *see monosymptomatic phobia.*

Simple schizophrenia   a form of the disorder in which there is a progressive deterioration akin to a *defect state*, in the absence of acute psychotic symptoms.

Sleep apnoea   a disorder occurring in some obese individuals and characterised by upper respiratory obstruction during sleep, in association with excessive snoring and nocturnal motor restlessness, which is followed by daytime drowsiness. Symptoms usually resolve with loss of weight, but when the periods of apnoea are severe, pulmonary hypertension can develop.

Sleep drunkenness   a disorder in which the subject is unable to awaken fully for several hours after rising, during which time he is irritable and confused.

Sleep paralysis   *see narcolepsy.*

Slow wave sleep   a phase of deep sleep characterised on the EEG by delta waves (low frequency high amplitude) (compare with *REM sleep*).

Small group psychotherapy   a form of psychotherapy usually conducted with 6–10 people. The group setting provides an opportunity to look at both interpersonal relationships and the dynamics of the group in terms of its social structure, interactions and the conflicts that develop within it. The most important therapeutic factor is the group itself, and its members gradually learn about their distorted views of relationships and maladaptive behaviour by disclosing personal difficulties and concerns, and discovering how to modify them accordingly (*see also group therapy*).

Social phobia   a persistent and irrational fear of situations in which an individual may be observed by others (e.g. restaurants or cinemas) and subsequently behave in an embarrassing or humiliating way (such as vomiting or fainting in public). As a result, the subject feels it necessary to avoid such situations.

Social skills training   a behavioural treatment used to help those who have difficulty in forming or maintaining relationships with others. Techniques include teaching the importance of non-verbal aspects of communication and role-playing commonly encountered social situations (*see also assertiveness training*).

Sociopathy   *see psychopathic personality disorder.*

Solvent abuse   the inhalation of chemical fumes from a wide variety of common domestic substances (including glues, plastic cements, paint thinners, petrol, hair lacquer and lighter refills) in order to produce an intoxicating effect.

Somatic passivity   a *first rank symptom of schizophrenia* in which the individual believes that he is a passive and reluctant recipient of bodily sensations imposed upon him by some external influence.

Somatisation disorder   *see Briquet's syndrome.*

Somnambulism   sleep-walking, which is often regarded as a *dissociative state*.

Special Hospitals   for the treatment, under conditions of special security, of mentally disordered patients who have dangerous, violent or criminal tendencies. There are four such hospitals in England (Broadmoor, Rampton, Moss Side and Park Lane) and one in Scotland (State Hospital, Carstairs).

Special Verdict (McNaughton's rules)   a psychiatric defence now rarely used in a court of law, most often applied when the accused is charged with murder. To be successful, it must be demonstrated that the accused was 'labouring under such a defect of reason from disease of the mind, as not to know the nature and quality of the act he was doing, or if he did know it, that he did not know what he was doing was wrong'.

Specific reading retardation a specific impairment of reading ability in children who otherwise have normal intelligence and are receiving adequate teaching. The reading age is 28 months or more below that expected.

Squeeze technique a form of *biofeedback* used in the treatment of *premature ejaculation*, which allows the development of control over the orgasmic reflex.

Standard unit of alcohol 1 standard unit of alcohol = 10 g of absolute alcohol = (approximately) half a pint of beer = one single spirit = one glass of wine = one small glass of sherry. A bottle of spirits therefore contains about 28 units, and a bottle of wine 7 units of alcohol.

Star chart a simple form of *operant conditioning* often utilised in the management of childhood disorders such as *enuresis* and *encopresis*. For example, in the case of bed-wetting, dry nights are rewarded by the child being allowed to stick a coloured star on a chart, while wet nights are ignored. It is a useful means of determining the frequency of the unwanted behaviour, and also helps to establish a reward system for the desired behaviour.

Stereotypic speech characterised by conversation which is punctuated by the constant repetition of words or phrases out of context. It may be a feature of *catatonia*.

Stereotypy a repetitive, non-goal directed action carried out in a consistent fashion, e.g. body-rocking or foot-tapping. It may be a feature of *catatonia*.

Stupor (akinetic mutism) a state in which there is absence of speech and movement, although consciousness is fully preserved. There may be a sudden change to a state of uncontrolled activity and excitement. If left to themselves, patients are unlikely to eat or drink and are often incontinent. The stuporose state is sometimes relieved by lowering levels of arousal (e.g. giving a benzodiazepine intravenously), or by the administration of *ECT*. Stupor can occur as a feature of *catatonia*, as well as in *organic reactions* and *functional psychoses*.

Sturge-Weber syndrome a rare disorder characterised by the presence of a naevus (port-wine stain) distributed variably over one-half of the face, neck and upper trunk. There is an associated underlying angiomatous growth involving the meninges on the same side as the external lesion, which may result in contralateral hemiparesis, convulsions and severe *mental retardation*. The mode of causation is unknown, although the condition may be genetically determined.

Subcultural mental retardation a limitation of intelligence partly due to inherited factors, but exacerbated by severe social and educational disadvantage.

Subdural haematoma can develop following relatively minor head injuries (especially in the elderly), sometimes trivial enough not to be remembered. The condition is characterised by a fluctuating level of consciousness, vague headaches, general slowness and difficulty with concentration or memory. Neurological signs are infrequent.

Sublimation a *defence mechanism* in which libidinal urges unacceptable to the self are channelled into acceptable behaviour.

Suicide an intentional, self-inflicted, life-threatening act which results in death.

Sulpiride a member of the *benzamide* derivative group of *neuroleptic drugs*.

Superego according to *psychoanalytical theory*, one of the important elements in developing personality; it represents an incorporation into the self of actual parental and social values, as well as being a manifestation of the fantasised standards, qualities and failings that the child attributes to his caregivers (*see also id and ego*).

Supportive psychotherapy a form of treatment using talking and listening, which attempts to carry or support the individual at a time when continuing stress is likely to result in a breakdown of functioning (*see also psychotherapy*). It aims to minimise disabling psychological symptoms and reduce anxiety by encouraging the ventilation of feelings, demonstrating empathy with the individual's worries and offering advice where appropriate. This is accomplished without necessarily trying to understand the fundamental origins of the presenting difficulties.

Systematic desensitisation an elaborate form of *graded exposure* in fantasy which is now largely obsolete.

Systemic lupus erythematosus a connective tissue disorder producing widespread inflammatory changes of blood vessels, with the extensive development of vasculitis and multiple microinfarcts. Psychiatric manifestations include *neuroses, psychoses* and *acute* or *chronic organic reactions*.

Tabes dorsalis a form of neurosyphilis, resulting in atrophy of the dorsal roots and posterior columns of the spinal cord, and characterised by ataxia, pain and paraesthesia of the lower limbs.

Tactile hallucination a false perception of touch, in the absence of an external stimulus.

Tardive dyskinesia an *extrapyramidal motor disturbance* associated with the use of *neuroleptic drugs*. Involuntary movements of the face, tongue and jaw occur which are socially embarrassing. Occasionally, muscles of the trunk and limbs are also involved.

Tay-Sachs disease an inherited disorder of lipid metabolism, which is more common among Jews, and is transmitted by an autosomal recessive gene. It is due to a deficiency of the enzyme hexosaminidase-A. Clinical features include *mental retardation*, a cherry-red spot on the macula, blindness, fits, spasticity and ataxia.

Testamentary capacity the ability of an individual to make a valid will, in that the testator must be of 'sound disposing mind'.

Tetrahydrocannabinol the active component of *hashish* and *marijuana* (*see also cannabis*).

Theory of social causation an hypothesis suggesting that the increased prevalence of mental disorder found among most migrant groups is due to the adverse effects of immigration.

Theory of social selection an hypothesis suggesting that the increased prevalence of mental disorder found among most migrant groups is due to the increased tendency of those with a predisposition to develop certain mental illnesses to migrate.

Therapeutic community a specialised unit offering a style of treatment (particularly for those with antisocial or psychopathic tendencies) in which modification of behaviour is attempted by peer pressure. This is applied through the process of living together in a democratic community that makes and implements its own rules and disciplines. In this way, the individual is encouraged to assume responsibility for his own actions, and to develop increased means of self-control over his behaviour.

Thiamine   vitamin B₁, a deficiency of which can lead to *Wernicke's encephalopathy* and *Korsakoff's psychosis*.

Thioxanthines   a group of *neuroleptic drugs* which includes clopenthixol and *flupenthixol*. They are often administered in the form of *depot preparations*. Flupenthixol also appears to have antidepressant properties in low dosage.

Thought alientation (delusion of the possession of thought)   the subject has the experience that his thoughts are under the influence of some outside force, or tha others are participating in his thinking (*see thought broadcast, thought insertion, thought withdrawal*).

Thought block   the objective manifestation of *thought withdrawal*, in which the subject is observed to stop in mid-sentence, and on resuming his conversation, might report that his mind was completely emptied of all thoughts.

Thought broadcast   a *first rank symptom of schizophrenia* in which the subject experiences his unspoken thoughts as being known to, or shared by, those around him, so that he believes they are not contained within his own mind.

Thought disorder (schizophrenic)   an indistinct abnormality of the construction and use of language, resulting from a basic disturbance of thinking. In its earliest stages, thought disorder may be apparent when the patient converses but the listener realises that he has understood little of what is being said (*see also concrete thinking, derailment, knight's move thinking, overinclusiveness* and *word salad*).

Thought echo   *see audible thoughts.*

Thought insertion   a *first rank symptom of schizophrenia* in which the individual experiences thoughts that he does not recognise as a product of his own mind, and which he believes have been put there by some outside force or agency.

Thought stopping   a behavioural treatment used in the management of *obsessions*. The subject is encouraged to relax and then ruminate, so that the obsessional thought is uppermost in his mind. At this point, the therapist shouts 'Stop!' and the patient must cease to ruminate. Eventually, he learns to internalise control.

Thought withdrawal   a *first rank symptom of schizophrenia* in which the patient experiences his thoughts as being taken out of his mind against his will by some external force or agency (*see also thought block*).

Tics   sudden, rapid, repetitive, non-goal directed movements, which although involuntary, can be suppressed with effort at the expense of mounting anxiety. They most commonly occur in the face and neck (as well as involving the vocal cords), and tend to be coordinated.

Token economy   a programme of behaviour modification, whereby in return for performing tasks such as bed-making or paying attention to personal hygiene, chronic patients receive tokens which they can later exchange for privileges, such as cigarettes and the right to watch television. This process has been used to help in the prevention of institutionalisation, by attempting to encourage motivation and activity.

Tolerance   the manner in which the body adapts to the repeated presence of a drug, so that the user has to increase the dose to achieve the original effect.

Topognosia   *see agnosia.*

Topographical disorientation   difficulty in finding one's way about, even in familiar surroundings. It may be a sign of organic brain disease.

Tort   a civil action brought in a court of law, such as for libel, slander or trespass.

Transcultural psychiatry the comparative study of mental disorder between different cultures.

Transference a process during *psychotherapy*, whereby the subject displaces or 'transfers' emotions derived from previous relationships in his life onto the therapist (*see also countertransference*).

Transient global amnesia a disorder, probably due to cerebral ischaemia, in which a sudden loss of recent memory occurs, accompanied by an inability to store new information, although recall of distant events and other cognitive functions are unaffected. Attacks usually last for several hours, after which memory function recovers completely, although there is an amnesic gap for the episode.

Transsexualism a rare disorder of gender identity in which the individual is certain of having been born into the wrong sex.

Transvestism (cross-dressing) a disorder of gender role behaviour which involves the habitual wearing of clothes of the opposite sex.

TRANX (Tranquilliser recovery and new existence) a self-help organisation for those dependent on, or withdrawing from *minor tranquillisers*.

Tremor a rhythmic, involuntary, alternating contraction of opposing muscle groups, which is fairly uniform in frequency and amplitude.

Tricyclic antidepressants a group of MARI antidepressants, which includes *amitriptyline* and *imipramine*, so named because of their chemical structure, which contains a three-ringed nucleus (*see also monoamine reuptake inhibitors*).

Tuberous sclerosis (epiloia) an inherited disorder transmitted by an autosomal dominant gene. Hard nodules of neuroglial cells are distributed throughout the substance of the brain, often resulting in the development of *mental retardation* and epilepsy. The clinical presentation is variable due to poor gene penetrance. Other features include a facial rash, fibromata, café-au-lait skin spots, phakomata of the retina, as well as muscle, fat and vascular tumours in the heart, lungs and kidneys.

Tumescence congestion and swelling, especially of the sexual organs.

Turner's syndrome a disorder arising from the absence of an X chromosome (karyotype XO). Physical abnormalities include short stature, with associated webbing of the neck and a valgus forearm deformity. Ovarian agenesis results in amenorrhoea, sterility and lack of female secondary sexual characteristics. One-third of cases develop coarctation of the aorta. *Mental retardation* is rare, and the condition is not incompatible with normal intelligence.

Twilight state a subjective alteration of awareness, so that emotionally significant experiences and perceptions have a dream-like quality. It may follow an epileptic seizure.

Twin studies an investigative procedure for assessing the influence of genetic and environmental factors in the causation of mental disorder by comparing concordance rates in monozygotic (identical) and dizygotic (non-identical) twins.

Unconscious mind according to Freud's topographical model, that part of the mind containing memories, thoughts, drives and conflicts which cannot be brought into awareness because of active *repression*.

Unilateral ECT administration of the treatment by application of the electrodes to one side of the head (*see also ECT*).

Unipolar affective disorder a condition in which an individual has experienced at least three episodes of *depressive illness*, with complete recovery in between, and none of *mania* (compare with *bipolar affective disorder*).

Vaginismus the involuntary spasm of the vaginal (and often adductor thigh) muscles in response to attempts at penetration. The cause is usually psychological, and often relates to guilt or anxiety about sex.

Verbigeration speech characterised by the continuous and senseless repetition of words or sentences (e.g one subject repeated the phrase 'the doors are all locked' for hours on end). It may be a feature of *catatonia*.

Visual agnosia *see agnosia.*

Visual hallucination a false visual perception in the absence of an external stimulus.

Von Recklinghausen's disease *see neurofibromatosis.*

Voyeurism sexual arousal and gratification obtained by watching others copulate, or by secretly observing women undressing or in the nude ('peeping Tom').

WAIS *see* Wechsler adult intelligence scale.

Waxy flexibility *see catalepsy.*

Wechsler adult intelligence scale (WAIS) a measure of *intelligence*, which assesses both verbal and performance skills. The WAIS consists of six verbal subtests which deal with words or numbers, and five subtests of performance. Verbal subtests include information (a test of general knowledge), comprehension (a measure of social awareness), arithmetic (assesses numerical reasoning), similarities (evaluates concept formation), digit span (a test of immediate and short-term memory recall) and vocabulary (a measure of expressive word knowledge). Performance subtests include digit symbol (a coding task), picture completion (a measure of attention to fine detail), block design (the arrangement of spatial patterns), object assembly (a jigsaw-type task) and picture arrangement (a measure of logical sequential thought processing). The full IQ score is derived from the combined scores of all the subtests.

Wechsler intelligence scale for children (WISC) a measure of *intelligence* for children, which assesses both verbal and performance skills (*see Wechsler adult intelligence scale* for further details).

Wernicke's encephalopathy the acute reaction to severe vitamin B_1 (Thiamine) deficiency, which is most commonly (but not exclusively) encountered in those who abuse alcohol and therefore have a poor nutritional intake. The principal clinical features are nystagmus, ophthalmoplegia (particularly of the lateral rectus muscle), ataxia, clouding of consciousness and peripheral neuropathy (*see also Korsakoff's psychosis*).

Wilson's disease an inherited defect of copper metabolism, transmitted by an autosomal recessive gene, which results in a deficiency of the enzyme caeruloplasmin. Excessive copper is deposited in the liver, kidney, basal ganglia and eye. Psychiatric manifestations include personality changes, affective and schizophrenic-like *psychoses*, as well as intellectual decline, sometimes progressing to *dementia*.

Windigo a rare culture-bound disorder seen in North American Indians which is regarded as a form of depressive psychosis. The subject has a delusional belief that he has turned into a cannibalistic monster, and subsequently may attempt to act on this conviction.

WISC *see Wechsler intelligence scale for children.*

Word salad a severe form of *thought disorder* in which the patient talks jumbled nonsense so as to be completely incomprehensible (also known as *schizophasia*).

Working through the re-experiencing of emotional conflicts during *psycho-therapy*.

XXX syndrome (superfemales) the presence of an extra sex chromosome is associated with mild mental retardation in a small minority of those affected. It does not produce any characteristic physical abnormalities.

XYY syndrome a disorder arising from the presence of an extra Y chromosome, affecting approximately 1 in 700 males. XYY males tend to be tall with normal fertility and secondary sexual characteristics. There is no definite association with *mental retardation*, and although it has been suggested that the syndrome is linked with a propensity towards criminal behaviour, this finding is not universally accepted.

INDEX